Occupation & Practice in Context

Gail Whiteford

&

Valerie Wright-St Clair

Foreword by Professor Elizabeth Townsend

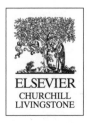

ELSEVIER
CHURCHILL
LIVINGSTONE

Sydney Edinburgh London New York Philadelphia St Louis Toronto

ELSEVIER

Churchill Livingstone
is an imprint of Elsevier

Elsevier Australia
30-52 Smidmore Street, Marrickville, NSW 2204

This edition © 2005 Elsevier Australia
(a division of Reed International Books Australia Pty Ltd)
ACN 001 002 357

National Library of Australia Cataloguing-in-Publication Data

---

Whiteford, Gail.
Occupation and practice in context.

Includes index
ISBN 0 7295 3753 6.

1. Occupations - Textbooks. I. Wright-St Clair, Valerie.

331.7

Publisher: Vaughn Curtis
Publishing Editor: Mary Maakaroun
Development Editor: Rhiain Hull
Cover and internal design by Tania Edwards Design
Edited, typeset and indexed by Puddingburn Publishing Services
Printed in Australia by Ligare Pty Ltd

Table of Contents

Foreword

Professor Elizabeth Townsend[1]

Occupation and Practice in Context is a landmark book on the context that shapes the practice of health professionals who are concerned with promoting people's participation in life. One can read this book forwards or backwards. The opening and closing chapters are preludes and postludes that alert the reader to the book's context of ideas, values and beliefs. In other words, the book is itself a context for raising issues and global professional challenges.

The ideas, values and beliefs expressed throughout *Occupation and Practice in Context* convey a congruent message about diversity as both a reality and a contextual force. The moral message is that social inclusion is good for us all. Whereas global management systems rely on the efficiencies of standardisation, uniform terminology, protocols and universal techniques, the authors illuminate the need to understand the complexity, differences and challenges of diverse human experiences in diverse cultural, economic, institutional, social and political contexts.

Readers who start at the beginning — at the prelude — will plunge into complexity theory, an interpretive wave that is overtaking systems theory. An exciting opening chapter by Whiteford, Klomp and Wright-St Clair presents complexity theory as a contemporary evolution of systems theory. Many professions embraced systems theory when it became popular starting in the 1960s. At that time, we needed to understand how the systems that had emerged through managerialism had formed a new world order. Systems theory helped to explain what professions, such as occupational therapy, called the *environment* in models of practice. Now *Occupation and Practice in Context* guides us to understand the complexity that characterises our 21st century world.

Readers who like to jump to the end of a book to see how it ends will discover a wonderful postlude on global thinking. Whiteford's closing chapter prompts reflections on the possibilities and limits of the Enabling State. With reference to

---

1 Elizabeth Townsend, Ph.D., O.T.(C), Reg. N.S., FCAOT is Professor and Director of the School of Occupational Therapy, Dalhousie University, Halifax, Nova Scotia, Canada.

the idea of a *third way* to work with globalisation, she considers how contexts limit or enable populations around to the world to achieve greater peace and fairness.

Occupation and Practice in Context sets a new standard. Typically, professional texts are profession-centred. In looking at a profession from within, texts have a tendency to be myopic. Typically, such works describe the theories, models and techniques of a profession *as the profession itself defines its own work*.

Instead, *Occupation and Practice in Context* is expansive. With a strong emphasis on practice, this is a publication to expand professional knowledge and skills for critically appraising the ideas, values and beliefs underlying professional work. To illustrate, instead of writing about methods for developing communication skills, Wright-St Clair and Seedhouse have written about the moral context of professional relationships. They make explicit the moral ground that shapes relationships in what they describe as a *taken-for-granted moral world*. Instead of teaching professionals how to assess randomised controlled trials as the only true evidence for practice, Whiteford challenges professionals to understand first how *knowledge and power shape the evidence we value* in making decisions. She highlights, for instance, the predominant biomedical orientation of evidence-based practice in today's health decisions. Chapparo and Ranka, instead of describing or comparing theories, examine *postmodernism's interests in diversity* as a foundation for interpreting theory as the intellectual context of health service delivery.

This is a thematic rather than a technical work. The theme of diversity comes particularly to light in two wonderful chapters that distinguish this as a text that prepares professionals to examine their own foundations. Mihi and Matiu Ratima have dared to privilege their first language, te reo Māori, in naming the subtitles of their chapter on indigeneous context. In doing so they embody the values of tangata whenua (indigenous peoples) in the writing itself. The authors place cultural diversity INSIDE a professional text. Instead of being named as clients, as the *other* in a professional text, their experience IS the text. Secondly, Michael Iwama, an occupational therapist, challenges his own profession to consider the epistemological construction of knowledge. Instead of writing about culture as an object of interest, he reminds professionals to learn the skills for understanding cultural relativism.

Beyond the generic theme of diversity, Whiteford and Wright-St Clair have used four themes to organise authors' contributions. Selecting randomly from the table of contents, one starts with the professional context of practice. For example, Hocking and Ness show us how international documents shape professional consistency worldwide. Allen, Oke, McKinstry and Courtney critique accreditation as a contextual force that shapes professionalism and accountability.

The theme of the organisational context of practice considers how systems determine practice possibilities. One chapter that particularly caught my eye is by Cusick and Lanin who examine the construction of allied health as a framework which defines the power and possibilities of health professions *other* than medicine. The sociocultural context of practice is also a theme. Selecting one to illustrate this theme, we can see that Wicks and Whiteford consider gender as context. The political and economic context is the final theme. As examples, O'Halloran and Innes consider the construction of work in contemporary society, juxtaposed against a chapter by Neumayer and Wilding on the commodification of leisure as an occupation.

An important question for the authors is: What will attract professionals to such a text? I believe that professionals will learn to critique their own work and life. There are lessons for critiquing and shaping practice relevant to front line practitioners, managers, policy makers, educators and researchers.

Whiteford and Wright-St Clair have put their fingers on the pulse of 21st century thinking in *Occupation and Practice in Context*. Their focus on context brings us face to face with globalisation and its impact on professions. This is a book that resounds with insights for us all. Written about and for health professionals concerned with promoting people's participation in life, *Occupation and Practice in Context* is a tremendous resource for any profession or citizen. With authors from various fields and parts of the globe, the book sets occupation-focused practice as a case in point on a world stage.

June 2004

Preface

It's difficult to pinpoint the exact moment in which the idea of a book is born, especially when, as the saying goes, there's a book in all of us just waiting for the right opportunity to be called into existence. Rather, we attempt here to chart some of the influences that led to its development. We also want to give you, the reader, an outline of what we believe the purpose of the book to be.

The personal experiences we have both had, especially as women, have undoubtedly influenced our world view and may be seen as foundational to the creation of *Occupation and Practice in Context.* We both believe quite strongly that understanding of self as a gendered, social and cultural being is the beginning point for overcoming ethnocentricity and working in partnership with others. In this regard, travelling and working in other countries and being with people from indigenous and differing cultural backgrounds, have been important in shaping our sense of self and other.

Being from a professional background, specifically that of occupational therapy, has also influenced our beliefs and hence the creation of this book. Occupational therapists are primarily concerned with issues of justice, participation and representation relative to what people *do* in society. Although there have been some periods of time in occupational therapy's history when concerns with social justice and inclusion were overshadowed with a preoccupation with pathology, things are changing. Occupational therapy, like many health professions, is claiming its autonomy and relevance to diverse groups of peoples. It is doing this through embracing multiple knowledge paradigms, through programs of focused enquiry, and through participation focused practice. It's an exciting and challenging time.

Finally, one of the broader influences that provided some impetus to the creation of this book was that of the meaning of citizenship in postmodern civil society. Over time, we have come to appreciate the influence of prevailing discourses on us as individuals and as community members. Increasingly we have come to realise the responsibilities we have as both citizen and professional to engage actively with (and hopefully influence) the larger discourses which shape our social, political and economic environments. In summary, all these influences relate to the contextual stages upon which our lives have been enacted over time.

Context is, of course, a central concern in this book. No communication, no interaction, no intervention that takes place between practitioner and client is context free. At any moment, the political, economic, organisational and sociocultural contexts in which we live and work impact upon daily practice in often invisible but important ways. Such is our belief in this as a truism, that we have structured the book correspondingly; that is, each of these contexts represents a discrete section. Our hope in this regard is to raise awareness of the interactive effects of context in order to inform "wise" professional practice.

If that sounds complex, then that's because it is. Accordingly, another objective of *Occupation and Practice in Context* has been to foreground understandings of complexity within professional practice. In the beginning of the book, we posit the suggestion that complexity theory should supplant [the limitations of] systems theory in professional preparation and education. Viewing causation interactively rather than atomistically, we suggest, creates new and exciting opportunities for how we conceptualise and approach working with individuals, families and communities. Indeed, complexity theory could well represent a "turning point" (to quote Fritjof Capra) in the disciplines in the same way it has revolutionized the basic sciences.

Finally, we have also aimed to further understandings of occupation within practice. Occupation, interpreted inclusively within this book as all things people do within the stream of time, should not just be the province of occupational therapists. Ultimately, all health interventions should be aimed at the achievement of wellness. This is because wellness is intimately connected with peoples' sense of meaning, connectedness and purpose in their lives regardless of levels of ability. To this end, we hope that the reader will gain some new insights into occupation as a complex, situated phenomenon.

In closing, we hope that you enjoy this book and find it stimulating and thought provoking. Though not intended as a blueprint for action, we also hope it may inform and guide changes in everyday practices that make a difference. Indeed, in a future in which *how* we address diversity and sustainability in multiple contexts will be essential to our common co-existence, evolution of theory and practice is probably requisite rather than voluntary.

Gail Elizabeth Whiteford
Valerie Wright-St Clair
September 2004

Contributing Authors

Rebecca Allen BAppSc(OT);
GDipOrgBehav; MBus; AccOT
Sub-Dean Learning & Teaching, Faculty of
Health Studies
Course Coordinator Occupational Therapy
School of Community Health
Charles Sturt University, Albury, NSW

Anita Barbara MOT, BOT
Lecturer, Occupational Therapy Program
School of Community Health
Charles Sturt University, Albury, NSW

Paul Brown PhD (Econ)
Senior Health Economist
Centre for Health Services Research & Policy
School of Population Health, University of
Auckland
Auckland, NEW ZEALAND

Christine J. Chapparo MA, PhD, DipOT,
OTR, FAOTA
Senior Lecturer
School of Occupation and Leisure Sciences
Faculty of Health Sciences
The University of Sydney, Lidcombe, NSW

Michelle Courtney BAppSc(OT),
GradDipHlthSci(Community Hlth);
AccOT; PhD candidate, La Trobe
University
Senior Lecturer
Occupational Science and Therapy
School of Health and Social Development
Faculty of Health and Behavioural Sciences
Deakin University, Geelong Waterfront
Campus, Geelong, VIC

Anne Cusick BAppSc(OT),
GradDipAppBehSc, MA (Psych), MA
(Interdisc Stud), PhD
Professor and Associate Dean (Academic)
College of Social and Health Sciences
University of Western Sydney
Campbelltown Campus
Penrith South, NSW

Natasha Lannin BSc (OT), PGDip (Case
Management)
Research Officer
College of Social and Health Sciences
University of Western Sydney
Campbelltown Campus
Penrith South, NSW

Clare Hocking PhD, MHSc (OT)
Senior Lecturer
Coordinator Postgraduate Studies
School of Occupational Therapy
Auckland University of Technology
Auckland NEW ZEALAND

Ev Innes PhD, MHPEd, BAppSc (OT),
AccOT, MHFESA
Senior Lecturer
School of Occupation and Leisure Sciences
Faculty of Health Sciences
The University of Sydney, Lidcombe, NSW

Michael Iwama PhD (Sociology), MSc
(Rehab Sci), BSc (OT), BSc (Kinesiology),
Associate Professor and Coordinator of the
Undergraduate Program
School of Occupational Therapy,
Dalhousie University, Canada;
Adjunct Associate Professor,
University of Queensland, Brisbane, Qld

Heather Jensen BAppSc (Biol), BAppSc (OT), MHlthSci (OT), GradCert Tert Teaching
Lecturer in Occupational Therapy
James Cook University
Townsville Qld

Marion Jones PhD; MEdAdmin (Hons); BA; RGON; FCONA
Associate Dean Postgraduate
Faculty of Health
Auckland University of Technology
Auckland New Zealand

Nicholas I. Klomp BAppSc, BSc(Hons), PhD
Professor and Head, School of Environmental and Information Sciences
Faculty of Science and Agriculture
Charles Sturt University, Albury, NSW

Michael Law MSc in Health, Population & Society, LSE
Research Associate
Centre for Health Services Research and Policy
School of Population Health
The University of Auckland Auckland NEW ZEALAND

Carol Elizabeth McKinstry BAppSc(OT); MHlthSci, AccOT
PhD candidate at La Trobe University
Manager in Quality Improvement and Risk Management, Vic
Bendigo, Vic

Nils Erik Ness
Associate Professor Occupational Therapy
Programme Leader Entry Level and Post Graduate Education in Occupational Science
Sör-Tröndelag University College
President of the European Network of Occupational Therapy in Higher Education (ENOTHE)
Sör-Tröndelag University College (HiST)
Ranheimsveien, Trondheim, Norway

Robert John Neumayer PhD (Leisure Studies)
Associate Professor and Head, School Of Community Health

School of Community Health
Charles Sturt University, Albury, NSW

David O'Halloran BAppSc (OT), MHlthSc (OT), AccOT
Regional Manager, Southern Tasmania
CRS Australia
Hobart, Tas

Linda E Oke Dip OT; MAppSci; AccOT
CEO, OT AUSTRALIA
Australian Association of Occupational Therapists
Fitzroy, Vic

Judy L. Ranka MA, BSc, OTR
Lecturer
School of Occupation and Leisure Sciences
Faculty of Health Sciences
The University of Sydney, Lidcombe, NSW

Matiu Ratima BA, MPhil
Whakatohea / Ngati Awa
Lecturer
Te Ara Poutama
Faculty of Māori Development
Auckland University of Technology,
Auckland, New Zealand

Mihi Ratima PhD, DPH, Dip Māori Development, BSc
Associate Professor
Division of Public Health and Psychosocial Studies
Faculty of Health
Auckland University of Technology
Auckland, New Zealand

David Seedhouse PhD
Professor of Health and Social Ethics
Division of Public Health & Psychosocial Studies
Auckland University of Technology
Auckland, New Zealand

Kit Sinclair PhD, MScPrac of Higher Ed, BScOT, OTR, FWFOT, FAOTA
Assistant Professor
Department of Rehabilitation Sciences
Hong Kong Polytechnic University Hung Hom
Kowloon, Hong Kong

Karen Stagnitti PhD
Senior Lecturer
Faculty of Health and Behavioural Sciences
Warrnambool Campus, Deakin University
Warrnambool, Vic

Yvonne Thomas Dip OT, MEd
Fieldwork Manager and Lecturer
Occupational Therapy
James Cook University
Townsville, Qld

Gail Elizabeth Whiteford PhD,
  MHSc(OT), BAppSc(OT)
Professor & Chair in Occupational Therapy
Director of RIPPLE, the Centre for Research
  in Professional Practice, Learning and
  Education, Head of Campus
Charles Sturt University, Albury, NSW

Alison Mary Wicks PhD, MHsc(OT),
  BAppSc(OT), AccOT
Freelance consultant, Occupational
  Perspectives
Nowra, NSW

Clare Wilding BAppSc(OT), MApSc(OT)
Lecturer in occupational therapy, Course
  coordinator, Bachelor of Social Science,
  Habilitation
School of Community Health
Charles Sturt University, Albury, NSW

Valerie Wright-St Clair MPH,
  DipProfEthics, DipBusStudies(Hlth Mgt),
  DipOT
Head, School of Occupational Therapy
Division of Rehabilitation and Occupation
  Studies
Faculty of Health
Auckland University of Technology
Auckland, New Zealand

The Professional Context of Practice

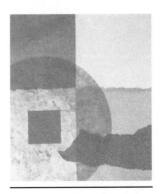

CHAPTER ONE

Complexity Theory: Understanding Occupation, Practice and Context

Gail Whiteford

Nick Klomp

Valerie Wright-St Clair

KEY WORDS

Complex systems
Connectivity
Occupation
Professional practice
Contextual influences

Chapter Profile

In this first chapter of the book, we explore both occupation and practice as context bound phenomena. We do this through an initial presentation of complexity theory as a contemporary evolution of systems theory and, as such, as an underpinning to the exploration of the contextual influences described in the four sections of the book; the professional; organisational; sociocultural and political/economic. The chapter presents a discussion of both occupation and professional practice as informed by complexity theory and considers the value therein. The chapter concludes with reflections on the challenges of practice in a rapidly changing global context in which complexity is a defining feature and in which diversity and sustainability are important considerations.

Introduction

It could be argued that reductionism in professional practice has served us well to date. The idea is simple: divide and rule. If you want to understand something complex, such as an organisation or work environment, break it down into its component parts and figure out how they all work. Historically, this approach has proved tremendously successful in science and technology. Over the course of four centuries, physicists and chemists have dissected matter into its components: molecules, atoms, protons, electrons and, most recently, quarks and muons. At every step of the way, they made important discoveries that helped us to better understand nature, whether it be the origins of the universe or the structure of DNA. And these discoveries led to all manner of practical applications, from aeronautics to biotechnology. In the face of such powerful methods, any other research approach could seem to be redundant.

Unfortunately, understanding complex human phenomena is not so simple. One reason, of course, is that no single approach can adequately address the enormity of variation possible within human systems. However, a much more important reason is that any given context is much more than the individuals that it comprises. Interactions do matter. The whole is much, much greater than the sum of its parts.

To understand complex systems — such as occupation and professional practice — understanding the components is clearly not enough (Kielhofner, 2000; Wilcock, 1998; Wilcock 2001). Strange things happen when you put individuals together to form a "system". They interact with their environment (their "context"). They interact with one another. And the effects of all these interactions can be unpredictable. They can be profound. Studying these effects — learning to understand them — that is what complexity research is all about.

Such challenges abound in understanding and addressing occupation and also in what we think of as professional practice. Occupation, or what people "do", is always bound by cultural, social, economic, historic and political forces (Whiteford, in press; Wilcock, 1998; Wilcock & Townsend, 2004). As such a socially (and, to some extent, individually) mediated phenomenon, occupation cannot be usefully considered within a reductionist paradigm, a reality acknowledged by a range of commentators from the profession of occupational therapy in what has been dubbed as a "renaissance of occupation" (Whiteford, Townsend & Hocking, 2000). Consistent with such a realisation has been a growing awareness of the need also to re-think practice that addresses people, their state of health/wellness and what they do everyday that influences this. An individual professional is the product of his or her society and education, practising in a discipline that is governed by currently accepted practice, embedded within a landscape dominated by social, cultural, political and economic influences. It is important that such a systems view is taken in attempting to understand both practice and occupation, because without such an approach, we may be guilty of simply studying the parts, and not the interactions that place them in context. Indeed, we need to understand the complexity that characterises these phenomena.

Complexity theory: An overview

"Complexity" is a term that may be used commonly, but has a specific meaning when we apply it to understanding systems. Perhaps the simplest description is to say that complexity is the richness and variety of structure and behaviour that arises from the interactions between the components of a system.

Despite the generality of the above definition, its relevance may not be obvious to many situations that we would regard as complex. Many systems that at first sight appear simple, can exhibit what is clearly chaotic behaviour. For example, an individual working in a professional organisation may appear to behave in a predictable way, with predictable outcomes for the organisation and profession. However, as we all experience in our professional lives, there are many confounding and conflicting factors that influence our occupational performance. Some of the factors that affect performance include the balance between personal and professional influences in a given day, or week; the influence of policies and funding on the directions of a profession or organisation or unit; the historical context and expectations in a given practice; and the interactions among managers and colleagues and the public. It is these interactions that make such systems so complex. In order to describe and address inherent complexity, the following categories are often employed within the literature. We present them briefly here for consideration.

The spatial scale

Many influences of practice and context come from sources outside the immediate profession. The global environment, governments of the day, competing organisations, current funding, public opinion and many other factors all affect context. Depending on the profession and context, a single decision by an individual may need to take into account the workplace, local community, the broader discipline, the national agenda and even the current practice globally.

The temporal scale

Many professions and the accepted practices within them have developed over time, that is, within an associated historical context. Accordingly, practices and decisions are relative to the historical context within which they were developed and would be different within a different social, political or knowledge environment. This has led to "time-blinkered" decisions in most professions.

The interaction of individuals

Nearly every practitioner has colleagues and bosses, clients and customers, assessors and critics. The operation of a given profession or practice many involve hundreds of people in a given day or week. However, it is not sheer numbers of individuals that make the context complex, but rather the enormous variety of ways in which they combine and interact. For instance, suppose that 100 people interact in any given context; then there are 4,950 possible pairs of interacting people (assuming all levels of an organisation can interact with each other and their clients on an equal basis). However, when we consider all combinations, the possibilities blow out to astronomical proportions. There are over 6 x 1019 ways in which groups of ten people could combine within a group of 100 people (that is a number greater than the age of the universe, in seconds!). Each combination will have different interactions, so could lead to different decisions or outcomes. This complexity increases further by orders of magnitude when the interactions of people and the physical environment within a system are considered.

Connectivity

The connectivity within a system determines the functionality of that system, so it is important to practitioners and managers, particularly in large organisations. What is connectivity? Two objects are "connected" if some pattern or process links them. Links arise either from static patterns (for example professional bodies, organisations and so on etc) or from dynamic processes (for example, exchange of information). Practitioners may be linked within a profession because they share the same knowledge, attended the same universities or work in the same organisations, as well as via their direct communications. There is a connection among them that will allow the flow of information and ideas. Clients, on the other hand, may share only a few links or connections with the entire health industry, perhaps via a single practitioner or a contact in one hospital.

An understanding of the implications of connectivity is leading to significant advances in disciplines as diverse as environmental management to social welfare. Studies of connectivity within the Swedish population have led to health authorities understanding the nature of the network of sexual interactions within the adult population. The research identified hundreds of "nodes" — mostly sex workers — that were internal to the sexual connectivity of the majority of the population. This will lead to informed and directed educational programs and health promotion to manage, for example, sexually transmitted diseases. This is a more efficient use of resources than the scatter-gun approach of attempting to reach all members of a community individually.

Human influence

In addition to making systems more complicated (or more difficult to manage), humans influence the management of systems by directing goals and agendas in ways that require decisions to be based on much more than knowledge of the profession or practice. This has led to the recent, rapid increase in the use of decision support models by managers (Klomp et al, 1997).

While these categories describe some of the features of complexity theory, they do not address the rationale for employing complexity theory in understanding occupation and practice per se. The next section then, provides a basis for the reader to understand why complexity theory is both useful and relevant in understanding not only the context bound issues presented in this book, but as a tool through which to make sense of the inherent dynamic nature of human phenomena.

Complexity, interconnectedness and knowledge generation

> ... [social institutions] are designed for specific purposes such as making money ... managing the distribution of political power, transmitting knowledge or spreading religious faith. At the same time, organizations are communities of people who interact with one another to build relationships, help each other and make their daily activities meaningful at a personal level.
>
> (Capra, 2003, p 87)

We need to understand complexity because so many crucial problems rely on us finding solutions to complex problems. The world is now so interconnected that it seems everything affects everything else. To manage people in one area, you need to understand their place in the larger context. As is discussed in the final chapter of this book, you also need to consider them in the context of globalisation; more often than not, processes in different countries are linked.

The paradox of traditional approaches to occupation and practice is that although they are dealing with inherently complex contexts, many individuals still act in ways consistent with reductionist methodologies. This is one of the core ideas discussed in chapter five as it relates to the determination of what constitutes a valid "evidence base" for practice. The emphasis is on finding simple explanations and straightforward cause and effect relationships. Interactions are viewed as an annoyance, not the heart of the process.

Indeed, institutions of higher learning are still culpable of reproducing such cognitive and methodological biases. Students obtain a grounding in the basic concepts of their chosen field, presented in discrete subjects or units, perhaps consistent with the current view of the profession. In an ideal program of study, there would be integrated subjects, as well as projects and other practical experience that draws on the various sub-disciplines. In the best university environment, the component disciplines would be delivered by leading researchers in their field. Not unnaturally, the tendency is for the experts in the field to focus narrowly within their own discipline.

This teaching strategy may be appropriate for narrow discipline areas, but results in many students being exposed to reductionist approaches as the dominant paradigm. Few, if any, discipline specialists venture beyond the boundaries of their own narrow research interests, and this bias is reflected in their teaching. The danger of this situation is that at the end of a course, the students conceptually have each discipline neatly allocated into an isolated box of knowledge. The reductionist culture is perpetuated not just by the structure of university courses, but also within the formalised structures of knowledge production and dissemination, such as professional journals and related publications.

The trend towards ever-narrower specialisations within professions has been driven partly by a tendency towards reductionism, but even more so by the sheer volume of knowledge. Today, it is almost impossible to develop deep expertise across a broad range of fields. However, the pace of increase in knowledge and information has become so fast, and the need for interdisciplinary approaches to problems so great, that graduates need the ability to synthesise ideas from many different disciplines.

People today tend to be temporary experts. What we need is not deep expertise about one particular field, but deep expertise about the particular issue or problem that is being dealt with at the time. And this deep knowledge may need to cut across a wide range of fields. But how is this possible? The answer is that we have to keep learning. Most educators stress that the most important skill needed today is to know how to learn. This is, of course, underpinned by an ability to think.

Systems thinking for complex situations

Most problems of any significance require the application of multiple disciplines. This is where an appreciation of multiple perspectives can ensure better communication at the outset, resulting in a solution to the actual problem experienced rather than on seeking a technical solution to the issue most easily addressed. A systems thinker would deal adequately with the social dimension of a problem (political, economic, human) rather than just the technical (Mant, 1997; Rimmington, 2001).

Mant described systems thinking as having the ability to examine a part in detail while maintaining an awareness of the whole. The systems thinker must be able to survey and understand the broader context and keep it in mind while looking at each component with a view to bringing understanding to the interconnections of individuals and disciplines. Indeed, some years ago Richmond (1977) insightfully described systems thinking as relating to the science and art of making inferences about behaviour through understanding structure. This echoed the earlier contributions of Forrester (1962) on the topic.

More recently, a systems orientation has been viewed as being inextricably linked to leadership. System thinkers apparently have "broad band intelligence" or "intellectual firepower", which Mant saw as a key attribute of leaders. There are similarities between the comparison of "narrow band intelligence" and highly focussed disciplinarianism and the contrast with the "broad band intelligence" of the systems thinker (Rimmington, 2000).

A single field of knowledge normally identified as the key attribute of a discipline or occupation is not enough to make a systems thinker (Gardner, 1993). Other intelligences concerned with linguistic, spatial, interpersonal and intrapersonal abilities are equally important attributes of a leader. Self-knowledge and interpersonal intelligence underpin proper appreciation of multiple perspectives, which in turn enable effective communication (Mackay, 1994) as well as higher order, constructivist learning (Driscoll, 1994).

Who is the best sort of person to lead such a team? Belbin (1993), developer of a widely used team-role modelling scheme, has identified the "long shadow" individual. This is a person who, more easily than others, can assume many different team roles and understand their significance, particularly at different stages of projects. Such a person is obviously invaluable when dealing with the complex matrix of discipline and team role specialities that may be found in the multi-disciplinary team. The contribution of this type of thinking, rather than the individual per se, is the focus of the next section.

The potential of complexity theory

> The use of complexity theory and the systematic analysis of first person conscious experience will be crucial in formulating a proper science of consciousness.
>
> (Capra, 2003, p 37)

Although still in its infancy, complexity theory has much to offer the human sciences; in particular, the emerging discipline of occupational science and the trans-disciplinary arena of practice. As is evident, in viewing people within multi-layered contexts, complexity theory offers a number of important considerations:

- it recognises the diversity of individuals;
- it recognises that individuals and processes interact to form complex systems such that no action should be viewed in isolation;
- it recognises that many processes are based on qualitative effects that need to be captured by symbolic rules, rather than by numeric formulae; and
- it recognises that in complex systems, no single model can be all-embracing, so different models may be needed for different purposes, whether it be explanation, prediction or control.

Still, a profession or organisation must strive to achieve sustainability and accountability, despite the inherent challenges in complex environments. In decision-making, the use of complexity theory will:

- recognise the need for simulation models, rather than simple models, which cannot always provide the outputs of complex systems;
- recognise that complex systems are often inherently unpredictable, so that we need to study scenarios instead;
- recognise that analytic methods cannot provide solutions to many complex problems and that we need to use adaptive methods instead; and
- recognise that patterns and relationships abound in complex systems, so exploratory methods, such as data mining, are increasingly important in research, but that all decisions must still be based on sound information.

Clearly, there is a natural alignment between the basic tenets of complexity theory and the epistemological foundations and chosen methodologies of the human sciences. The potential for this alignment to inform and guide developments is significant. In the next sections, however, we examine just how complexity theory can be utilised or incorporated into the two main areas of focus in this book, namely occupation and professional practice.

Using complexity theory to understand and address occupation

> Communities need occupations that generate social as well as economic capital ... individuals need community supports for occupational experiences of positive independence, respect, connectedness and resource sharing.
>
> (Christiansen & Townsend, 2004, p 167)

Occupation as a concept is the subject of confusion and misinterpretation, depending on where you come from in understanding it. To the person on the street, occupation refers to a job, or work of some form. To governments, occupations as a type of job are classified and grouped, and rates of "occupational participation" refer to how many people are employed within these categorised groupings. In occupational therapy, however, occupation has a very different meaning. Occupational therapists have, through historical research, analysis and in-depth critical professional dialogue, come to understand occupation as *all* the things that people do within the stream of time. Wilcock, whose scholarly work into the origins and meanings of occupation has made a significant contribution to the conceptual terrain in this area, recently proposed an encompassing definition of occupation:

> Occupation encompasses all the things that people do, is part of their being and integral to their becoming whatever they have the potential to become. Occupation has a biological purpose in that it is the mechanism by which people, throughout time, have acquired all they need to accomplish in order to be safe and feel good.
>
> (2001, p 10)

From this definition, occupation becomes something central to the existence of individuals and groups of people; the very fabric of everyday doing that enables them to survive, and hopefully thrive. However, when we pause to consider a phenomenon so central to human existence, we must also consider its inherent complexity. All occupation takes place in a context. That is, no action is independent of the social, cultural, historic, political and economic contexts in which it occurs. These contextual forces, to a greater or lesser extent, shape the form and performance of the occupation as well as the meaning ascribed to it by an individual or group.

Given this growing appreciation of occupation as a complex, socially mediated phenomenon, there have been a number of divergent perspectives applied through which to understand it more fully. Examples include discussion of occupation as: culturally relative (discussed by Iwama in chapter 13); a gendered construct (discussed by Wicks in chapter 11); a form of colonisation (McKinley, 2002); a communitarian necessity (Townsend & Christiansen, 2004); the basis of civil society (Thibeault, 2002); and as an economic concern (Wilcock, 2001).

Such perspectives represent a powerful development in the way we think about, and therefore approach, everyday "doing". Since World War I, with a move towards rehabilitation, doing or occupation became increasingly understood within bio-medical and biomechanical paradigms. This predicated an atomistic orientation to doing; that is, examining the component parts of the body as though it were a machine. By fixing a part of the machine through prescribed and predetermined interventions, it was theoretically possible to have it "functioning" again, at least to its capacity. Viewed thus, the individual's inner world and the external social world were not especially relevant.

The humanist movement of the seventies was the crucible of change with respect to such narrow constructions of occupation. Numerous professional groups were advocating the valuing of people as individuals with social and cultural iden-tities. Holism emerged at this time as a value, if not a reality, in health and human services. In particular, the profession of occupational therapy began to challenge the dominant paradigm of biomedicine and present its own unique constructions of occupation as a broader, more complex phenomenon. There were a number of key figures involved at this time including Gail Fidler and Elizabeth Yerxa, but it was Gary Kielhofner (1985) who first began articulating the value of systems theory to understanding the dynamism and situatedness of occupation. Subse-quently, a general systems perspective has underpinned most major theoretical developments in the field.

As may be evident, then, systems thinking has informed the development of the concept of occupation and practices aimed at enabling it for some time. However, given the more recent evolution of systems thinking within complexity theory, we propose in this chapter that complexity theory has much to offer an expanded appreciation of occupation. This is because, as previously suggested, complexity theory acknowledges the interconnectedness of people and events. It addresses the interactivity of contexts and the potential chaotic effect on people's behaviour. It provides a vehicle for understanding how the actions of an individual resonate with, or impact upon, others. Finally, we suggest that complexity theory may provide the most appropriate means through which to describe occupation within communities because of its centralisation of connectivity. This idea is fundamental, for, what are communities if not essentially connected through what each member does and its impacts on others?

While the potential of complexity theory to inform and guide understandings of occupation may be exciting, a considered program of scholarship and research is requisite to such a development. If this is to occur, there must be a concomitant development of understandings of practice from this perspective also. This is the focus of the next section.

Applying complexity theory in professional practice

> Harder to capture are the material, social, discursive and historical conditions that shape and sometimes disfigure practice; the requirement for practical deliberation and exploratory Faction that are, or should be, the stock trade of the wise practitioner; and the need for continuing public discourse in open public spheres to justify and transform practice in the light of changing material, social, discursive and historical conditions.
>
> (Kemmis, 2004, p 22)

Extensive literature now exists on complexity science and how complexity theory applies to health, health systems and health-care organisations (Albrecht, Freeman & Higginbotham, 1998; Arndt & Bigelow, 2000; Dershin, 1999; Plsek & Greenhalgh, 2001; Plsek & Wilson, 2001; Zimmerman, 1999). However, an interpretation is needed to understand how the theory and fundamental ideas apply to practice. To do this, an assumption is made that the same thinking about organisations as complex adaptive systems can be applied to what goes on in practice. In this sense, practice is what occurs at the interface between the person or persons seeking health care or disability support and the people providing the care or service. Before proceeding, it is worth considering the notion of practice itself.

"Practice" is a word that exists as part of the everyday language of health professionals. Inherent is a sense of intuitive knowing about what it is and who does it. In general, the user of the word practice does not need to explain what is meant and others do not need to ask. Historically, it originates from the Latin word *practica*, meaning a "frequently repeated or customary action; habitual performance; [or] a succession of acts of a similar kind" (Dictionary.com, 2004). While the original meanings still apply in today's world, it has developed to also mean "the carrying out or exercise of a profession or occupation ... the method of action or working ... the practical aspect or application of something as opposed to the theoretical aspect ... [and] in reality" (Brown, 1993, p 2317). Put simply, practice is what is done. The practitioner therefore is "a person involved in the practice of an art, profession, or occupation ... a practical or professional worker" (Brown, p 2318). The practitioner is the doer. This seeming dichotomy between knowing and doing is discussed later in the chapter.

Over the last few decades, in the context of the impacts of scientific discovery, population mobility and migration, globalisation, information technologies and knowledge economies, much has been written about the increasing complexity, and degree and rate of change within the health-care context (Fish, 1998; Higgs & Titchen, 2001; Albrecht et al, 1998). Similarly, understandings of health and health problems are now understood as complex phenomena, not able to be understood as direct cause and effect relationships between things. Drawing this idea through to understanding practice in a changing, complex and uncertain world, it is logical to conclude that practice itself is subject to the same forces and dynamics. Therefore, being an effective practitioner in this current world demands different ways of knowing and doing than in previous more stable environments (Miller, Crabtree, McDaniel & Stange, 1998; Wilson & Holt, 2001).

Looking at employment advertisements for practitioners suggests that the traditional knowledge, skills and attributes for defined fields of professional practice are no longer enough. Organisations are looking for dynamic practitioners who are adaptable and flexible and who can think on their feet in the face of challenging situations. One advertisement for a health, safety and environment field manager reflects the attributes commonly sought in seeking strong analytical skills, a desire to see changes and good problem-solving skills ("Got what it takes?", 2004). Practitioner attributes suited to the complex practice context seem at least as important as the knowledge and wisdom of technical practice.

Practice in a zone of complexity

Earlier in this chapter, complexity was defined as the richness and variety of structure and behaviour that arises from the interactions between the components of a system. In accepting that consumers and practitioners are inherent components of a health system, and the inherent subtleties and complexities of entering into and sustaining helping relationships, it may be said that practice occurs at the very edge of chaos (Lindberg, Herzog, Merry & Goldstein, 1998). Higgs and Titchen (2001) suggest that in this context "health professionals seek to practise and generate knowledge in confusing circumstances and at local and global levels" (p 526). While the expression "knowledge for practice" suggests that knowledge and practice are somewhat separate, "knowledge arises from and within practice, and practice is the purpose of knowledge" (Higgs & Titchen, p 526).

When actualised within any one context, a synergistic effect is produced which is greater than the separate components. Therefore, the particulars of each and every situation mean the interplay between practice knowledge and practice is relational and contextually constructed. Practice occurs in the "zone of complexity" (Zimmerman, 1999, p 46). That is, no two practice occurrences can be the same. Much of what exists in practice is unseen and may only be appreciated through engaging in a deliberative process of enquiry and reasoning. This means that practice cannot be understood or learned by breaking it down into its component parts. While scientific knowledge is one consideration within a professional reasoning process, professional practice is a craft embracing a combination of "intuition, sensitivity, imagination and creativity" (Fish, 1998, p 24).

Practice as an art form

The notion of "practice artistry" has been posited as a useful means of thinking about context specific practice and professional reasoning in complex, uncertain environments. Language and ideas from the arts are applied to professional practice. This emergent thinking suggests practitioners, like artists, must learn to see, interpret and make new meaning things (Fish, 1998). Practice artistry involves "knowing how to make professional judgements and improvise in uncertain and messy situations, where neither ends nor specific means can be pre-specified" (Fish & Coles, as cited in Higgs & Titchen, 2001, p 528). Some of the ways of working

13

in the complex zone of practice have been suggested as asking questions that assist in throwing new light on seemingly familiar situations or basic practice assumptions, using metaphors to communicate complex ideas (Hayle, 2004) and using intuition and muddling through with the client in shaping the practice reality (Wilson & Holt, 2001).

Practice in a complex, uncertain world must be constructed through an emergent process. All of its intricacies cannot be fully analysed or known beforehand. However, each encounter promises a journey into the unknown and therefore the promise of emergence of new understandings grounded in practice.

Conclusions

> Without context, words and actions have no meanings at all. This is true of not only human communication in words, but of all communications whatsoever.
>
> (Bateson, 1979, p 4)

In this chapter, we have considered the basic tenets of complexity theory and why it may be useful in developing our understandings of occupation and practice. The reason for this is because complexity theory addresses: *context*; the dynamic interactive effects between parts of systems; the inherent connectivity that exists between people and events in time and space; and the essential unpredictability of human interactions. We considered some of the recent developments in the conceptual domains of both occupation and professional practice and the apparent goodness of fit between the key issues underpinning each as well as the essential features of complexity theory. In conclusion, this chapter has argued that, in order to understand and meaningfully address the future challenges of what people do and our professional actions relative to this in a sustainable manner, complexity theory has much to offer.

References

Albrecht, G., Freeman, S. & Higginbotham, N. (1998). Complexity and human health: The case for a transdisciplinary paradigm. *Culture, Medicine and Psychiatry, 22*, 55–92.

Arndt, M. & Bigelow, B. (2000). Commentary: The potential of chaos theory and complexity theory for health services management. *Health Care Management Review, 25*(1), 35–38.

Bateson, G. (1979). *Mind and nature: A necessary unity*. London: Flamingo.

Belbin, R. M. (1983). *Team roles at work*. Oxford: Butterworth-Heinemann.

Bossomaier, T. R. J. & Green, D. G. (2000). *Complex Systems*. Cambridge: Cambridge University Press.

Brown, L. (Ed.). (1993). *The new shorter Oxford English dictionary: On historical principles*. Oxford: Clarendon Press.

Capra, F. (2003). *The hidden connections: A science for sustainable living*. London: Flamingo Publishers.

Coverney, P. & Highfield, R. (1995). *Frontiers of complexity. The search for order in a chaotic world*. London: Faber & Faber.

Dershin, H. (1999). Nonlinear systems theory in medical care management. *The Physician Executive, 25*(3), 8–16.

Dictionary.com (2004). *Webster's Revised Unabridged Dictionary 1998*. Retrieved 3 May 2004, from http://dictionary.reference.com/search?q=practice

Driscoll, M. P. (1994). *Psychology of learning for instruction* (2nd ed.). Boston: Allyn & Bacon.

Fish, D. (1998). *Appreciating practice in the caring professions: Refocusing professional development and practitioner research*. Oxford: Butterworth-Heinemann.

Forrester, J. W. (1961). *Industrial Dynamic*. New York, NY: Productivity Press.

Gardner, H. (1983). *Frames of mind. The theory of multiple intelligences*. New York: Basic Books Inc.

Got what it takes? (2004, May 8–9). Situations Vacant. *New Zealand Herald*, p C25.

Hayle, N. K. (2000). *From chaos to complexity: Moving through metaphor to practice*. Retrieved 3 May 2004, from http://www.southernct.edu/chaos-nursing/chaos4.htm

Higgs, J. & Titchen, A. (2001). Rethinking the practice–knowledge interface in an uncertain world: A model for practice development. *British Journal of Occupational Therapy, 64*(11), 526–533.

Kemmis, S. (2004). Knowing practice: searching for saliences. Paper presented at the conference Participant Knowledge and Knowing Practice, Umea, Sweden March 26–27.

Kielhofner, G. (1985). *A model of human occupation*. Baltimore: Williams & Wilkins.

Kielhofner, G. (1997). *Conceptual foundations of occupational therapy* (2nd ed.). Philadelphia: F. A. Davies.

Klomp, N. I., Green, D. G. & Fry, G. (1997). Roles of technology in ecology. In N. I. Klomp & I. D. Lunt (Eds), *Frontiers in Ecology: Building the Links*, pp 299–309. Oxford: Elsevier Science.

Liljeros, F., Edling, C. R., Amaral, L. A. N., Stanley, H. E. & Aberg, Y. (2001). The web of human sexual contacts, *Nature, 411*, 907–908.

Lindberg, C., Herzog, A., Merry, M. & Goldstein, J. (1998). Life at the edge of chaos. *The Physician Executive, 24*(1), 6–21.

Mackay, H. (1994). *Why don't people listen? Solving the communication problem*. Sydney: Pan Macmillan Australia.

Mant, A. (1997). *Intelligent leadership*. Sydney: Allen & Unwin.

McKinley, E. (2002). Brown bodies in white coats: Māori women scientists and identity. *Journal of Occupational Science, 9*(3), 109–116.

Miller, W. L., Crabtree, B. F., McDaniel, R. & Stange, K. C. (1998). Understanding change in primary care practice using complexity theory. *Journal of Family Practice, 46*(5), 369–377.

Plsek, P. E. & Greenhalgh, T. (2001). The challenge of complexity in health care. *British Medical Journal, 323*, 625–628.

Plsek, P. E. & Wilson, T. (2001). Complexity, leadership, and management in healthcare organisations. *British Medical Journal, 323*, 746–749.

Rimmington, G. (2001). Systems thinking and leadership in agriculture science. *Agriculture Science, 13*(4), 28–31.

Thibeault, R. (2002). Occupation and the rebuilding of civil society: Notes from the war zone. *Journal of Occupational Science, 9*(1), 38–47.

Townsend, E., & Chistiansen, C. (2004). The occupational nature of communities. In C. Christiansen & E. Townsend (Eds), *Occupation: The art and science of living*, pp 141–172. Upper Saddle River: Prentice Hall.

Townsend, E. & Wilcock, A. (2004). Occupational justice. In C. Christiansen & E. Townsend (Eds), *Occupation: The art and science of living*, pp 243–273. Upper Saddle River: Prentice Hall.

Whiteford, G., Townsend, E. & Hocking, C. (2000). Reflections on a renaissance of occupation. *Canadian Journal of Occupation, 67*(1), 61–69.

Whiteford, G. (in press). Understanding the occupational deprivation of refugees. *Canadian Journal of Occupational Therapy*.

Wilcock, A. (1998). *An occupational perspective of health*. New Jersey: Slack.

Wilcock, A. A. (2001). *Occupation for health (Vol 1): A journey from self health to prescription*. London: British College of Occupational Therapists.

Wilson, T. & Holt, T. (2001). Complexity and clinical care. *British Medical Journal, 323*, 685–688.

Zimmerman, B. (1999). Complexity science: A route through hard times and uncertainty. *Health Forum Journal, March–April*, 42–46.

CHAPTER TWO

The Moral Context of Practice and Professional Relationships

Valerie Wright-St Clair
David Seedhouse

KEY WORDS

Taken-for-granted moral world
Professional ethics
Human relating
Moral competence
Occupational therapy values
Moral reasoning

Chapter Profile

The contextual landscape for health practice is increasingly articulate about human and consumer rights, professional accountability and demonstrable ethical competence. Fundamentally, the practice context ought to be understood as a moral context. This chapter aims to make visible the taken for granted moral context of the everyday world of practice for health professionals. In particular, the lens is focused on aspects of the day-to-day relating between practitioners and clients, and the gap between the rhetoric of the ideal and the reality in practice. Initially, the moral dimensions of human relating are explored. This provides a foundation from which to consider the relevance of professional codes of ethics in guiding practice decisions. It is argued that practitioners need to develop new modes of reasoning and relating that go beyond the intuitive, or a reliance on codes of ethics, in seemingly unproblematic and troubling situations.

Finally, a case example drawn from contemporary practice is used to illuminate the arguments posed in the chapter. As a logical way forward, the foundations theory of health is presented as a framework for guiding moral decision-making. While research findings and case examples in occupational therapy are used, the ideas in this chapter are applicable to the world of health professional practice in general.

Introduction

By virtue of being human, we live as part of families, communities and societies. Human-to-human relating therefore makes up the very fabric of people's co-existence. In striving to live together harmoniously and cooperatively, moral understandings are shared ideas that guide us towards being thoughtful and considerate in how we are and what we do in our everyday worlds. Capra (2003) describes morality as "a standard of human conduct that flows from a sense of belonging" (p 187). Learning moral competence is thus an imperative in understanding human relationships. Some relationships in society take on special responsibilities. The idea of a "helping relationship" has informed professional understandings about the moral values and obligations that health practitioners hold towards their clients. By their very nature, helping relationships are entered into by persons seeking assistance to achieve a positive health or life change. While technical competence of the health practitioner is important, the effect of intervening in another's life may be essentially influenced by the characteristics and quality of the relationship and the health professional's skill in relating (Lloyd & Maas, 1993).

Ethics, as an idea and a concern, has held a place in popular professional culture for several decades. Increasingly, ethical concerns about extraordinary biomedical cases are thrust into the public arena and capture the imagination of professionals and laypersons alike. While such conversations are necessary for moral development in the delivery of health care, they serve to conceal that which exists in the ordinary dimensions of practice. Accordingly, the nature of morality and ethics is generally misunderstood in the professional context. In the tide of high-profile ethical debates and growing public expectations for morally-competent practitioners, codes of ethics are typically generated by professional groups and endorsed as universal statements of communal ethical principles. Practitioners' endorsement of the codes supposedly acts to promote and guide the espoused standards of professional behaviour. But despite their popularity, professional codes of ethics in themselves are impotent guides for moral reasoning in the everyday practice world.

Practice in the moral landscape

For centuries, moral philosophers have debated how we ought to live our lives in relation to others. Regardless of people's particular moral commitments, if we wish to be moral we must constantly consider how we are, and what we do, in the world. Rachels' (2003) explanation of morality as being, at a minimum, "the effort to guide one's conduct by reason" (p 14) goes part of the way to defining what morality might mean as an everyday concept for health practitioners. However, in its simplicity, Rachel's definition reduces the idea of moral ways to being a solely intellectual pursuit. It suggests that deciding what to do is a rational process. It is silent on the idea that wise decision-making for practitioners engaged in a helping relationship may essentially emerge from a mix of feeling and thinking (Mayeroff, 1971). Knowing how to respond in a given situation may be founded in the practitioner's gaining a sense of who the client is and a receptivity to apprehend how things are understood by him or her (Noddings, 1984).

Morality, therefore, is not something that exists as a quantifiable measure in the human environment. Rather, morality exists in people's experienced, subjective worlds. It is a dynamic construction in the everyday, interactional world of human relating. Some relationships, by their very nature and circumstance, are defined by particular qualities and expectations. The nature of the purposive relationship between health practitioners and those who seek assistance from them is one that receives considerable attention in society. The responsibility of health professionals to be considered in their relationships with clients is more morally, and in many cases more legally, binding than casual, social relationships. While practitioners' technical competence is important, the effect of intervening in others' lives is essentially influenced by their skill in relating and the characteristics and quality of their relationships with clients (Lloyd & Maas, 1993; Van Amburg, 1997).

Codifying morality

Professional codes of ethics are typically embraced as a panacea to avoid or correct wrongdoing. They publicly name and thus attempt to encourage the moral competence of the profession's members. As such, the codification of moral obligations and their enforcement is often claimed as characteristic of being a bona fide profession (Beauchamp & Childress, 2001). While upholding the benefits of a code of ethics may be intuitively appealing, attempting to capture the complexity of professional morality in a codified form is where the idea starts to encounter difficulty. By their very nature, professional codes of ethics contribute to a shift in emphasis from morality being considered as integral to relating in the everyday practice world towards being something that directs decisions about how to act, particularly in ethically challenging situations. Three reasons are suggested why codified ethics contribute to this distortion.

The invisibility of moral dimensions

First, the commonplace nature of morality means it is consigned to the routine, habitual ways of being and acting in the world. It is something that is everywhere (Christiansen, 2001; Seedhouse, 2000). Morality is, therefore, taken for granted and invisible to the everyday eye unless something happens to bring it into sharp relief. Practitioners naturally go about their everyday business of being with and acting in relation to clients, their families and others around them without continuous reflection and reasoned consideration. Relating becomes instinctive. In other words, the practitioner's usual habits in communicating and reasoning are enacted in routine ways. This is not to suggest the majority of day-to-day interactions and decisions are immoral or that health professionals are not well intended. Rather, it means that the subtleties of relating can and do mostly happen without conscious reflection and deliberation.

If we accept that "ethics is a pervasive phenomenon of human life ... [then] every human action that can affect one or more of us has ethical content" (Seedhouse, 2000, p 181). Therefore, a commitment to consider seriously the everyday, routine ways of relating would illuminate things not usually thought about. At one level, at least, this is happening. The escalation of interpretive studies within the health care context, particularly those exploring the lived experiences of consumers and their families, is giving new voice to that which has been unseen and likely thought of as not existing. Diekelmann's (2002) recent collection of studies illustrates how interactions and practices in health care settings implicitly embody oppression and violence. Serious reflection and deliberation on the ordinary events in practice is put forward as one means of practitioners understanding how clients receive and experience them (Smythe, 2002). Similarly, Christiansen (2001) suggests that when therapeutic encounters fail, practitioners are inclined to underestimate, or dismiss as inconsequential, the effect on their client's sense of self and self-efficacy.

Being receptive towards the idea that clients may experience a sense of harm through their everyday interactions with them may enable health practitioners to start new conversations that challenge conventional understandings about the moral dimensions of relating in practice.

The fascination in extraordinary events

A second reason why the moral dimensions of human relating may remain hidden in the practice world seems to rest on the predictability of everyday events. Things seemingly go well when there are no indicators to the contrary. But unseen things can and do go wrong and the unpredictable can occur. Biomedical ethics and the study of professional morality (Purtilo, 1999) have thrived within a context of increasingly sophisticated, technological advances in health care. Alongside these advances have been escalating levels of public scrutiny and consumer autonomy. Professional and public attention is drawn towards the extraordinary and often unpredictable moral events. A consciousness of the everyday moral dimensions of practice seems lost in the background.

Heightened public expectations for health professionals to be ethically competent and ethically accountable adds valence to the understanding that professional morality and health ethics exist almost exclusively within the realm of significant moral events and hard cases (Foto, 1998; Wright-St Clair, 2001). In the face of mounting public pressure to respond to the unpredictable and the dramatic, it could seem unproductive for professionals to turn their attention to the commonplace matters of relating to and being with clients. Even if the everyday dimensions of morality are uncovered, "habitual ways of viewing things may keep [health practitioners] from gaining new understanding" (Wright-St Clair, p 188).

19

Morality exists in Codes of Ethics

The third reason posited for everyday morality being unseen in the practice context is the standard conception of professional morality as existing in codes of ethics. Professional codes of ethics are supposedly created with the intention of communicating the scope of moral responsibilities and morally acceptable actions to the profession's members. As a public relations effort, codes of ethics may be purported as an enforceable means of directing practitioner's behaviour, protecting consumer's rights, and amending specific ethical concerns about the practice (Scott, 1998). A look at codes of professional ethics available on the Internet shows conformity with Scott's ideas. The codes' purpose statements primarily spell out behaviourally-focused objectives. They claim to tell "the practitioner what to do" (Occupational Therapy Association of South Africa, 2000, p 1), describe, promote and/or maintain the highest, proper or acceptable standards of professional conduct (American Occupational Therapy Association, 2000; Canadian Physiotherapy Association, 2001; College of Occupational Therapists, 2000; New Zealand Medical Association, 2002; New Zealand Society of Physiotherapists, 2003; World Medical Association, 2002; World Federation of Occupational Therapists, 2002), define the "essentials of honourable behaviour" (American Medical Association, 2001, p 1), set the "profession's non-negotiable ethical standard" (American Nurses Association, 2001, p 2), provide a basis for "professional and self reflection on ethical conduct" (Australian Nursing Council, 2000, p 1), guide the "pursuance of ... professional practice" (Australian Association of Occupational Therapists, 2001, p 2), and act as an aid and guide to "ethical decision making" (New Zealand Occupational Therapy Board, 1998, p 3).

Although codes of ethics are primarily promulgated as serving clients' best interests, the professional group's self-interest is covertly served by protecting "the profession itself and its position in the public mind" (Corbett, 1993, p 117).

A focus on moral competence

In the process of reducing the notion of professional morality to a list or coded set of moral attributes, rules or principles, the abstractions and complexity of both the taken for granted and the dramatic events in practice seem lost. Whereas the obligation to maintain clinical competence gets a strong voice in professional documentation and standards of practice, ethical codes are predominantly mute on the matter of moral competence, lending credence to the idea of the ethics myth. Within this mythical realm, practitioners believe that the codified ethical rules will guide resolution when the out-of-the-ordinary or crises occur (Seedhouse, 2000).

The evidence suggests that codes of ethics are indeed failing to deliver on their promise. Research findings now offer "extensive documentation on the lack of concordance between such guidelines and the experience of 'real' dilemmas" (Barnitt & Partidge, 1997, p 178). Rich modes of questioning and deep reasoning are seemingly superseded by the directive, authoritarian voice of codes of ethics. Nonetheless, with or without ethical codes, good practitioners can do bad things and vice versa. Any attempt at scripting moral competence will be enigmatic. No simple formula exists for building good arguments or evading deficient ones

(Rachels, 2003) in the moral context. This means professional groups may be wiser to shift their focus from constructing codes of ethics as lists of moral principles to considering how their members can:

1. gain enriched understandings about the ways of being in the world;

2. understand the nature of knowledge;

3. come to know about things moral; and

4. build competence in the ways of engaging in moral decision-making with regard to everyday encounters and practice concerns.

Codes of ethics as a statement of philosophical and professional values

Professional codes of ethics may fail to deliver on their promise to promote or guide moral conduct and moral judgements in the professional context but they could stand as a public statement of the group's philosophy and its inherent values.

Occupation-focused practice: Philosophy and values

Enabling people to participate in their human and ecological environments is a central aim of occupation-focused practice in the health, disability and social arenas. While such a focus is not the exclusive domain of occupational therapists, occupational therapy practice is essentially occupation-focused practice. In order to illustrate application of the ideas developed in this section, reference is made to occupational therapy where necessary.

One central tenet of occupation-focused practice is that human engagement in occupations of significance is important to health. That is, people's healthfulness is influenced by doing the things they want and need to do within their socially and culturally-defined contexts. Emerging from humanist foundations, occupation-focused practice is based on understanding the person as "active, capable, free, self-directed, integrated, purposeful, and an agent who is the author of health-influencing activity" (Yerxa, 1992, p 79). The recent adoption by a range of professional groups of the term "client-centred practice" in essence captures these theoretical ideas (Townsend, 1993), containing the promise of a therapeutic encounter that bears all the hallmarks of the notion's philosophical underpinnings. While the term "client-centred" may be a sincere effort to say something about professional values, a shift to thinking about "person-centred" practice would go some way towards embracing broader moral understandings of clients as autonomous persons.

Thus, in order to be grounded in the philosophical underpinnings and be meaningful as a codified statement of professional values, the moral principles of beneficence and respect for autonomy ought to be evident in any code of ethics informing occupation-focused practice.

The meaning of beneficence and autonomy

The principle of beneficence "establishes an obligation to help others further their important and legitimate interests" (Beauchamp & Childress, 2001, p 166). What is good for the person must therefore be defined and interpreted in context. In any occupation-focused practice encounter, the important and legitimate interests in the client's experienced world ought to be centred to practice, being aimed towards achieving occupational benefits for him or her.

The principle of respect for autonomy establishes an obligation to value, in attitude and actions, the person's capacity and right to "hold views, to make choices and to take actions based on personal values and beliefs" (Beauchamp & Childress, 2001, p 63). Although the concept of autonomy is at times criticised as being inherently individualistic, richer understandings of autonomy are also used. Autonomy is understood to be relational and contextual, consistent with people's social connectedness. Occupation-focused practice is concerned with enabling people as autonomous persons, and not simply acknowledging their right to make autonomous choices. As such, respecting autonomy also embraces an obligation to help develop or maintain the person's capacities as an autonomous agent. The person's understandings of, and reflections on, values and beliefs in shaping and living out a life plan are central.

A critical reflection on Occupational Therapy Codes of Ethics

A review of eight occupational therapy codes of ethics reveals atomistic representations of beneficence and respect of autonomy, and a failure to contextualise the ideas within the profession's collective philosophical consciousness. Two of the codes are entirely silent on the notion of beneficence. Only one of the codes reviewed addresses an obligation to assist the client to achieve his or her desired outcomes. The remainder typically represent beneficence as an obligation to be concerned about the client's welfare, or to be client-centred and needs-focused in practice decisions.

All of the codes say something about autonomy but they mostly refer to the obligations of respecting the client's right to make autonomous choices, giving information, having the client as an active participant in decisions, or respecting the client's right to refuse. Notions of the client as an autonomous person are typically reduced to obligations such as promoting dignity, privacy and safety, or not discriminating against the client on the basis of personal characteristics.

While codes of ethics refer to autonomy as a principle, occupational therapists in practice are more likely to talk about promoting independence, but are they the same thing? Russell, Fitzgerald, Williamson, Manor and Whybrow (2002) propose that practitioners' understandings about independence have shifted away from simply meaning a physical self-reliance in doing things towards meaning autonomy, or self-determination. However, research shows the everyday language of independence tends to focus on clients learning to do things for themselves and regaining skills in daily living activities (Barnitt, 1998; Barnitt & Partridge, 1997; Hasselkus & Dickie, 1990; Hasselkus & Dickie, 1994; Russell et al).

The generality with which the principled statements are described in the occupational therapy codes of ethics reviewed, means they could be written for any health professional group. If codes of ethics are to stand as statements of a profession's philosophy and values at least minimally, then interpretations of the moral principles and language in context are needed.

A gap between the ideal and the real

In practice, the fact that codes of ethics fall short of their espoused promise is probably unimportant. It is likely that most practitioners intuitively identify moral concerns and want to do the right thing without conscientiously reading and attempting to apply the principles embedded in a code of ethics. Nevertheless, studies exploring the identification of ethical issues and ethical reasoning in practice illustrate that practitioners from a range of disciplines know and intuitively integrate their profession's philosophical underpinnings in their language and what they attend to (Barnitt, 1993; Barnitt, 1998; Barnitt & Partridge, 1997; Hasselkus & Dickie, 1990; Hansen, Kamp & Reitz, 1988; Uden, Norberg, Lindseth, & Marhaug, 1992).

Uden et al's study revealed philosophical differences in nurses' and physicians' approaches to moral reasoning, with ethical content frequently surrounding issues of power or powerlessness, responsibility and the right to decide. Similarly, Barnitt and Partridge (1997) explored physiotherapists' and occupational therapists' moral reasoning by analysing stories about a recent "ethical dilemma" experienced in practice (p 182). They found physiotherapists primarily used a biomedical frame of reference and forms of diagnostic reasoning, and emphasised how the diagnosis was arrived at and the implications for treatment. Conversely, in their stories, occupational therapists used a psychosocial or humanistic frame of reference, narrative forms of reasoning, and emphasised the social context and background to the issues described. In particular, distress was experienced when the client's wishes to do everyday occupations conflicted with the therapist's judgement about safety, or when the therapist's recommended interventions were rejected.

When practitioners' and clients' worlds collide

Russell et al (2002) found that practitioners' concerns in relation to older adults' independence commonly arose from a sense of responsibility for client safety. They suggest a caveat is constructed wherein clients are "*allowed* to be independent (autonomous decision-makers) as long as they are *safe* to do so ... in the opinion of the therapist" (Russell et al, p 375). Similarly, Barnitt (1993) found that ethical issues for practitioners commonly surfaced when "their moral rule was challenged" either by clients or team members (p 211). Similar findings were revealed in a later and more extensive questionnaire-based study in which occupational therapists and physiotherapists were asked to write about an ethical dilemma. Many of the practitioners described making difficult, "risky" judgements around clients' readiness for discharge. In particular, the dilemmas described safety issues in relation to older adults going home, and clients continuing to do activities the therapists considered were unsafe (Barnitt, 1998).

While practitioners are reported as valuing good communication with clients and families and gaining a genuine understanding of their needs and wishes (Hasselkus & Dickie, 1994), a number of studies point to a gap between what therapists believe, the rhetoric of the ideal and the reality of everyday practice (Barnitt, 1998; Barnitt & Partridge, 1997; Hasselkus, 1991; Russell et al, 2002; Townsend, 1993; Van Amburg, 1997). Hasselkus (1991) interviewed family caregivers of older adults receiving occupational therapy and clearly illustrated encounters where the caregiver's experiences were at odds with the profession's espoused values. The data revealed instances of carers changing the treatment regimes set by therapists because things didn't fit their day-to-day reality or match the carer and client goals.

In critically considering why clients and caregivers increasingly report their experience of health care services as depersonalising, Van Amburg (1997) lays some of the blame at the feet of codes of ethics and the promulgation of moral rules defining professional role boundaries. He points to moral edicts for practitioners to "avoid those relationships or activities that interfere with professional judgement and *objectivity* [italics added]" (p 187), reasoning that collaboration is absent in professional objectiveness, resulting in disengaged and depersonalised relationships with clients. The paradigm underpinning professional role boundaries in moral practice ought to be founded in forming authentic, caring relationships and not based on positivist, biomedical values for objectivity (Van Amburg).

The gap itself may not be a major cause for alarm as morality is not about understanding how things are, but about being considered and making reasoned responses. Being moral is about continuously considering how things ought to be. It is therefore suggested that the solution lies in practitioners holding a rich awareness of the moral dimensions of practice, a genuine mindfulness of the complexity in everyday environments and professional relating, a deep reflection on the intuitive ways of being and acting, an openness to receive alternative views and a commitment to thoughtful, considered reasoning.

Closing the gap through considered reasoning

The unique combination of characteristics in each and every practice situation means that the factors constituting a reason in one instance may not do so in others. As such, any movement towards a solution lies in practitioners seeking a rich awareness of the other's subjective meanings and aspirations and a commitment to continuous, considered reasoning. Barnitt and Partridge (1997) observed that practitioners seemed less threatened and experienced less uncertainty when confronted with seemingly familiar situations. This suggests that practitioners may be unreceptive to the unique characteristics inherent in each situation having developed more fixed, less-considered modes of reasoning. Serious reflection and open deliberation is not easy. It takes courage and open-mindedness to consider the complex dimensions of the seemingly banal moral encounter. Yet, not to do so suggests a serious gap in moral competence and a perpetuation of instances that may inflict an everyday violence on those practitioners wish to protect from harm.

To illustrate a way forward when a practitioner and client, or client's family member, disagree on what ought to be done, a case example from contemporary practice is presented and interpreted.

Moral reasoning in practice

The following is an edited story received from a New Zealand occupational therapist in response to a request for an "example of an ethical concern taken from real life". It relates to a difficult, though not unusual, experience in which service providers and services users disagreed about what should be done. The story highlights the gap between the understandings and values held by the practitioner and client, or in this case the client's husband. It is presented as a means of illustrating how the practitioner's professional code of ethics failed to inform a defensible solution to the issues. Following this, an occupationally-focused philosophy of health and a process of moral reasoning are presented as a rigorous and considered way forward in working through the complexities of the situation. The client is given the name of Mrs Mitchell.

Mrs Mitchell is 82 years old. She lives with her husband in a large, three-level house on a rural property. Mr Mitchell, also in his 80s, has a tertiary education and has kept himself fit and active in his retirement. While Mrs Mitchell has been primarily responsible for the housekeeping and meals, she is used to working hard having raised four children. Their adult children now live out of the district or overseas, with the closest and eldest daughter being eight hours' drive away.

It came as a surprise to everyone, family and neighbours alike, when Mrs Mitchell collapsed and was taken to hospital by ambulance. She had experienced a subarachnoid haemorrhage. Mrs Mitchell's previous good health was a likely contributor to the medical team deciding she was stable enough for discharge home after ten days in hospital. At this point, a referral was sent to the occupational therapist for assessment of her home environment prior to discharge the following day. The medical staff then requested a cognitive assessment. Accepting the referral, the therapist planned to assess how well Mrs Mitchell managed with her everyday self-care and then take her home to evaluate how well she managed her usual daily occupations in her own, familiar environment. She set up a meeting with Mr and Mrs Mitchell to explain the recommended assessments and invited the social worker. Before the meeting, nursing staff approached the therapist to say the eldest daughter wished to bring her mother to convalesce with her, in line with the family's wishes.

In the meeting to discuss the pre-discharge assessments, Mr Mitchell expressed his frustration. He was convinced that being in hospital was prolonging his wife's recovery. He felt boredom was causing her to be lethargic, sleepy and confused at times. Mr Mitchell was forthright in his insistence that he could manage everything without assistance. He expressed doubt that the assessments would be of any use and a concern that they might simply act to delay his wife's return home. However, he finally consented to the assessments going ahead.

Results of the self-care assessment showed Mrs Mitchell was unsteady with walking, needing one assistant, and was unable to manage her medications herself. In the cognitive assessment, Mrs Mitchell presented as having pre-senile dementia with difficulties of memory, reasoning, judgement and orientation. At this point, the therapist questioned whether it was safe for her client to go home. She recommended transfer to an assessment, treatment and rehabilitation unit and communicated the results to Mr Mitchell, as requested. In spite of his wife saying she did not want to go, Mr Mitchell still felt she would do better at home and chose to discharge her, making his wife walk to the car. The next day, the occupational therapist visited Mrs Mitchell at home and was concerned to find she had been moved into, and slept alone, in a cottage adjacent to the family home as she couldn't manage the stairs. Mrs Mitchell had not taken any medication since her discharge the previous day.

Identifying the concerns

The therapist reflected on the following concerns:

1. Mr Mitchell seemed to misunderstand what the service could offer.

2. Mr Mitchell seemed more driven by a distrust of the system rather than a concern about his wife's recovery.

3. Mr Mitchell wrongly interpreted his wife's sleepiness as being due to boredom.

4. Something else may be behind Mr Mitchell thinking that home rather than hospital was the best place for his wife's recovery.

5. Mrs Mitchell may be expected to do all her usual work, including cooking, at home rather than be allowed time for recovery and rehabilitation.

6. The "family's wishes" as expressed by the daughter conflicted with the husband's wishes.

7. The therapist still felt a "duty of care" towards Mrs Mitchell in spite of a hostile exchange with the husband and asked a colleague to attend the next home visit.

Considering the practical options

One way forward in thinking through the best course of action is for the practitioner to consider the practical options presented by the circumstances. They might be:

1. leave Mrs Mitchell and her husband to sort out their own affairs;

2. continue to visit and offer support to Mr and Mrs Mitchell;

3. arrange for Mrs Mitchell to stay at her eldest daughter's home, if convinced she would be better supported there; or

4. advocate for Mrs Mitchell to remain in health or social services care.

Which of these options is ethical? Which one is the most ethical? Are any of them unethical? What would help answer these questions? Will reference to either a professional code of ethics or the application of one or more moral principles (or both) guide the ethical resolution of such issues? Despite the popularity of professional ethics, making reference to moral codes and principles can be counter-productive. The following section illustrates why.

Codes of Ethics are inadequate

Codes of ethics and ethical principles are inadequate for proper decision-making, a fact that is very easy to demonstrate. Extracts from a current code of ethics (New Zealand Occupational Therapy Board, 1998) are used as a means of illustrating the argument in relation to Mrs Mitchell's situation.

> [Practitioners] shall respect the autonomy of people receiving their service, acknowledging the client's role, and sharing power and decision making.

Which people? Presumably, Mrs Mitchell since she is the only person in receipt of any service. However the code goes on to state that:

> [Practitioners] shall work with clients and their family/whanau or carers to determine goals and priorities.

Immediately, a difficulty is encountered. Now it seems that Mrs Mitchell's autonomy is not paramount after all — rather it is the client (Mrs Mitchell) *and* the family who must determine goals and priorities. But who defines "family"? The practitioner must do so, sharing power and decision-making. So a solution is no closer. The problem remains the same; whose wishes to respect, whom to involve in the decision-making and how much power to share? Returning to the code:

> [Practitioners] shall have the needs of the client as the focus of their practice.

The picture changes again. The priority is no longer the client and the family; it is to meet the needs of the client. But which needs of Mrs Mitchell? The need to be at home? The need for medication or therapy? The need for safety? Who defines the needs; Mrs Mitchell, Mr Mitchell, Mr and Mrs Mitchell together, Mrs Mitchell's daughter, the therapist, a psychiatrist, the police, or everybody?

The next principle guiding the relationship with the person receiving services specifies that:

> [Practitioners] shall base their intervention and perform their duties on the basis of accurate and current information.

Unfortunately, in Mrs Mitchell's case, the information is confused and conflicting. While the ethical principles sound appealing at first glance, they offer no help to Mrs Mitchell's therapist. Indeed, it is suggested that such codes are unlikely to offer help to practitioners who have to decide in *any* circumstances where there are different options about how best to proceed. Would more general considerations of moral principles help?

Moral principles are inadequate

Two decades ago, two American academics, Beauchamp and Childress (1994), published the "four principles approach" to medical ethics, the principles being:

- beneficence or the obligation to provide benefits and balance benefits against risks;
- non-maleficence or the obligation to avoid the causation of harm;
- respect for autonomy or the obligation to respect the decision-making capacities of autonomous persons; and
- justice or the obligations of fairness in the distribution of benefits and risks.

The idea has proved widely influential in both teaching and writing about medical and health ethics, particularly among medical clinicians and nurses. However, the four principles idea is deceptively simple. By using these principles, either singly or in combination, a practitioner is supposed to be able to arrive at a satisfactory answer to any moral problem in his or her work. It is acknowledged that practitioners may need additional interpretations and specifications and further rules, such as in regard to keeping confidences, but essentially the four principles are thought by their advocates to provide an adequate framework for all moral deliberation in health care.

Gillon (1994) offers full support for this principled approach claiming that regardless of a practitioner's philosophical, political, religious or moral stance, a commitment to the four, prima facie moral principles will guide ethical decision-making in most, if not all, of the moral issues arising in the health care context (prima facie meaning a principle is binding unless it conflicts with another moral principle in a given case). If it does conflict, then a choice must be made between them. However, the principled approach does not claim to provide a method for doing so. Instead, it offers a common set of moral commitments, a common moral language and a common set of moral issues to be considered in particular cases. While the principles have been criticised as reducing moral reasoning to a checklist of values, perhaps more importantly they fail to give a theoretical guide to how the principles work together in generating clear, coherent and specific rules or how to deal with a conflict of principles (Clouser & Gert, 1990).

Because the principles lack detail, they can be used by almost anyone to defend almost anything. Each of the principles is open to such wide interpretation that it is indefensible to state, "I am following principle X" without further explanation of what X is taken to mean. And if you can articulate what you mean more exactly, you will find you have gone beyond the principles anyway. So thoughtful reflection on moral priorities renders the four principles redundant. In moral reasoning, matters of meaning and purpose must be addressed. Philosophical questions should therefore be determinedly pursued in order to develop an underlying theory capable of supporting moral and practical conclusions.

Practical philosophy can provide the solution

What can be used to provide the best solution to the moral concerns posed in the story about Mrs Mitchell? Resorting to codes of ethics and ethical principles has been discounted as inadequate. Such arguments may simply obscure what is really going on; that is, the use of subjective values and preferences in deciding what to do. There is also nothing to be gained in searching for the most ethically-correct solution, since there may be no such thing. What can be done, however, is to develop theories of purpose. Such theories explain why health work is important and provide practical guidance on their implementation. It is theories of purpose that offer a considered way forward in the complex moral context of health practice. The "foundations theory of health" (Seedhouse, 2002) is one such theory. It focuses on peoples' occupations, enabling participation in chosen environments as the purpose of working for health. It can be applied to individuals or groups and therefore embraces a broad understanding of both population and personal health.

Foundations Theory of Health

Starting from philosophical foundations, the application of the foundations theory of health might shed new light on what to do in Mrs Mitchell's case.

Essentially, a health practitioner using this approach is committed to the view that work for health is work to create autonomy, or enable a person to do the things he or she wants or needs to do (Seedhouse, 2002). Autonomy is created by building up a person or group's basic foundations for participation and achievement in their life world. The four main boxes in the model represent the central conditions for leading a fulfilling life and enhancing potentials. They represent persons having:

1. basic needs met including nutrition, shelter and sense of purpose in life;

2. access to a range of information in relation to things that influence the person or person's life and life choices;

3. skill in assimilating the information and understanding how it applies to them and the confidence to make a reasoned decision; and

4. a sense of place and belonging in the environment and community.

The fifth box represents the temporary, or long-term, additional supports needed in particular life circumstances. Supports may be health or social services such as medicine, nursing and occupational therapy, or removing environmental barriers to community participation, and so on (Seedhouse, 2002).

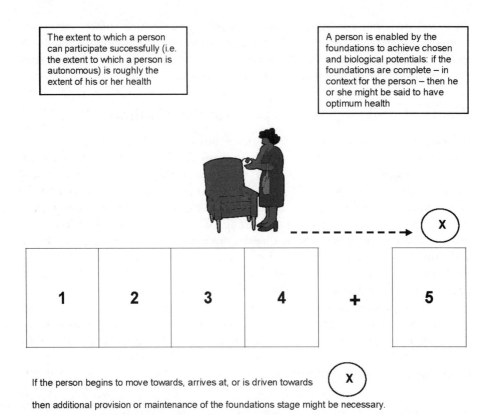

The extent to which a person can participate successfully (i.e. the extent to which a person is autonomous) is roughly the extent of his or her health

A person is enabled by the foundations to achieve chosen and biological potentials: if the foundations are complete – in context for the person – then he or she might be said to have optimum health

If the person begins to move towards, arrives at, or is driven towards X

then additional provision or maintenance of the foundations stage might be necessary.

Figure 2.1   Foundations Theory of Health

Adapted from: *Total health promotion: Mental health, rational fields and the quest for autonomy.* D Seedhouse (2002), p 95. Copyright John Wiley & Sons Limited. Reproduced with permission.

The figure on the foundations can be a person, a family, a larger group, a nation or even larger. It is for the health practitioner to decide whom this figure represents and therefore the focus of services. There is no getting away from this first step. The selection of the figure is a matter of choice, a preference of either the person, the practitioner, the funder or the service. And there are no binding rules to guide this decision, although the practitioner is fundamentally guided by the desire to build autonomy.

Building Mrs Mitchell's foundations for health

Consider what the picture means for Mrs Mitchell alone, Mr and Mrs Mitchell, or the wider family and so on, in order to see if there is a compelling reason as to how one selection is likely to benefit (with regard to autonomy) much more than any other. Once the figure on the platform is understood, things become clearer. Let's say the figure is chosen to be Mrs Mitchell. The evaluative nature of the decision must be acknowledged and the selection justified as fully as possible. Next, the basic foundations are considered and any gaps identified. If certain aspects are lacking, what may be needed to reconstruct them for Mrs Mitchell is considered. What are her basic needs? Are they being met from her perspective? Does she need more information about what is possible? Can she communicate what she wants and needs to do in her life? Does she need protection and quiet in order to decide? If her current cognitive processing means she cannot decide what will best promote her autonomy with reference to the foundations, then who should decide? Does she need the support of friends from outside her family?

While there is no simple direction forward with Mrs Mitchell, or in any other situation, answers can begin to emerge when the practitioner's questioning and reflection are guided by a theory of health. Application of the theory helps to make the complexities and the context explicit from a given philosophical perspective. Most importantly, the health practitioner is able to construct a picture in context and articulate the reasons for making choices about how to proceed consistent with a theoretical foundation.

Conclusion

Understanding morality as existing within human relating sets the foundation for interpreting the practice context as a moral context. In doing so, the moral dimensions of practice, usually hidden, are illuminated. This new way of seeing can enable practitioners to uncover the complexities inherent within the seemingly ordinary events in the everyday world of practice. Intuitive ways of thinking about, and acting towards, everyday events can then be replaced by a commitment to reflective, considered reasoning. By presenting a real practice vignette, this chapter has critically considered and rejected professional codes of ethics and principled arguments as adequate guides to moral reasoning. Instead, the thoughtful use of an occupationally-focused theory of health that can be applied to individuals or groups in their subjective life context is suggested as a way forward. Its implementation is centred on defining and building the foundational platform from which the person or persons can be enabled to participate in the things they want and need to do in life. This philosophical approach is not an answer in itself. It is a method of uncovering the complexities and considering contextualised choices. Rather than fall back on empty principles or rules, practitioners and their collective professions are encouraged to be morally thoughtful.

References

American Medical Association. (2001). *AMA Principles of medical ethics*. Retrieved 18 April 2004, from http://www.ams-assn.org/ama/pub/category/2512.html

American Nurses Association. (2001). *Code of ethics for nurses with interpretive statements*. Retrieved 18 April 2004, from http://www.nursingworld.org/ethics/code/ethicscode150.htm

American Occupational Therapy Association. (2000). *Occupational therapy code of ethics*. Retrieved 15 August 2003, from www.aota.org/general/coe.asp

Australian Association of Occupational Therapists. (2001). *Code of ethics*. Retrieved 15 August 2003, from www.ausot.com.au/promotional_items.htm

Australian Nursing Council. (2000). *Code of ethics for nurses*. Retrieved 18 April 2004, from www.anc.org.au/02standards/_docs/codes/code_ethics

Barnitt, R. (1993). What gives you sleepless nights? Ethical practice in occupational therapy. *British Journal of Occupational Therapy, 56*(6), 207–212.

Barnitt, R. (1998). Ethical dilemmas in occupational therapy and physical therapy: A survey of practitioners in the UK National Health Service. *Journal of Medical Ethics, 24*(3), 193–200.

Barnitt, R. & Partidge, C. (1997). Ethical reasoning in physical therapy and occupational therapy. *Physiotherapy Research International, 2*(3), 178–192.

Beauchamp, T. L. & Childress, J. F. (2001). *Principles of biomedical ethics* (5th ed.). Oxford: Oxford University Press.

Canadian Physiotherapy Association. (2001). *Canadian Physiotherapy Association code of ethics and rules of conduct*. Retrieved 18 April 2004, from http://www.physiotherapy.ca/ethics.htm

Capra, F. (2003). *The hidden connections: A science for sustainable living*. London: Flamingo.

Christiansen, C. (2001). Ethical considerations related to evidence-based practice. *American Journal of Occupational Therapy, 55*(3), 345–349.

Clouser, K. D. & Gert, B. (1990). A critique of principalism. *The Journal of Medicine and Philosophy, 15*, p 232.

College of Occupational Therapists. (2000). *Code of ethics and professional conduct for occupational therapists*. Retrieved 15 August 2003, from www.baot.org.uk/public/practice/code.code.htm

Corbett, K. (1993). Ethics and occupational therapy practice. *Canadian Journal of Occupational Therapy, 60*(3), 115–117.

Diekelmann, N. L. (Ed.). (2002). *First, do no harm: Power, oppression, and violence in healthcare*. Madison, USA: The University of Wisconsin Press.

Foto, M. (1998). Change, commitment, and ethics: Where do we stand? *The American Journal of Occupational Therapy, 52*(2), 87–89.

Gillon, R. (1994). (Ed.). *Principles of Health Care Ethics*. Chichester: John Wiley & Sons.

Hansen, R. A., Kamp, L. & Reitz, S. (1988). Two practitioners' analyses of occupational therapy practice dilemmas. *American Journal of Occupational Therapy, 42*(5), 312–319.

Hasselkus, B. R. (1991). Ethical dilemmas in family caregiving for the elderly: Implications for occupational therapy. *American Journal of Occupational Therapy, 45*(3), 206–212.

Hasselkus, B. R. & Dickie, V. A. (1990). Themes of meaning: Occupational therapists' perspectives on practice. *The Occupational Therapy Journal of Research, 10*(4), 195–207.

Hasselkus, B. R. & Dickie, V. A. (1994). Doing occupational therapy: Dimensions of satisfaction and dissatisfaction. *American Journal of Occupational Therapy, 48*(2), 145–154.

Lloyd, C. & Maas, F. (1993). The helping relationship: The application of Carkhuff's model. *Canadian Journal of Occupational Therapy, 60*(2), 83–89.

Mayeroff, M. (1971). *On Caring*. New York: Harper and Row Publishers.

New Zealand Medical Association. (2002). NZMA *Code of ethics*. Retrieved 18 April 2004, from http://www.nzma.org.nz/about/ethics.html

New Zealand Occupational Therapy Board. (1998). *Code of ethics for occupational therapists*. Retrieved 15 August 2003, from http://www.regboards.co.nz/occtherapists/pdfs/CodeofEthics.pdf

New Zealand Society of Physiotherapists. (2003). *NZSP code of ethics*. From http://www.physiotherapy.org.nz/index02/publications/code_of_ethics.html

Noddings, N. (1984). *Caring: A feminine approach to ethics and moral education*. Berkeley: University of California Press.

Occupational Therapy Association of South Africa. (2000). *Occupational therapy code of ethics*, Retrieved 15 August 2003, from www.occupational-therapy.co.za/codeofethics

Purtilo, R. (1999). *Ethical dimensions in the health professions* (3rd ed.). Philadelphia: WB Saunders and Company.

Rachels, J. (2003). *The elements of moral philosophy* (4th ed.). Boston: McGraw-Hill.

Russell, C., Fitzgerald, M. H., Williamson, P., Manor, D. & Whybrow, S. (2002). Independence as a practice issue in occupational therapy: The safety clause. *American Journal of Occupational Therapy, 56*(4), 369–379.

Scott, R. (1998). *Professional ethics: A guide for rehabilitation professionals*. Baltimore: Mosby.

Seedhouse, D. (2000). *Practical nursing philosophy: The universal ethical code*. Chichester: John Wiley & Sons.

Seedhouse, D. (2002). *Total health promotion: Mental health, rational fields and the quest for autonomy*. Chichester: John Wiley & Sons.

Smythe, E. (2002). The violence of the everyday in healthcare. In N. L. Diekelmann (Ed.), *First, do no harm: Power, oppression, and violence in healthcare*, pp 164–203. Madison: The University of Wisconsin Press.

Townsend, E. (1993). 1993 Muriel Driver Lecture: Occupational therapy's social vision. *Canadian Journal of Occupational Therapy, 60*(4), 174–184.

Uden, G., Norberg, A., Lindseth, A. & Marhaug, V. (1992). As cited in R. Barnitt, & C. Partidge, (1997). Ethical reasoning in physical therapy and occupational therapy. *Physiotherapy Research International, 2*(3), 178–192.

Van Amburg, R. (1997). A Copernican revolution in clinical ethics: Engagement versus disengagement. *American Journal of Occupational Therapy, 51*(3), 186–190.

World Federation of Occupational Therapists. (2002). *Code of ethics for occupational therapists*. Retrieved 15 August 2003, from www.iit.edu/departments/csep

World Medical Association Inc. (2002). *International code of medical ethics*. Retrieved 18 April 2004, from http://www.iit.edu/departements/csep//Publicwww/codes/coe/World_Medical_Association

Wright-St Clair, V. (2001). 2000 NZAOT Frances Rutherford Lecture. Caring: The moral motivation for good occupational therapy practice. *Australian Occupational Therapy Journal, 48*, pp 187–199.

Yerxa, E. J. (1992). Some implications of occupational therapy's history for its epistemology, values and relation to medicine. *American Journal of Occupational Therapy, 46*(1), 79–83.

CHAPTER THREE

Knowledge, Power, Evidence: A Critical Analysis of Key Issues in Evidence Based Practice

Gail Whiteford

KEY WORDS

Empiricism
Evidence
Knowledge generation
Qualitative research
Reflective practice
Research paradigms

Chapter Profile

This chapter critically analyses important, yet relatively unexplored issues, within the evidence based practice discourse. The chapter opens with an exploration of the rise of evidence based practice (EBP) in health and then examines some problematic features of the current evidence based practice dialogue, including:

- the predominant biomedical orientation of EBP;
- the representation and valuing of qualitative research as evidence;
- the value and role of reflective professional practice; and
- the economic and managerial implications of how EBP is framed.

The chapter concludes with a consideration of future challenges and possible professional responses, arguing for inclusive approaches to evidence and the importance of professional autonomy and reflective processes in evidence based practice.

Introduction

"Evidence", and "evidence based practice" as an idea, have dominated our professional terrain for a number of years now. Consistent with this development, there has been a small explosion of related learning materials, courses, texts, databases and a corresponding demand from clinicians and managers to gain the skills to become more evidence based in their practice or in their service, despite some very real resource challenges that may militate against it. However, while such focus and activity at the skills end associated with evidence based practice have arguably enhanced understandings of research utilisation, there has been precious little time and attention given to the very important philosophical and epistemological questions that relate to evidence based practice such as:

- what forms of research are considered as constituting valid and valued evidence and why?
- how does knowledge generation in professions relate to utilisation of research evidence?
- what are the implications of how evidence based practice is interpreted and understood for the profession?

Focusing on these questions is of particular importance as they uncover issues of power and control, cause us to consider how we understand experience and reality, and, most importantly, prompt us to reflect on how knowledge is constructed, valued and infused into practice. Clearly, these are issues that should concern us both as individuals and as professionals at large, as autonomy, identity and self-determination are at stake. This chapter considers these important issues and the implications they have for health professions now and in the future. In order to understand the complexity and inter-relatedness of these issues, the chapter begins with an exploration of the emergence of evidence based practice and how it is currently being interpreted.

The rise of evidence based practice

Evidence based medicine and its relationship to evidence based practice

> Medical knowledge that is the product of the clinical gaze, establishes an authoritative "truth" about the body and the person. And, as such, definitions and identifications that emerge from observations of the physical movements and behavior produce power.
>
> (Samson, 1999, p 9)

While it has become popular to start with contemporary evidence based medicine (EBM) as the beginning point in tracing the origins and rise of what we understand as evidence based practice today, we can link its conceptual origins to the 17th century. Enlightenment thinking, with its attendant features of

35

secularism, objectivity, rationalism and reductionism (Samson, 1999; Taylor & White, 2000) have, to a greater or lesser extent, influenced the development of medicine and medical research over time. Cartesian dualism, the legacy of Descartes' conceptualisation of body as machine and psyche as distinct and separate, is often identified as a hallmark of Enlightenment thought and has influenced Western perceptions of health for a number of centuries. This dualist construction differed markedly from the more holistic understandings of health in the Middle Ages (Wilcock, 2001) and was one that championed the intellect, indeed:

> ... whereas the mind (as the new soul) was sacred, the body (became) ... mere matter, operating according to the laws of mechanics. With the body constituted as both separate from our human essence and purely material, the way was cleared for the medical understanding of illness and disease as primarily physical in nature.
>
> (Samson, 1999, p 4)

As is evident from a contemporary perspective, such an orientation ultimately became problematic in understanding the complexity of health as it has failed to address what we now understand to be a dynamic interconnectedness between mind, brain, body, spirit and environment in the experience of health and well-being (Capra, 2003). However, such mechanistic, cause and effect constructions lead to claims of "objective knowledge" as a basis for practice which privileged the subsequent growth and power of medicine (Foucault, 1999) and served as the foundation of the development of medical research over the centuries (Dubos, 1960).

Given this historic tradition of empiricism in Western medicine, the rise of evidence based medicine as a movement strongly oriented to positivist methodologies is unsurprising. Indeed Sackett et al (2000) attribute this orientation as a defining quality of a figure they consider one of the pioneers of EBM, Pierre Louis of revolutionary France, who "sought the truth" through systematic observations of patients (p 2). Generally speaking, however, Sackett and his colleagues, along with other commentators, identify the antecedent of contemporary evidence based practice as developing at McMaster University in Canada with its formal creation occurring in 1992. Not long after, a definition of evidence based medicine as "the process of systematically finding, appraising and using contemporaneous research findings as the basis of clinical decisions" was proposed by Rosenberg & Donald (1995, p 1122). From a relatively modest beginning, the growth of the evidence based medicine movement has subsequently been described as internationally phenomenal in quantitative terms (Sackett et al).

Several authors point to the development of evidence based practice (EBP) as emerging from, and being strongly influenced by, this "phenomenal" rise of evidence based medicine (EBM). Law (2000), for example, sees the two as being strongly linked with the only difference being a technical one of orientation; that is, EBM is legalistically about the discipline of medicine, whereas EBP is identified as being an extrapolation to all arenas of health including rehabilitation, and is thus a more suitable term (Brown & Rodger, 1999). Hamer (1999) points to a more developmental sequence of events. She suggests that, in fact, the framing of evidence based medicine was quickly experienced as too narrow in orientation and that evidence based practice emerged as an attempt to broaden its applicability to other disciplines. She describes the naming of evidence based practice as constituting "an amalgam of the terminology of science and professional practice" (p 6). Other descriptions of the relationship between EBM and EBP include that of Taylor, who states simply and categorically that "EBP has its roots in EBM" (2003, p 91) to that of Clarke, who suggests a more complex and power-driven relationship involving "a transition from EBM, evolving from one discipline to … rhetorically enveloping all other health professionals" (Clarke, 1999).

Clearly then, EBM and EBP are historically, professionally and ideationally related. However, the nature of this relationship, in terms of the tacit epistemological and ontological issues that EBM has exerted on the discourse and practice of EBP, has received too little attention, especially in the occupational therapy literature. Indeed, the focus in the literature has overwhelmingly leant towards functionalism — that is, "how do we *do* evidence based practice" — rather than considered interrogation of evidence based practice as a construct or vigorous debate regarding the tacit values informing the development of the EBP dialogue internationally. This is despite some very real tensions between practice-generated knowledge and research-derived knowledge and the still too evident gap in research utilisation (Brown & Rodger, 1999; Cusick & McClusky, 2000). The next section explores some of these tensions with a focus on how qualitative research is represented and valued as a form of evidence.

Critically analysing the evidence based practice discourse

Paradigms of knowledge: Representation and valuation of qualitative research

> The rise in evidence based practice over the past decade has led to an ever increasing emphasis on research centering on hypothesis testing.
> (Williams, 2002, p 109)

In the last section, the historical development of medical research was identified as having been strongly influenced over time by the tradition of Western empiricism. Accordingly, the development of EBM has also been grounded in, and influenced by, this tradition. In light of critical scrutiny, what becomes evident is that empiricism is also tending to dominate as a prevailing research paradigm in the development of the EBP discourse and its translation into practice. This is not surprising when considered in the context of the larger historic, economic and political moment in which we find ourselves, that is, one that has become increasingly concerned with rational and instrumental processes despite the demands of complex social problems clamouring for attention from diverse, trans-disciplinary perspectives. This has been described variously as a new "methodological conservatism" (Lincoln, 2003); a form of managerial hegemony (Parsons, 2003); and as being indicative of a society "unreasonably dominated by the cognitive frameworks of science to the extent that other potential forms of knowledge are downgraded" (Higgs & Titchen, 1995, p 526).

Let's consider then, how the values associated with empiricism are reproduced and reinforced in such a way that, even tacitly, they influence the terrain of the evidence based practice discourse. Certainly, one of the most obvious means is through linguistic constructions of evidence in descriptions such as "levels of evidence" or "hierarchies of evidence".

In most texts on evidence based practice, the beginning sections orientate the reader to these identified levels or hierarchies of evidence (established initially within EBM), and, although wording may differ slightly, the constructions are similar to that which follows:

- **Level/type 1:** Evidence obtained from systematic reviews of relevant and multiple randomised controlled trials (RCTs) and meta analyses of RCTs

- **Level/type 2:** Evidence obtained from well designed RCTs

- **Level/type 3:** Evidence obtained from well designed non-randomised controlled trials — experimental studies

- **Level/type 4:** Evidence obtained from non-experimental research

- **Level/type 5:** Respected authorities/opinion based on clinical experience, descriptive studies or reports of expert committees (Madjar & Walton, 2001).

So, what is problematic about such a construction? A key issue is that of reification. This refers to a process through which something is accorded greater value than something else, and is represented accordingly within a discourse. Reification is often subtle, however, because language and culture are so powerfully linked, the impacts can be pervasive and enduring, particularly in how professional epistemologies are shaped over time (Whiteford & Wilcock, 2000).

Through presenting an absolute hierarchy of evidence in which qualitative research is represented at the bottom (along with expert opinion, an issue which will be addressed later in this section), a clear valuation of one knowledge paradigm over another — of empiricism over interpretivism — is represented. In translation, it sends an unambiguous message to the reader that numerical data derived through experimental means are more important than narrative data derived through naturalistic means. As has been suggested, definitions and constructions of what counts as evidence represent tacit assumptions and ideologies (Estabrooks, 2001; Madjar & Walton, 2001) and the phenomenon of ordering a hierarchy of evidence does exactly this: reinforces a historic and ideological tradition of the supposed superiority of empiricism and the scientific method. As should be evident, this is potentially oppressive to a whole tradition of research and knowledge construction and, in effect, represents an absolute rather than pluralistic approach to what counts as evidence. It also represents a fiction, an illusory belief that "research methods and techniques provide secure paths to truth and certainty" (Kemmis & McTaggart, 2001, p 15). Rather, human research is characterised by complexity, fallibility and messiness (Tickle-Dingen, 2000).

One additional problem arises when such hierarchies are reproduced in the prevailing discourse around evidence based practice and when statements are made, such as that by Sackett, that it's better to avoid the non-experimental approaches as they may lead to "false positive conclusions" (1997, p 4). This is that a clear message about what type of knowledge is valued is being sent to a variety of audiences — that is, that derived through measurement. These audiences include clinicians, managers and funders of services. For clinicians, it has the effect of devaluing a knowledge tradition that may be central to their profession and diminish the importance of a rich and relevant source of data — that derived through qualitative means. For managers and funders, a clear distinction becomes evident between those interventions which can provide the "gold standard evidence" over those that cannot or whose services and interactions are not conducive to measurement through a randomised controlled trial approach or experimental research. This is where issues of power and control become evident in the dynamics of how evidence is framed, a point made stridently by Jones & Higgs when they suggest that:

> ... if the evidence of evidence based practice is restricted to information available from select quantitative studies fulfilling stringent criteria, for example randomized controlled trials, then this paradigm shift has significant consequences in terms of the scope of practice strategies that would be justifiable under the new regime of RCT evidence. For some health professionals whose decisions traditionally go beyond pathophysiological considerations, this shift in what is deemed evidence could create very real dilemmas concerning "credible" practices.
>
> (Jones & Higgs, 2000, p 309)

In order to address this issue of representation, the notion of a construction of evidence as a continuum, as opposed to a hierarchy (Humphris, 2000), is more appropriate. Such a continuum would, in equal measure, represent practice based knowledge and expertise alongside research generated from differing paradigms and approaches. Then, depending on the nature of the problem/area being considered, a "goodness of fit" between the question and the type of research could be ascertained or ordered. For example, if I wanted to address an issue relating to medication levels, RCT-type research may well be appropriate and more valuable to me in that arena than descriptive research. However, if I was attempting to understand what the best practices are in supporting people with chronic mental illnesses in independent community living — a complex, socially situated concern — I would be looking to qualitative research findings inclusive of consumer perspectives, triangulated with other data to best inform me. In this way, hierarchies of evidence may still be useful, but only relatively, that is in relation to the nature of the question rather than as an absolute construction for all arenas of enquiry. In summary, "level of evidence is not an inherent attribute of a design or methodological approach alone, but is (also) dependent on the question for which evidence is being sought" (Williams, 2002, p 111).

Paradigms of knowledge: Arguing for a pluralistic approach to understanding complex health phenomena

> … the exclusion of qualitative methods is like playing a round of golf with one club.
>
> (Murphy & Dingwall, 2001, p 166)

One of the associated problems with presenting a hierarchy of evidence as an absolute rather than relative construction is that, despite acknowledgement that there are other forms of research, the emphasis falls predominantly on RCTs (Clarke, 1999; Taylor & White, 2000; Madjar & Walton, 2001; Williams, 2002). However, despite such emphasis that presupposes methodological superiority, a question that requires careful examination is whether randomised controlled trials (RCTs) are really the best method in understanding health phenomena especially in the arenas we work in as allied health professionals. First, RCTs are conducted with clearly defined and delimited populations and often exclude for example, people with cognitive or communication problems (Jones & Higgs, 2000). Additionally, the process of data analysis that controls for difference and excludes extreme scores creates a picture of a so-called "average patient", a construction that bears little resemblance to the real people with real problems encountered in the everyday world of practice. Another feature of RCTs is that, in order to produce findings that can be generalised, not only are individual differences in clients controlled for, but so is context. The task of the health practitioner then, is to re-contextualise the findings with respect to their own client group and setting. This may be particularly difficult in a challenging context, such as in a remote or resource-poor setting, or when working with people whose cultural and social beliefs may preclude the so-called "gold standard" intervention. De-contextualization also carries with it the risk that attendant moral and ethical issues in health and health care are subverted, creating a "moral tension" with respect to the design and conduct of RCTs (Christiansen, 2001; Lilford et al, 2001). As has been suggested, much of what comprises the human experience of health *cannot,* and, from an ethical perspective, *should not* be measured (Madjar & Walton).

Qualitative research represents a distinct epistemological and ontological tradition and as such deserves a more equitable representation in the EBP discourse. To be fair, select texts and scholarly articles on EBP include sections on qualitative research. For example Taylor's (2000) text "Evidence Based Occupational Therapy" includes a chapter on qualitative research, as do other works. However, where such inclusions follow the presentation of hierarchies of evidence, the tacit message remains that qualitative research is necessarily considered secondary to systematic reviews and randomised controlled trials. Indeed, in some representations, qualitative research is described only as adjunctive to quantitative methods, rather than as a distinct tradition in its own right (Muir Gray, 2001).

Such inequitable representation and valuation of qualitative research in the evidence based practice discourse represents a potential threat to knowledge development in the health professions. In occupational therapy, for example, the profession has only recently arrived at a point of developing its own unique epistemological foundation of occupation, which has been identified as being best understood through naturalistic means (Yerxa, 1991; Townsend, 1996; Clark et al, 1997; Wilcock, 1998; Wicks & Whiteford, 2003). However, the emergence of an EBP discourse in which a positivistic orientation is dominant (Hamer, 1999; Morse, 2001; Williams, 2002) potentially devalues narratively-derived knowledge. Accordingly, if health professionals fail to challenge current constructions of evidence and fail to argue for greater visibility and valuation of qualitative approaches, this historic development could represent a retrograde impact on our professions collectively.

In championing the case for qualitative research as a valid and valuable form of evidence to inform practice, it is important to highlight both its distinctiveness and how it allows us to address different types of questions related to health, wellness and, in occupational therapy, to occupation itself. First, qualitative research approaches are context specific and capture context-bound narratives. This is important in assisting us to address the "life world" of the people we work with and the myriad of influences upon it, as well as in understanding the context relatedness between what people do and the state of their health. In occupational therapy, for example, developing deep understandings of the complexities of how contextual forces interact to influence what people do in communities, must (or should) be one of the main projects of the profession internationally. An excellent example of such research was Townsend's (1998) study into mental health service delivery in Atlantic Canada. The study used an institutional ethnography design to inquire into occupational therapy service delivery for people with mental illnesses and sourced data from multiple sources. The data was then interpreted relative to institutional and provincial mental health policy. It remains a landmark study in its critical highlighting of contextual complexity and its analysis of the power relationships inherent in organisational structures which impacted on both occupational therapy practice and the experience of service recipients.

Secondly, qualitative approaches offer an "emic" or "insider's" perspective and experience. This is crucial in understanding the meaning constructions of the individual, group or community in relation to specific health-related concerns. Such health-related areas may range from chronic unemployment to youth suicide to living with HIV to aged care. Enquiry into meaning constructions relative to practice should be fundamental (Kemmis & McTaggart, 2000), especially in people-oriented professions, and numerous examples have emerged with this focus in recent times. One of the most engaging works in this arena has been Hasselkus' (2002) scholarly work on occupation in which data generated from

41

phenomenological interviews with occupational therapists provides insights into the meanings of occupations in people's lives. Jackson et al (1998) also emphasised the meaning of occupation in their landmark well elderly study in California, while Christiansen et al (1999) undertook a study which focused on meaning constructions through engagement in personal projects. These are all examples of how situated meaning is best elucidated through narrative means.

A third important feature of interpretive research is that it is "iterative" in nature, allowing for new and sometimes highly unexpected findings to emerge. As compared to a hypothetico-deductive approach, qualitative research, through its exploratory approach and data responsive processes (Llewellen, 1999), is particularly important in sensitive areas of research. Touringy's (1998) study of inner city youth in Detroit stands out as a cogent example of the value of qualitative research in informing health-care practice. Her study, which originally was oriented towards HIV/AIDS educational programs instead uncovered a practice by Afro American youths actively to "choose" to acquire HIV, knowing the consequences. This shocking finding pointed to extreme existential issues linked to socio-economic milieu, including hopelessness, despair and committing suicide.

Finally, though power relations are part of any research project (Carmody, 2001), the power relationship in qualitative research approaches (especially participatory action research) allows for greater opportunities for participants/informants to have ownership or control over data and findings, hence becoming stakeholders in potential changes emerging from the research. This differs from quantitative methods which, in operationalising concepts in order to measure them, frames them from the perspective of the researcher, leading to the question "whose voice is speaking?" (Olson, 2001, p 261). An excellent example of a study which seeks to empower through actively involving participants as research partners and stakeholders is Gwynn's (2003) research into type 2 diabetes and indigenous communities. Framed theoretically as an issue of occupational justice, Gwynn addresses the historical background of colonisation alongside the attendant cultural, socio-economic and political dimensions in her ethnographic study situated in NSW, Australia. Through the process of philosophically and theoretically "situating" the project and giving voice to indigenous community members, Gwynn's study has an expected outcome of empowerment through the conjoint development of a school-based program for children. Clearly, such an outcome in such an important and sensitive area, could only have been addressed through rigorous qualitative means.

Wick's (2003) in-depth narrative study of the life histories of older rural women is another example of research as a process for building social capital. Through the process of being engaged with other women in focus groups and then in individual interviews, the women generated a self-help orientation to their daily lives and actively networked with each other after the research formally concluded. Such outcomes are heartening and reinforce the concept of research as praxis (Lather, 1986). Given the many inequities that continue in the health status of subpopulations around the globe today, research which not only generates data to serve as an evidence base for practice, but which also empowers through its process and outcomes, has to be seriously considered as the option of choice in many areas.

While all these characteristics of qualitative research support the case for its inclusion in generating research that both informs and serves as a basis for practice, there are some specific issues that need to be addressed with respect to how this is done. One of the primary issues is how the "quality" of qualitative research can be evaluated. While it can be relatively straightforward to detect major methodological or analytic flaws in quantitative research through interpretation of the numerical values presented, it can be a more demanding task to evaluate qualitative studies and their findings. This is because published qualitative studies are text rich, and address (or should address) the complex fabric which represents the philosophical, theoretical, contextual and ethical dimensions of any interpretive study. Additionally, the description of the research is made even more dense through the inclusion of reflexive commentary which "situates" the researcher which should appear along with the presentation of finely-grained data illuminating the phenomenon being studied. Such density predicates a more in-depth interaction between reader and text, requiring a reasonably demanding level of familiarity with the conceptual underpinnings of not only qualitative research as a paradigm, but also of the specific approach utilised. In my experience as an educator working with different groups of allied health professionals in understanding qualitative research, I have found that the general perception of published qualitative research is that, at best, it is challenging. At worst, it is perceived to be jargon laden and exclusive. In order to address this gap between perception and understanding, guidelines for evaluating qualitative research can be useful. One of the best summaries of published guidelines for reviewing qualitative research has been produced by Kuzel and Engel (2001) whose orientation is grounded in the tradition of pragmatism, and they approach qualitative research evaluation from this perspective. Additionally, the web-based tool developed for reviewing qualitative studies at McMaster University (http://www.fhs.mcmaster.ca/rehab/ebp) is useful for critiquing published qualitative works in a systematic manner.

In summary, the conduct of all research should be guided by the nature of the research question. The approach and method should represent the best fit with the problem or issue of concern. The same principle then, should apply to the utilisation of research as evidence, a principle that is especially important if we truly centralise consumers' perspectives. In this respect, qualitative and quantitative research should be represented and valued equally as providing an important evidence base for practice. Qualitative research, as I have argued here, has a particularly vital role to play in illuminating understandings of the dynamism of health, wellness, doing and meaning in context and is arguably more closely aligned with the epistemic foundations of the health professions collectively.

Ultimately, we need to be mindful that health care:

> ... is essentially a human oriented practice and there are many dimensions to being human which should be reflected in the diversity of evidence gained and valued ... there also has to be acknowledgement that any evidence is only a tool, which ultimately requires human judgment.
>
> (Clarke, 1999, p 189)

Given then, that judgment is crucial in the understanding, interpretation and utilisation of evidence, how are everyday practice judgments arrived at? The answer is through reflective processes and reasoning which, alongside issues of accountability, is the focus of the next section.

Paradigms of knowledge: Reflection, reasoning and evidence in the era of accountability

> The idea that professionals can be shaped by evidence legitimized by managers and funding bodies and by coercive policies that mandate action on the basis of evidence, belies the complexity of professional work.
>
> (Davies, 2003, p 101)

> The second assumption is ... that good workers use research; it resembles a blaming the victim stance.
>
> (Estabrook, 2001, p 281)

As suggested earlier in this chapter, the primary orientation of the EBP discourse in the health professions has been geared toward "doing" evidence based practice. Accordingly, much time is seemingly devoted to how and where to search for evidence, and how, for example to conduct systematic reviews. However, identifying and evaluating evidence is only one part of what is, in actuality, a highly complex process in which professional knowledge, experience, reasoning and reflection are incorporated into decision-making in everyday practice. Because of this complexity, an in-depth exploration of the elements of this process and their interconnectedness is beyond the scope of this chapter. I do, however, wish to identify some key concepts with respect to types of knowledge, reasoning and reflection and then move on to a consideration of these in the context of institutional accountability.

What constitutes legitimate knowledge in the professions has been a topic of heated debate and discussion throughout the ages. Controversy over the topic of knowledge generation was, for example, a hallmark of the life of Socrates and his followers. However, as a continued discourse in the form we know it, discussion and dissent over professional knowledge constructions have been active for around half a century (Parry, 2001). There is general agreement in the literature that there is a distinct difference between "knowing that" and "knowing how", more formally classified as propositional and non-propositional knowledge. In health, the work of Higgs & Titchen, along with other linked authors, represents an extended scholarly investigation into the relationship between these forms of knowledge and practice. Higgs & Andresen (2001) describe propositional knowledge as arising from theory and research, including scientific and procedural knowledge. In their model, non-propositional knowledge has been developed to represent two distinct categories: professional craft knowledge and personal knowledge. They contend that the interaction between these sets of knowledge is dynamic and suggest that in practice, professionals draw upon all knowledge sources in a fluid way to guide everyday decision-making. Titchen & Esser (2001) expand these categorisations and attempt to describe the relationship between them and what they term "knowing in practice" (p 52). The main distinction in their model is the identification of critical reflection as the foundation of non-propositional/craft knowledge.

Critical reflection and reflective practice have become legitimised as a concept (Gamble et al, 2001) in the health profession literature to the point where it is now considered to be central to health-care practice. In the UK, for example, the Quality Assurance Agency for Higher Education outlined in its benchmark statement for health-care programs, professional competencies in reflection as including:

- *self-reflection* on the extent and limitations of the role of the health care practitioner in a variety of settings;

- the ability to *reflect critically* on their overall performance and take responsibility under supervision for varying action in the light of this; and

- being reflexive in the formulation of *problems* and identification of *solutions* (Brown & Esdaile, 2003, p 123).

The identification of such competencies serves both to centralise reflection in everyday actions as well as distinguish us as professionals, as distinct from technicians. However, the framing of evidence based practice in some contemporary descriptions tends to minimise the role of reflective processes, having the potential impact of reducing practice to a technical instrumentality of the sort eschewed by Schön (Parry, 2001). In the profession of occupational therapy, models which:

- highlight the complexity of clinical reasoning, such as the work by Chapparo and Ranka (2000);

- centralise reflective reasoning and its relationship to theory and practice (Mitcham, 2003);

- represent evidence as only *one* element alongside ethics, environment, experience and expectations (Pollock & Rochon, 2002); and

- embrace imagination and creativity (Denshire, 2002)

serve as important contributions to the valuation and inclusive representation of what constitutes occupational therapy knowledge. Further illumination of the complex interactions between self, types of knowledge, reasoning and action needs to be prioritised in the profession's research agenda, in other words, capturing the "occupational therapy way of knowing". This is because acknowledging and legitimising the profession's unique epistemic foundations and the knowledge embedded in the everyday actions of an occupational therapist in a range of contexts and settings, is crucial if the profession is to claim its own distinct professional terrain. It is particularly crucial in the context of what has been dubbed the "era of accountability", an era that potentially represents some threats to professional autonomy.

The move towards greater levels of accountability in health care can be interpreted as both relative to current and future demographic changes which challenge health-care budgets and to growing managerial hegemony. In the former context — one in which health services are reconfiguring themselves as a response to demographic changes, a difficult process always underpinned by tacit social values (Muir Gray, 2001) — greater demands for accountability by funders of providers may be interpreted at least as an understandable, perhaps pragmatic response. However, in the latter context — one in which the value system of the "new managerialism" has become the prevailing ideational framework in health care — new accountability demands may be viewed by professionals as being indicative of several covert agendas, one of which is control. Onora O'Neil, in the 2002 Reith lecture series, suggests that the new culture of accountability essentially aims to control "perfectly" institutional and professional life. As O'Neil argues, the systems and structures utilised to measure and record performance have been inherited from financial systems (and, inherently, capitalist ideology) and have not translated well to the human service domain. Indeed, new accountability demands have eroded autonomy and made it difficult for a profession in any arena to achieve "its proper aim", an aim "not reducible to meeting set targets and following prescribed procedures and requirements" (O'Neil, 2002, p 3).

The other covert agenda of managerialism and the new accountability is the delimiting of professional knowledge and, therefore, institutional power, through a unidimensional focus on cost effectiveness. While some commentators have denied that viewing evidence based practice as a cost saving measure is a myth (Law, 2002), others contend that the emergence of evidence based practice cannot be separated from the fiscal agenda of managerialism (Taylor & White, 2000; Muir Gray, 2001; Davies, 2003). Paradoxically, it seems that the knowledge base of professionals is at once relied upon *and* undermined by managerial framings of evidence based practice (Davies). This has been described as a process in which the "efficient choice" message is promulgated, assuming autonomy and choice in the identification and utilisation of research, whereas, in reality, autonomous action is delimited in most contemporary institutions (Estabroks, 2001).

Clearly, it is the responsibility of all professionals to be actively and critically engaged in the dialogue of accountability. We need to ask the question of new data gathering requirements, "Whose purpose does this serve?" and in doing so maintain our focus on our clients and their needs. In occupational therapy in particular, we need to continue to champion the cause of the people we have traditionally served, that is those often living at the margins of society with little voice or representation (Wilcock & Whiteford, 2003). This is particularly important in the prevailing context of accountability when social and community-based programs are attracting greater scrutiny with respect to a concern as to their cost effectiveness as opposed to their societal value.

Evidence based practice: Future challenges

> The proponents of evidence based practice propose an unproblematic relationship between research and practice and also amongst policy, research and practice.
>
> (Davies, 2003, p 98)

As Davies suggests, the prevailing tenor of the evidence based practice discourse seems characterised by somewhat simplistic, context-free notions of the relationship between research, professional knowledge and experience, and practice. Perhaps the beguiling simplicity of the project of EBP thus framed is what has given it such great appeal. Perhaps it is because so much is apparently at stake: those that can demonstrate their ability to be "good" evidence based practitioners in a highly competitive environment will succeed. However, it is precisely because there is so much at stake that we need be more active in our interaction with both the evidence based practice dialogue and its translation to everyday practice. As the popular phrase suggests, "for every complex problem, there's a solution that's neat, simple, and wrong". Using a delimited approach with essentially positivistic overtones is not the way forward for us to address the serious, complex, situated problems relating to health, wellbeing and occupation now and in the future. The challenge for the health professions lies in tackling the following issues with some urgency:

- broadening the professional dialogue around EBP to shift the focus from "how do we do it" to "why" and "what will it mean to how we practice — ethically and morally as well as pragmatically";

- challenging absolute, empirically-driven hierarchical constructions of evidence as inappropriate;

- arguing for, and adopting, a pluralistic perspective of what constitutes evidence, that is from multiple sources and paradigms as matches the type of question being asked;

- emphasising practice as a (non-reducible) complex phenomenon in which experience, non-propositional knowledge, reasoning and reflection interact along with research generated evidence in everyday decision-making;

- acknowledging that EBP has emerged within an historic, socio-political context and, as such, needs to be critiqued in relationship to the accountability requirements of a managerial ethos;

- considering that power relationships between medicine and allied health practitioners as well as between allied health practitioners themselves are, and will continue to be, influenced by how EBP is framed and implemented.

Conclusion

In this chapter, some of the key issues surrounding evidence based practice have been considered and critically discussed. These have included:

- the empirical/positivistic orientation of EBP discourse;

- the representation and valuing of qualitative research and the adequacy and ethics of randomised controlled trials;

- the complexity of practice as including reasoning, reflection and being based on non-propositional knowledge as well s research evidence; and

- finally, that evidence based practice needs to be understood within the prevailing political and economic climate in which it has emerged.

Recommendations for the future, in the form of issues that all health professions need to address as a matter of some urgency, closed the chapter.

References

Brown, G. & Esdaile, S. (2003). Enhancing reflective abilities: Interweaving reflection into practice. In G. Brown, S. Esdaile & S. Ryan (Eds) *Becoming an advanced healthcare practitioner*, pp 118–144. Edinburgh: Butterworth-Heinemann.

Brown, T. & Rodger, S. (1999). Research utilization models: Frameworks for implementing evidence based occupational therapy practice. *Occupational Therapy International, 6*, 1–23.

Capra, F. (2003). *The hidden connections*. London: Flamingo.

Carmody, M. (2001). Dangerous knowledge: The politics and ethics of research. In H. Byrne-Armstrong, J. Higgs & D. Horsfall (Eds) *Critical moments in qualitative research*. Oxford: Butterworth-Heinemann.

Chapparo, C. & Ranka, J. (2000). Clinical reasoning in occupational therapy. In J. Higgs & M. Jones (Eds) Clinical reasoning in the health professions, pp 128–137. Oxford: Butterworth-Heinemann.

Christiansen, C., Backman, C., Little, B. R. & Nguyen, A. (1999). Occupation and wellbeing: A study of personal projects. *American Journal of Occupational Therapy, 53*(6), 91–100.

Clark, F., Carlson, M. & Polkinghorne, D. (1997). The legitimacy of life history and narrative approaches in the study of occupation. *American Journal of Occupational Therapy, 51*(4), 313–317.

Clarke, J. (1999). Evidence based practice: A retrograde step? The importance of pluralism in evidence generation for the practice of healthcare. *Journal of Clinical Nursing, 8*, 89–94.

Cusick, A. & McClusky, A. (2000) Becoming an evidence based practitioner through professional development. *Australian Occupational Therapy Journal, 47*, 159–170.

Davies, B. (2003). Death to critique and dissent? The policies and practices of new mangerialism and of 'evidence based practice'. *Gender and Education, 13*(1), 91–103.

Denshire, S. (2000). Imagination, occupation, reflection: Ways of coming to understand practice. *Unpublished Master's thesis,* School of Occupation and Leisure Sciences, University of Sydney.

Dubos, R. (1960). *The mirage of health*. London: Allen & Unwin.

Estabrooks, C. (2001). Research utilization and qualitative research. In J. Morse, J. Swanson & A. Kuzel (Eds) *The nature of qualitative evidence*, pp 275–298. Thousand Oaks: Sage Publications Inc.

Foucault, M. (1999). Spaces and classes. In C. Samson (Ed.) *Health studies: A critical and cross cultural reader*, pp 22–35. Oxford: Blackwell.

Gamble, J., Chan, P. & Davey, H. (2001). Reflection as a tool for developing professional practice and expertise. In J. Higgs & A. Titchen (Eds) *Practice Knowledge and Expertise*, pp 121–127. Oxford: Butterworth-Heinemann.

Gwynn, J. (2003). Occupational justice and chronic disease in Australia indigenous people. *National Conference of the Australian Association of Occupational Therapists*, April 2003, Melbourne.

Hamer, S. & Collinson, G. (1999). *Achieving evidence based practice: A handbook for practitioners*. Edinburgh: Ballière Tindall.

Hasselkus, B. (2002). The meaning of everyday occupation. Thorofare: Slack.

Higgs, J. & Andresen, L. (2001). The knower, the knowing and the known: Threads in the woven tapestry of knowledge. In J. Higgs & A. Titchen (Eds) *Practice Knowledge and Expertise*, pp 10–21. Oxford: Butterworth-Heinemann

Humphris, D. (2000). Types of evidence. In S. Hamer & G. Collinson (Eds) *Evidence Based Practice: A handbook for practitioners*. Edinburgh: Baillière Tindall.

Jackson, J., Carlson, M., Mandel, D., Zemke, R & Clark, F. (1998). Occupation in lifestyle redesign: The well elderly study occupational therapy program. *American Occupational Therapy Journal*, *52*(5), 326–336.

Jones, M. & Higgs, J. (2000). Will evidence based practice take the reasoning out of practice? In J. Higgs & M. Jones (Eds) *Clinical Reasoning in the Health Professions* (2nd ed,), pp 307–315. Oxford: Butterworth-Heinemann.

Kuzel, A. & Engel, J. (2001). Some pragmatic thoughts about evaluating qualitative health research. In J. Morse, J. Swanson & A. Kuzel (Eds) *The nature of qualitative evidence*, pp 114–138. Thousand Oaks: Sage Publications Inc.

Lather, P. (1986). Research as praxis. *Harvard Education Review*, *56*(3), 257–275.

Law, M. (2002). *Evidence based rehabilitation*. Thorofare: Slack.

Llewellen, G., Sullivan, G. & Minichiello, V. (1999). Sampling in qualitative research. In V. Mininchiello, G. Sullivan, K. Greenwood & R. Axford (Eds) *Handbook for research methods in the health sciences*. Sydney: Addison Wesley.

Madjar, I., & & Walton, J. (Eds). (2001). What is problematic about evidence? In J. Morse, J. Swanson & A. Kuzel (Eds) *The nature of qualitative evidence*, pp 28–45. Thousand Oaks: Sage Publications Inc.

Mitcham, M. (2003). Integrating theory and practice: Using theory creatively to enhance professional practice. In G. Brown, S. Esdaile & S. Ryan (Eds) *Becoming an advanced healthcare practitioner*, pp 64–98. Edinburgh: Butterworth-Heinemann.

Muir Gray, J. (2001). Evidence based healthcare: How to make health policy and management decisions. Edinburgh: Churchill Livingstone.

Olsen, K. (2001). Using qualitative research in clinical practice. In J. Morse, J. Swanson & A. Kuzel (Eds) *The nature of qualitative evidence*, pp 259–273. Thousand Oaks: Sage Publications Inc.

O'Neil, O. *A question of trust. 2002 BBC Reith Lectures*. Cambridge: Cambridge University Press.

Parry, A. (2001). Research and professional craft knowledge. In J. Higgs & A. Titchen (Eds) *Practice Knowledge and Expertise*, pp 109–206 Oxford: Butterworth-Heinemann.

Pollock, N. & Rochon, S. (2002). Becoming an evidence based practitioner. In M. Law (Ed.) *Evidence based rehabilitation: A guide to practice*. Thorofare: Slack.

Rosenberg, W. & Donald, A. (1995). Evidence based medicine: An approach to clinical problem solving: *British Medical Journal*, *310*, 1122–1126.

Samson, C. (1999). Biomedicine and the body. In C. Samson (Ed.) *Health studies: A critical and cross cultural reader*, pp 22–35. Oxford: Blackwell.

Sackett, D. L. (1997). Foreword. In *The Evidence Based Medicine Workbook*. R. A. Dixon, J. F. Munro & P. B. Silcocks (Eds), pp vii–viii. Oxford: Butterworth-Heinemann.

Sackett, D. L. (2000). *Evidence based medicine: How to practice and teach EBM*. Edinburgh: Churchill Livingstone.

Taylor, C. (2003). Evidence based practice: informing practice and critically evaluating related research. In G. Brown, S. Esdaile & S. Ryan (Eds) *Becoming an advanced healthcare practitioner*, pp 90–117. Edinburgh: Butterworth-Heinemann.

Taylor, C. & White, S. (2000). *Practicing reflexivity in health and welfare: Making knowledge*. Buckingham, UK: Open University Press.

Titchen, A. & Ersser, S. (2001). The nature of professional craft knowledge. In J. Higgs & A. Titchen (Eds) *Practice Knowledge and Expertise*, pp 35–41. Oxford: Butterworth-Heinemann.

Townsend, E. (1996). Enabling empowerment: Using simulations vs. real occupations. *Canadian Journal of Occupational Therapy*, 63(2), 114–127.

Townsend, E. (1997). *Good intentions overruled*. Toronto: University of Toronto Press.

Tickle-Dengen, L. (2000). What is the best evidence to use in practice? *The American Journal of Occupational Therapy*, 54(2), 218–221.

Tourigny, S. (1998). Some new dying trick: African American Youths "choosing" HIV/AIDS. *Qualitative Health Research*, 8(2), 149–167.

Whiteford, G. & Wilcock, A. (2001). Centralising occupation in occupational therapy curricula: Imperative of the new millennium. *Occupational Therapy International*, 8(2), 81–85.

Wicks, A. (2003). Understanding occupational potential across the life course: Life stories of older women. *Unpublished Doctoral thesis*. Charles Sturt University.

Wilcock, A. (1998). An occupational perspective of health. Thorofare: Slack.

Wilcock, A. (2001). *Occupation for health (Vol 1): A journey from self health to prescription*. London: British College of Occupational Therapists.

Wilcock, A. & Whiteford, G. (2003). Occupation, health promotion and the environment. In L. Letts, P. Rigby. & D. Stewart (Eds) *Using Environments to Enable Occupational Performance*, pp 55–70. Thorofare: Slack.

Williams, B. (2002). The role of qualitative research methods in evidence based mental health care. In S. Priebe & M. Slade (Eds) *Evidence in mental health care*. New York: Brunner-Routledge.

Yerxa, E. (1991). Seeking a relevant, ethical and realistic way of knowing for occupational therapy. *American Journal of Occupational Therapy*, 54(3), 1–17.

CHAPTER FOUR

Theoretical Contexts

Chris Chapparo
Judy Ranka

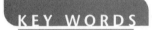

KEY WORDS

Health

Theory building

Theory

Occupation

Chapter Profile

Along with changes in social and practice contexts, health care workers have been compelled to rethink the focus of service delivery. This chapter frames theory and theory building as the intellectual context of health service delivery. The theoretical context is considered in relation to general theories of health and disability, theoretical approaches to practice and personal theories. Initially the chapter presents a macro (overarching) theoretical view of the health and disability context and its place in theory prior to considering a micro (individual) view of context and its specific impact on practitioners in context. The understandings are interpreted in relation to occupational therapy. In particular, postmodernism is discussed as a critical reappraisal of modern modes of thought, beliefs and conviction.

Introduction

At the beginning of the 21st century, it is argued that we are witnessing the emergence of a new age of uncertainty for human services in health and disability for which we need new theories, new forms of practice and an associated language (Corker & Shakespeare, 2003). Globalisation, new communication technologies, the techno-industrialisation of war, privatisation of social systems such as health and education and the advent of universal consumerism are only a few of the transformations that have had a profound effect on human services. Within this context of uncertainty and change, the task for health workers and researchers is to engage in problem solving with people who experience ill health or disability, their families and carers (Chapparo & Ranka, 2000). Interventions are characterised by increasing social complexity and expectations of collaboration among multiple individual and institutional stakeholders. Health-care workers have been compelled to engage in the process of theory building as they rethink the focus of service delivery. This process involves constructing conceptual models that explain or guide practice within this complex social web (Higgs & Jones, 2000). The success of theory-building processes in health is questioned, with many authors suggesting that the theory base to service delivery for people with ill health and disability is at best inadequate (Corker & Shakespeare; Losardo & Notari-Syverson, 2001) and at worst, non-existent (Oliver, 1996). Twentieth century views of health and disability appear too narrow with an inability to account for the variation in beliefs and customs of diverse cultures and the complexity of adaptation to these changing conditions.

The purpose of this chapter is to frame theory and theory building as the intellectual context of health-care service delivery. The profession of occupational therapy is used as one example of how contemporary social change and thinking in the postmodern age impacts on the focus of theory development that underpins specialist service delivery. Although traditionally identified as a health-care profession, contemporary occupational therapy services extend across a number of public and private service systems that include health, education and welfare. Similar to other health-care professions, theory-building processes that attempt to define the central concept of the profession — occupation — are simultaneously creating equivalent and corresponding forms as a profession (occupational therapy) and as a discipline (occupational science) (Royeen, 2003; Yerxa, 1997; Zemke & Clark, 1996).

Theory: A conceptual context for health workers

Theories are conceptual systems or frameworks used to organise knowledge (Creek & Feaver, 1993). Theory building is considered requisite to the production of knowledge in any profession (Henderson, 1988). Theories are not reality, but intellectual structures that are created to guide, control or shape reality for some particular purpose. Theory building is the process of creating a language for the specific purpose of explicating and sharing ideas. As with all living language systems, constant change and evolution is expected. When the purpose, structure and complexity of the theory vary, so does its language. The process of theory building occurs in stages over long periods of time, from conceptualisation to formal theory development and validation (Hardy, 1985). It is not a linear process, but rather iterative and circular, depending on where the process starts. Few theories are complete, so various theory typologies and hierarchies have been proposed (Mosey, 1996) that identify the stage to which a theory has been developed (Dickoff, James & Weidenbach, 1968) or the type of theory-building process used (Meleis, 1991; Sieg, 1988). This has resulted in some confusion in the literature about the exact usage and meaning of the term "theory" and generated substitute words such as meta-theory, model and framework to delineate the scope and completeness of a formal theory (Mosey).

In this chapter, the term theory is used loosely to mean the articulation and communication of a conceptual image of health and ability or conversely, ill health and disability, its components and the way those components are connected. In occupational science and therapy, theory is the articulation and communication of a conceptual image of occupation in relation to health and ability, its component parts and the way those parts might be connected. Occupational therapy practitioners sometimes question the importance of theory (Chapparo, 1997), instead wanting to get on as quickly as possible with "the facts" or "the evidence" (Javetz & Katz, 1989; Law & McColl, 1989). In truth, we all theorise whether or not we realise it, interpreting facts in the light of theories that give those facts the meaning that we seek (Schön, 1983). Theorising forms a constant mental background upon which our actions are based. Formal theory building is simply a more thorough and carefully explicated form of the informal or "tacit" theorising (Fleming, 1991; Schön) used by all health-care workers or the "naïve" theorising that lay people use as part of their everyday life. As Meleis (1991) reports, any time we delineate and link concepts to describe, explain, predict or prescribe, and then communicate and use these concepts in a number of situations, the beginning of a theory is formulated.

Impact of health and disability theories on occupational therapy

Theories that are used by health workers are constructed out of specialised knowledge and consist of three broad areas. First, general theories dealing with views on the nature of ill health and disability form a broad base that biases the focus and scope of any service delivery. These broad theoretical perspectives drive administration of health programs, health policy, people and social systems. Secondly, theory that is specific to a discipline such as occupational therapy is used to drive specific approaches to service delivery. Thirdly, all health professionals construct their own tacit or personal theories, forming the final "filter" through which decisions are made about what the problem is, what can be done about it and the style of social interaction that occurs between them and their clients (Chapparo, 1999). All three theoretical perspectives are used to inform practice in occupational therapy and contribute to the knowledge base, or "intellectual context", upon which decisions are made about a range of health care issues for individuals, groups or communities (Higgs & Jones, 2000).

Health care systems have been described as "soft systems" (Checkland, 1981), where the goals may be unrecognisable and the outcomes ambiguous. Interactions within soft systems reflect the theoretical positions of the people, organisational strata and the system itself. In Australia, three overarching theoretical positions that relate to definitions of health and ability appear to drive contemporary policy and service delivery for people with ill health and disability. These are:

- health as the absence of illness, disease and disability;
- health as personal ability and adaptation; and
- health and ability resulting from equality and social opportunity.

Each theoretical perspective has been abstracted from a number of theories and synthesised to present the central constructs that influence service delivery. Each perspective outlined below has its own strengths and weaknesses, characterised by hidden values and assumptions that implicitly organise service delivery. All occupational therapists work in contexts that support one or other of these theoretical positions. They find themselves creating modes of service delivery that are congruent with the prevailing soft system theory (Chapparo, 1997), often not realising that the theoretical underpinning of the institution contributes to their view of the people they serve.

Health is the absence of illness, disease and disability

Three theoretical perspectives of ill health and disability combine to form what has been referred to as "the medical model" (Sherry, 2002; Wilcock, 1998), a powerful and prevailing theoretical context that views health and ability as the absence of disease and handicap. This theoretical perspective has driven the focus of Australian health-care policy and delivery for decades (Willis, 1983). First, the view that health and ability are *ideal states*, characterised by the *absence of illness* and *perfection*, is central to the medical model. Seedhouse (1986) described how this view of health has always been part of "human dreams" (p 30), creating an image of a desired "end point" that does not match the reality of the human condition, or real world context. Secondly, the theory that *health is physical and mental fitness needed for daily tasks* supports the specific view that illnesses and diseases resulting in disability and handicap must be absent for "normal" social function (Oliver, 1996; Seedhouse). This perspective has supported the belief that people with disabilities are unable to function within a society that views ability as perfection unless they become more normal. Normal social functioning is the desired end point. Interventions that focus on restoration, amelioration and measurement against an artificial "norm" are consistent with this theoretical position. Thirdly, is the theory that *health is a commodity that can be lost, bought, received or sanctioned*. Fundamental to this theory is the notion that health and ability can be reduced to individual components and restored by component parts when required. Health is conceptualised as a phenomenon that exists *apart* from people and can be lost and recaptured given the "right" sort of intervention. Seedhouse describes how this theoretical perspective provides the rationale for contemporary health-care practices that are bought and sold, a means for the receiver and an end for the provider (p 29). In occupational therapy, private practice is a thriving contemporary service delivery system that has its foundations in this theoretical perspective.

Together, these three theories contribute the core elements to what is referred to as the "medical model" that functions on the following assumptions (Petersen, 1994; Sherry, 2002):

1. People do not normally demonstrate symptoms of ill health as it is conceptualised.

2. People become ill or disabled because of a deviation from the biological norm.

3. Emotional or physical changes make people aware that something is wrong.

4. Problems that are identified by health workers will be accurate and relevant.

5. Intervention will lead to recovery and "cure".

The assumption that illness and impairment are the root causes of problems people may experience leads to interventions (policy and practice) that focus on solutions to obtain perfection, such as prevention (maintaining perfect state), cure (obtaining perfection), disease containment (for example pain management), rehabilitation, amelioration and palliation (obtaining a normal state). Attitudes consistent with these theories of health and ability are prevalent across a broad range of health professionals (Sherry, 2002) indicating their pervasive influence.

Clear parallels can be made between the medical model of health and ability and the development of occupational therapy theory. During its early years, occupational therapy expanded services within a variety of medical facilities, theoretically aligning notions of occupation with the absence of disease and disability. There was a clear focus on isolated cause and effect principles of illness. Growing pressure from medicine for a more scientific rationale for practice (Licht, 1947; Wilcock, 1998) resulted in specialised interventions which generated explanations of human occupation that paralleled medical explanations of disease and disability (Chapparo & Ranka, 2000; Kielhofner, 1992; Kielhofner & Burke, 1977). In concert with contextual expectations, clients' problems with daily occupations were reduced to components, and expressed in terms of physical or psychiatric diagnosis rather than occupational need (Spackman, 1968). Even occupations themselves were broken into units such as activities of daily living and assigned a hierarchy of performance importance culminating in independence. This type of reductionist focus persists today and is found, not only in occupational therapy services in clinics and hospitals, but in educational and community settings where assessment of occupational performance is based on measurement of ability against what are considered "normal standards" (Losardo & Notari-Syverson, 2001).

Just as medical research and clinical practice have been used to construct multiple "mini-theories" to guide health practices, occupational therapy mini-theories relating to the nature of component parts of occupation and the effects of intervention on larger units of occupation contribute to our understanding of occupation as a whole. Theory in the form of practice frameworks have been distilled and abstracted from much wider theories to generate physical (Trombly & Radomski, 2002), sensory (Ayres, 1972), cognitive (Radomski, 2002) and psychosocial (Solet, 2002) approaches that explain and guide practice. Examples of these practice frameworks and their link to theories of health and ability are illustrated in Figure 4.1 (see next page). Contemporary literature often refers to the practice emanating from these component theories as "bottom-up" as opposed to "top-down" approaches that are purported to consider the whole client situation. To discard these components from theoretical views of occupation would reduce the understanding of occupational experience for clients who wish to focus on specific components of their occupational wellbeing. However, focusing on these components to the exclusion of a larger view of occupation would result in a limited theoretical view of occupational existence.

The impact of health as perfection theory is reflected in contemporary literature that laments the lack of appropriate evidence on which to base health policy and practice. The current evidence debate demonstrates the dominance of reductionist science across health and disability services. For example, Australia's National Health and Medical Research Council (2000) outlined three dimensions to evidence: strength (level or study design; bias minimisation; statistical precision), size of effect and relevance. Assumptions that underpin this view of evidence subscribe to the theoretical position that health is a universal perfection and can be measured the same way for all people; that ill health and disability can be reduced to small units of measurement that accurately reflect a larger problem; and that what scientists choose to and are able to measure is relevant to people who experience ill health and disability. The evidence based medicine movement uncritically adopts these dimensions to evidence and exercises considerable influence within the health sciences. The influence upon occupational therapy is clear. Contemporary literature is again exhorting a preferred research design, the systematic review of randomised control trials as the favoured approach in all study contexts, reminiscent of scientific dogma that "derailed" (Shannon, 1977) the focus of occupational therapy in the 1950s, 1960s and 1970s. Implicit in this approach is the theory that ill health and disability can be reduced to individual factors, pushing researchers towards positivist experimental methods, precisely defined outcomes and relying heavily on statistical analysis (Sibthorpe & Dixon, 2001). This theoretical context calls for and favours randomised controlled trials, even when we know that within the context of something as complicated, multifaceted and dynamic as human occupation, they are difficult to conduct and often unhelpful in terms of the information they produce.

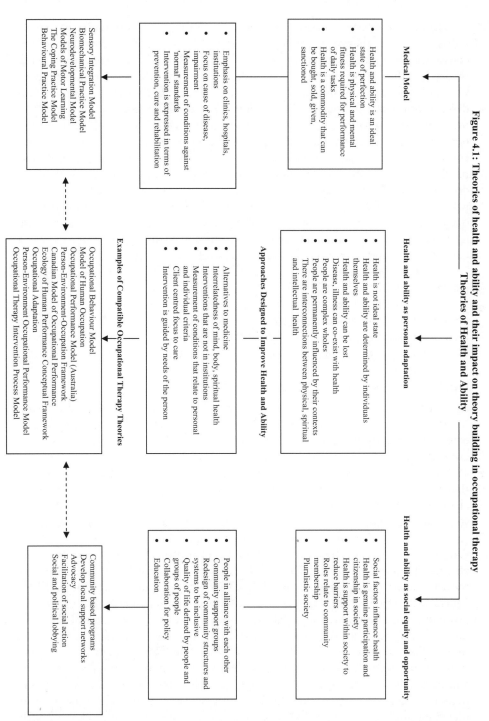

Figure 4.1: Theories of health and ability and their impact on theory building in occupational therapy

The impact of health as perfection theory on Australian health policy is evident. Policy makers, argues Walt (1998), are most receptive to research findings that construct theoretical positions acknowledging political exigencies. Otherwise, theory is either reconstructed or discarded to suit the decision-making process. Often devoid of a comprehensive theory base, Sibthorpe and Dixon (2001) describe how governments tend to develop health policy in the form of "soundbite interventions" (p 4) which are characterised by reductionist and easily-measured outcomes. Examples would include such measures as length of hospital stay, community access to high-tech medical facilities and specific physical and psychological outcomes of medical intervention, as opposed to measuring the degree to which meaningful engagement in personal, social and occupational patterns is obtained and maintained through life. In turn, the policy context determines the resources, scope and mode of service occupational therapists are able to offer. Unfortunately for occupational therapists, the determinants of health contained in most theories of occupational and social health and wellbeing are "highly contingent upon the context of the study and fly in the face of political palatability" (Sibthorpe & Dixon, p 3).

The medical model is not without merit. It has been responsible for considerable achievements in medicine. There will always be a need for intervention regimes that focus on the difficulties associated with medical disease, illness and impairment (Sherry, 2002; Sibthorpe & Dixon, 2001).

Health as personal ability and adaptation

Against the background of dissatisfaction with a material, technologically-driven society, a more critical conception of human society, referred to as postmodern, emerged in the twentieth century (Wilcock, 1998). Postmodernism represents a critical reappraisal of traditional modes of thought, beliefs and conviction (Waters, 1985). As with any sector of society, the health system and the health professions that work within that context have been affected to a greater or lesser degree by changes resulting from postmodern thought. Traditionally-held views of social structure including medicine were criticised by postmodernists as monologic, representing as universal, a particular European, masculine view (Callinicos, 1990; Carter, 1993; Harvey, 1989; Norris, 1992; Rose, 1989). The view of health as the absence of disease, for example, has been criticised by postmodernists as a totalising meta-narrative, obscuring other possible narratives (Mattingly & Fleming, 1994; Morse & O'Brien, 1995; Mosey, 1985; Oliver & Barnes, 1998). In articulating postmodern thinking, Waters (1986) describes a deepening suspicion of the rigid dichotomies between objective reality and subjective experience, fact and imagination, secular and sacred, public and private. Rather than permanence, stability and constancy as societal values, change, growth, innovation, modification and personally-directed alternative lifestyles have become the rule for the last four decades (Riggar et al, 1989). In health care, this social change has seen the rise and increasing social acceptance of alternative and personally-directed modes of health care. In occupational therapy theory, this reappraisal is expressed in advancing the interactionist views of occupation (Ranka, 1997) whereby occupation is theoretically represented as person-centred, systemic, multifaceted, temporal and complex. This view is based in humanism, bringing some contemporary theories of occupation into sharp conflict with health practices aligned with medical models of health and disability (Chapparo & Ranka, 2000; Griffin, 1988).

Based on humanistic notions propounded by postmodern theorists, in which humans express free will and a capacity to pursue self-improvement actively (Wilcock, 1998), occupational therapy theorists of the early postmodern era began to question the entrenched medical model and the reductionist direction of occupational therapy at the time (Reilly, 1969). Theories that defined occupation as the personal capacity to engage in desired occupation emerged, emanating from a broader humanist emphasis on the individual need and interaction within specific environments. Basic to a humanist position is that human dignity depends upon self-determination (Seedhouse, 1986). Humanism resists and counteracts dogmatism, and acknowledges that practical knowledge is important. With respect to health and disability, humanism proposes that health is a personal goal and that people should be free to obtain this goal through their own efforts. Humanists posit that people are complex, physical, emotional, intellectual and spiritual beings and that the whole is not equal to the sum of the parts. As reported so eloquently by Wilcock, a rediscovery of earlier humanist theories of occupation as health and adaptation (Meyer, 1922) was spearheaded by Reilly in the middle of the twentieth century and was based on the "sensitivity, adaptability, durability, and creativity of humans in tune with their environments" (p 200). Reilly (1969) initiated the first formal theory of occupation as health, termed "occupational behaviour", which promoted the view of occupational behaviour as the entire continuum of play and work. Occupation was the central construct of the model and it explicated the way occupation could be used by people to obtain behavioural change (Reilly, 1974). Occupation was at once a means to an end and an end in itself. Emphasis was placed on the centrality of the individual, and the individual's ability to cope with changes in personal ability and life situation, thereby establishing the first formal client-centred view of practice in occupational therapy (Van Duesen, 1988).

One seminal extension of Reilly's work is Kielhofner's Model of Human Occupation (1995), which evolved within the context of occupational therapy. This model focuses on purposeful activities and their central place in the experience of living. Human occupations are described as housing multi-dimensional components, and performance is embedded within individual physical and cultural environments. Humans are viewed as open systems. The humanistic roots of this theory of occupation are clear in the assertion that occupation is governed by three sub-systems that would appear closely aligned to self-determination and adaptation: volition, habituation and performance. Far less emphasis has been assigned to the role of the environment (Haglund & Kjellberg, 1999). Assessments that have evolved from this model consider strengths and difficulties in occupational behaviours that are necessary to fulfil life roles such as worker, parent or friend. Intervention seeks to develop, remediate or enhance individual performance. Success in occupational performance is considered inherently organising and related to feelings of mastery, competence, acceptance and sense of identity. Other early theories of occupation that are aligned with the health as human adaptation theory, emphasising individualism, include the following. Fidler (1981) linked "doing" with competence, mastery, adaptation and self-esteem, constructing an early model of occupational performance. Mosey (1986) articulated a set of philosophical assumptions about the individual need for occupational balance and realisation of occupational potential. From a neurobiological framework, Moore (1975) linked Reilly's concepts of occupational behaviour with biological science, proposing that patterns of occupational performance experienced as successful are outcomes that express the central nervous system demands for maintenance of homeostatic balance. Individual differences in central nervous system function and structure drive individual, multiple and highly variable relationships with our environment. Moore's perspective is extended further in Wilcock's theory of an occupational brain (1998).

Of more importance in the postmodern shift away from medical theories of health and disability, Reilly's model was applicable to both "well" and "sick" (Laukran, 1977). "Wellness" was identified as the extent to which people were able to engage in chosen occupations. Consistent with the humanist view, health and ability are not thought of as absolute (Seedhouse, 1986). Health and ability through occupation, according to Reilly's theory, is a personally-constructed task. Just as it is possible for disease and occupational wellness to coexist, so it is possible for the absence of disease to coexist with occupational ill health.

The influence of individual environments on human behaviour is a feature of humanist theory, such that the totality of a person is not considered to be separate from his or her context. In her theory of occupational behaviour, Reilly reinforced the importance of context on human performance. Reilly extrapolated two major concepts from humanism — the importance of individual self-determination and the relationship between people and their real world context — and aligned them with the concept of occupation. In doing so, Reilly not only constructed a theory of occupational behaviour, but also planted the seeds of person-environment-occupation constructs that are central to contemporary theory building that explains occupation and occupational performance.

Person-environment-occupation models

It is not within the scope of this chapter to describe each person-environment-occupation theory in detail. Readers are directed to the literature for more comprehensive, and perhaps alternative descriptions of each (Christiansen & Baum, 1997; Fisher, 1998; Trombly & Radomski, 2002; Schkade & Schultz, 1992). The following three examples of person-environment-occupation models have been used to describe how Reilly's concepts have been translated into contemporary notions of occupational performance through theory building. The Person-Environment-Occupational conceptual framework (Law, Cooper, Strong, Steward, Rigby & Letts, 1996), the Ecology of Human Performance conceptual framework (Dunn, Brown & McGuigan, 1994) and the Occupational Performance Model (Australia) (Chapparo & Ranka, 1997). These three models were generated independently across three different countries and cultural contexts and although they show definitive and structural differences, they all focus on similar constructs.

The Person-Environment-Occupation model (PEO) (Law et al, 1996) illustrates a transactive approach to understanding a person's occupational performance. Occupational performance is characterised as the transaction between the person, the environment and the occupation, as shown in Figure 4.2. The environment includes physical, social, political, economic, institutional, cultural and situational contexts that can enable or disable performance (Law, 1991). Occupation refers to the activities and tasks that people do to carry out their daily lives in concert with life-roles.

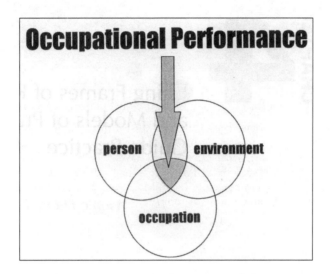

Figure 4.2: A Person-Environment-Occupation Model: A transactive approach for occupational performance (Law, Cooper, Strong, Stewart, Rigby & Letts, 1996)

The Ecology of Human Performance model (Dunn, Brown & McGuigan, 1994) is based on similar constructs, outlining person, task and context variables and stating that the interaction among these three variables determines a person's performance range as illustrated in Figure 4.3. In this model, the person is recognised as a product of genetic endowment together with sensory, cognitive and psychosocial abilities and experiences. The context incorporates physical, social, cultural and temporal aspects of the environment. For these theorists, tasks are those selected by people based on interest and skill which are supported within particular contexts. These tasks designate a performance range as depicted in Figure 4.3. When a person has limited skill or a restricted environment, the performance range is narrowed. Occupational therapists work to expand the performance range to include more tasks using a number of intervention strategies.

The Model of Occupational Performance (Australia) (Chapparo & Ranka, 1997) (Figure 4.4) explicates similar constructs in more detail. Differences between this model and the models already described include the following. Performance, according to this model, extends the usual concept of performance as doing to the

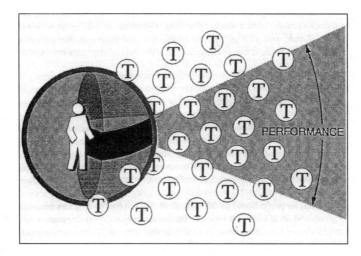

Figure 4.3: Schemata for the Ecology of Human Performance Framework

This figure depicts how people (figure) are embedded within unique contexts (circle) with an infinite variety of tasks around them (T). The thick black line indicates how people "look through" their contexts when choosing the tasks they need or want to do (Dunn, Brown & McGuigan, 1994, p 600). Performance is the resulting range of tasks that people do (arrows). The performance range can be broad or narrow, depending on the skills and abilities of people and the amount of environmental support available.

purposeful way in which someone acts or reacts in particular situations. Action or reaction might be physical, mental or emotional change. Purpose implies desire or motivation. Performance, in this theory, is also assumed to go beyond "doing" to incorporate "knowing" and "being", concepts fundamental to humanism. Eight major constructs form the theoretical structure of this model, enabling occupational therapists and others to appreciate the importance of smaller units of occupation when necessary. The person in relation to occupational performance is described through the constructs of occupational performance roles, areas, components and core elements. Life-roles, referred to in other models, are more specifically defined as occupational roles. Component functions are conceptually linked to everyday tasks and routines or self-maintenance, rest, leisure and work, prompting a theoretical shift from reductionist views of component performance in medicine to a more holistic view of occupation. The authors stress, however, that all constructs work as an integrated and dynamic whole and that it is not possible to "functionally separate, reduce or understand" them as individual elements (Chapparo & Ranka, 1997, p 11). In this model, the person is not necessarily an individual, but may be a group, community or society thereby moving away from notions of individuality and self-determination that may be alien to societies whose sociocultural identity is collective rather than individualistic (Manstead & Hewstone, 1995). The external environment in this model contains similar elements to those outlined above but includes two further constructs, time and space.

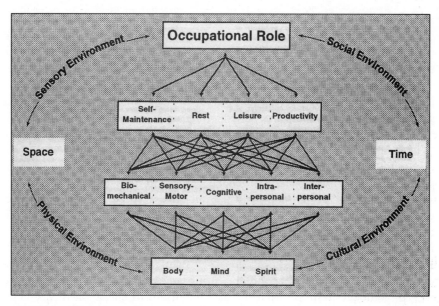

Figure 4.4: The Occupational Performance Model (Australia) (Chapparo & Ranka, 1997, p 23)

Complexity theory

Contemporary models of occupation as health and adaptation often describe the relationship in terms of a complex system. Following on from Kielhofner's (1995) use of systems theory to describe relationships within the Model of Human Occupation, contemporary theories of occupation (Gray, Kennedy & Zemke, 1996) and occupational performance (Chapparo & Ranka, 1997) are turning to non-linear systems theory to explain the individuality of occupational existence further (Royeen, 2003). Dynamic systems theory presupposes the evolving nature of a process across time. Such occupational complexity refers to the many variables surrounding occupational performance in context and the way they affect one another. In linking occupational complexity to chaos theory, Royeen describes how the concept transcends the parallel and distributed processing simple systems that have been used to explain occupational performance processes (Kielhofner). As illustrated in the Occupational Performance Model (Australia), occupational complexity is conceptualised by arrows as systems or networks within networks that are arranged and organised into an overall system that changes according to variations within the person or from the environment. No one arrow or construct has logical precedence over another.

There is considerable theory building to be done to develop this concept further and apply it in a meaningful and practical way to occupational therapy. Perhaps Royeen (2003) comes closest to explicating this when describing the processes involved in occupational performance as the "web of life" (p 616). The promise of occupational science is to stretch the narrowly defined occupations as "activities of daily living", or "work" or "leisure", into a theory of occupation that adequately describes the larger richness and diversity of occupation for all. How occupations enfold into one another and across the lifespan was a question raised by Reilly half a century ago, and is only just begun to be answered today. Using the language of chaos theory, the task of occupational science is to identify and delineate the complexities of occupational webs and the key "control" variables. The task of occupational therapy would be to implement planned-for, force-creating adaptations of control parameters impinging on occupational webs that are specifically designed to promote health and ability (Royeen, 2003).

There is clear evidence of attempts to integrate views of health as personal ability and adaptation into health service delivery through client-centred approaches (Law, 1998). There is general agreement that health worker/client interaction can be characterised by mutual tolerance, respect, freedom to choose a course of intervention and support for those choices; in short, competence in social and cultural interaction about health and disability. Often however, these views, although clearly espoused by health workers, are not carried out. More often than not, disagreements within service delivery systems and among health workers, clients and families about what the presenting problem is, and how it should be managed, gradually diminish even the best intentions to engage in theory-based, humanistic, client-centred health practice (Chapparo, 1997).

Models of inquiry that are being used by health researchers to explore the many individual interpretations of health and disability within contemporary Australian society find their roots in humanism, originating largely from outside the field of medicine. Emanating from a common assumption that health and disability are not words with a single uncontroversial meaning, research using qualitative methods has contributed to our understanding of health and disability as multifaceted and highly personal concepts. Discourse analysis, which has its origins in the analysis of text comprehension and conversation, has been extended into medicine (for example, Patel & Frederiksen, 1984) and occupational therapy (Crepeau, 1991). Phenomenological methods, where the focus is on understanding the individual ways people experience life situations, have been applied to medicine (Ramsden, Whelan, & Cooper, 1989) and occupational therapy (Mattingly & Fleming, 1994). With the increasing acceptance of qualitative methods, researchers in health science have begun to be receptive to new forms of inquiry that stress the interpretative aspect of health and disability experience. Ethnographic researchers have begun to generate multiple descriptions of experiences of ill health and disability. This type of research takes into account the context of experience, realising that without this context, reports of human behaviour are meaningless. Although interpretative research has had a long history in education (Glaser & Strauss, 1967), its acceptance in health and disability fields has come considerably later and has yet to be fully completed.

Health and ability result from equality and social opportunities

Studies from the field of social science confirm the persistence, and indeed widening, of social gradients of health among sociocultural groups (ACROD, 1999; Australian Early Childhood Association, 1999; Bowers, Esmond, Lutz &

Jacobson, 2003; Deafness Forum of Australia, 1999; Eckersley, Dixon & Douglas, 2001; Edgar, 2001; Ethnic Disability Advocacy Centre, 1999; Mental Health Coordinating Council, 1999; National Caucus of Disability Consumer Organisations, 1999; National Ethnic Disability Alliance, 1999; Organisation for Economic Co-operation and Development, 2001; Schorr, 1991; Swales, 2000; Winter, 2000). Various authors question the sophistication of contemporary theories of health and wellbeing, describing theoretical dichotomies between medical and social models (Eckersley et al). Questions arise as to why, in an increasingly "evidence-based" world, little evidence is being used to construct theories that are capable of guiding health policy and practice on a larger scale (Sibthorpe & Dixon, 2001).

Development of social theories of health and disability has been central to redefining the terms (Shakespeare, Gillespie-Sells & Davies, 1996). Grouped together, these theories have been referred to as "social disability theory". This theory is based on the distinction between impairment and disability. Impairment refers to medical conditions that inhibit health while disability refers to the social reactions to impairment, particularly experiences of discrimination, oppression, social exclusion and marginalisation (Oliver & Barnes, 1998; Peters, 2000). Unlike the medical model, this social model encompasses positive social identities at an individual and collective level for people with ill health and disability (Swain & French, 2000). The impact of social disability theory on policy is potentially dramatic but yet to be fully realised. It moves the focus away from impairment to disability by defining disability as a rights issue, and locating the cause of disability in exclusionary social, economic and cultural barriers. The theory asserts that the complexity and multiplicity of social restrictions experienced by people with disabilities means that they often experience ill health (Sherry, 2002).

Although development of a social model of disability significantly advanced our understanding of disability, some assumptions underlying the model raise questions for occupational therapy. For example, it is based on the assumption that some people are clearly identified as "disabled" or "non-disabled". In reality, lived experiences of disability and ill health are more complex. There are groups of people who refuse to identify as disabled. These have included for example, people with learning difficulties (Chappell, 1998), people with hidden chronic illness (Vickers, 2001) and people with hearing loss (Corker, 1998).

Along similar lines, the structure-agency theory adopted by sociologists and anthropologists posits that lifestyle patterns may be differentially adopted, thereby creating differently patterned conditions of health risk and health needs for different social environments. Despite evidence supporting this view, interventions at both individual and population levels are rarely based on an integrated appreciation of both social and medical theories of causation. Fragmented service delivery, lack of coordination between health, education and social services, allocation of resources to crisis management and acute care rather than planned universal service delivery and poor overall coherence and comprehensiveness is experienced across the whole health-care sector and can be partly attributed to a theoretical void (Keating & Hertzman, 1999; Leutz, 1999). Understanding of social environments in their own right, separately from individual medical factors, is paramount to construction of a theory of overall health and wellbeing that is able not only to drive policy, but to integrate professional practice across disciplines, settings and services.

Social and occupational justice

Health and ability for all is conceptualised as a social justice issue, so it is not simply the concern of people with disabilities or those who are ill (Fawcett, 2000; Sherry, 2002; Veatch, 1990). In extrapolating theories of social justice to occupational therapy, Wilcock (1998) and Townsend (CAOT, 1997) place practice in the realm of public health and outline the following theoretical constructs that would promote social and occupational health for all:

- a balance of wellbeing maintained through occupation;
- enhancement of unique capacities and potential;
- occupational and social support and justice for all people and communities; and
- politically-supported and socially-valued occupational opportunity.

In reality, social justice is a theoretical vision of everyday life in which "people can choose, organise and engage in meaningful occupations that enhance health, quality of life and equity in housing, employment and other valued aspects of life" (CAOT, 1997, p 182).

Only time will reveal the extent to which theories of social and occupational justice will develop the course of occupational science and therapy practice. Research supporting this view of occupation and health is scarce. As suggested by Wilcock (1998), occupational therapists will not only have to change the focus of practice to make the transition to public policy, but will have to change the focus of research as well. Exploration of the impact of short-term illness on long-term health and ability, exploration and description of occupational wellness (balance, satisfaction, value and opportunity) and the effects of various social and ecological environments on the development of occupational existence are just some examples of the larger research questions that remain unanswered. Interventions building on social justice and disability theory will have to address structural factors in communities rather than behaviours in individuals, as traditionally seen in occupational therapy. Public policy will have to become an everyday working arena for occupational therapists who have clear theoretical views of occupation as it "fits" with social need, from the smallest component to the broadest concept.

Common features

Although differences exist between each of the theories presented, there are commonalities among them. First, health and ability do not have a single meaning and within each theory, there is no undisputed example of health. As Seedhouse suggests (1986), this is demonstrated by the fact that all of them are legitimate and relevant to different situations. Similarly, all occupational therapy models are plausible and have legitimacy, depending on their relevance to a particular client situation. Just as people's health cannot be fully understood in isolation from what they do in their lives, human occupation cannot be fully understood in isolation from the context in which it is performed. Although there is potential for theoretical conflict between the theories listed, a common factor is that all strive to promote health, ability and human potential. So too, all models of occupation and therapy seek to remove obstacles to desired performance. Figure 4.1 shows a hypothesised relationship between each of the theories presented and between theories of health and occupational therapy theory. Each theory has been condensed and is an oversimplification of the conceptual ideas supporting it. The dotted lines between each type of occupational therapy model suggests that there is conceptual and practical movement between different models and that the conceptual framework from which therapists operate changes according to their knowledge, perception of the problem and client need. This probably reflects the fact that in health, as in occupational therapy, there is no comprehensive theory, requiring a pluralistic rather than a monistic theoretical approach (Mosey, 1985). In contemporary health care, there is no single principle that can define health, disability, occupation or occupational therapy. Each theoretical approach discussed in this chapter contributes a distinct and different view of human experience of health and ability. Perhaps this is the fundamental element of an intellectual context for practice — a pluralistic approach that allows the conceptual freedom to expand, change and progress, unencumbered by one tradition, authority or ideology. Perhaps the key to theory and theory building is the ability to analyse our theoretical underpinning, develop new theories and consider alternative theories. As Mosey (1985) suggested, perhaps a pluralistic theoretical view of health, ability and occupation, while uncomfortable for some, may help meet the varying needs of people who seek our help.

Conclusion

This chapter has presented a view of theory as an intellectual or conceptual context for health care in general and occupational therapy in particular. Three overarching theoretical positions of health and ability were identified: health and ability as the absence of disease and impairment; health as personal ability and adaptation; and health and ability as social equity and opportunity. Theory and theory building in occupational therapy were paralleled with each of these overarching theories and a picture emerged of a pluralistic theoretical approach. Theories of medical science, humanism and social justice that have the capacity for conflict have been harnessed by occupational therapy theorists and converted into practice models to guide therapy. The theory-building process indicates that within the science of occupation and the practice of occupational therapy, integration of concepts from each theoretical position may be possible.

References

ACROD. (1999). *ACROD — Submission — Reference group on welfare reform.* From http://www.facs.gov.au/internet/facsinternet.nsf/aboutfacs/welfaresubmissions3.htm

Australian Early Childhood Association. (1999). *Submission to Department of Family and Community Services reference group on welfare reform.* From http://www.facs.gov.au/internet/facsinternet.nsf/aboutfacs/welfaresubmissions3.htm

Ayres, A. J. (1972). *Sensory integration and learning disorders.* Los Angeles: Western Psychological Services.

Bowers, B., Esmond, S., Lutz, B. & Jacobson, N. (2003). Improving primary care for persons with disabilities: The nature of expertise. *Disability and Society, 18*(4), 443–455.

Callinicos, A. (1990). *Against postmodernism: a Marxist critique.* London: Polity Press.

CAOT. (1997). *Enabling occupation: An occupational therapy perspective.* Ottawa, CA: Canadian Association of Occupational Therapists.

Carter, B. (1993). Losing the common touch: A post-modern politics of the curriculum? *Curriculum Studies, 1*(1), 149–156.

Chapparo, C. (1999). Working out: Working with Angelica — Interpreting practice. In S. Ryan & E. McKay (Eds), *Thinking and reasoning in therapy: Narratives from practice*, pp 31–50. UK: Stanley Thornes.

Chapparo, C. (1997). *Influences on clinical reasoning in occupational therapy. Unpublished Doctoral thesis.* Ryde, NSW: Macquarie University.

Chapparo, C. & Ranka, J. (2000). Clinical reasoning in occupational therapy. In J. Higgs & M. Jones (Eds), *Clinical reasoning in the health professions* (2nd ed.), pp 128–137. Oxford: Butterworth-Heinemann.

Chapparo, C. & Ranka, J. (1997). *Occupational Performance Model (Australia): Monograph 1.* Lidcome, Australia: University of Sydney.

Chappell, A. (1998). *Nothing about us without us: Disability oppression and empowerment.* Berkeley, CA: University of California Press.

Checkland, P. B. (1981). *Systems thinking: System practice.* New York: John Wiley & Sons.

Christiansen, C. & Baum, C. (1997). *Occupational therapy: Enabling functional well-being* (2nd ed.). Thorofare: Slack.

Corker, M. (1998). *Deaf and disabled or deafness disabled?* Buckingham: Open University Press.

Corker, M. & Shakespeare, T. (2003). Mapping the terrain. In M. Corker & T. Shakespeare (Eds), *Disability/Postmodernity: Embodying disability theory*, pp 1–17. London: Continuum.

Creek, J. & Feaver, S. (1993). Models for practice in occupational therapy: Part 1, defining terms. *British Journal of Occupational Therapy, 56*(1), 4–6.

Crepeau, E. B. (1991). Achieving intersubjective understanding: Examples from an occupational therapy treatment session. *American Journal of Occupational Therapy, 45*(1), 1016–1025.

Deafness Forum of Australia. (1999). *Submission to reference group on welfare reform*, 17th December 1999. From http://www.facs.gov.au/internet/facsinternet.nsf/aboutfacs/welfaresubmissions3.htm

Dickoff, J., James, P. & Weidenbach, B. (1968). Theory in a practice discipline: Part 1: Practice oriented theory. *Nursing Research, 17*(5), 415–435.

Dunn, W., Brown, C. & McGuigan, A. (1994). The ecology of human performance: A framework for considering the effect of context. *American Journal of Occupational Therapy, 48,* 595–607.

Eckersley, R., Dixon, J. & Douglas, B. (2001). *The social origins of health and well-being.* Cambridge, UK: Cambridge University Press.

Edgar, D. (2001). *The patchwork nation: Re-thinking government — rebuilding community.* Sydney, NSW: HarperCollins Publishers.

Ethnic Disability Advocacy Centre. (1999). *EADC's response to the discussion paper — the challenge of welfare dependency in the 21st century.* From http://www.facs.gov.au/internet/facsinternet.nsf/aboutfacs/welfaresubmissions3.htm

Fawcett, B. (2000). *Feminist perspectives on disability.* Harlow: Pearson Education.

Fidler, G. (1981). From crafts to competence. *American Journal of Occupational Therapy, 35,* 567–573.

Fisher, A. (1998). Uniting practice and theory in an occupational framework. *American Journal of Occupational Therapy, 52,* 509–521.

Fleming, M. H. (1991). The search for tacit knowledge. In C. Mattingly & M. H. Fleming. *Clinical reasoning: Forms of inquiry in a therapeutic practice*, pp 22–34. Philadelphia: F. A. Davis Company.

Glaser, B. & Strauss, A. (1967). *The discovery of grounded theory.* Chicago: Aldine.

Gray, J. M., Kennedy, B. L. & Zemke, R. (1996). Application of dynamic systems theory to occupation. In R. Zemke & F. Clark (Eds), *Occupational science the evolving discipline*, pp 309–324. Philadelphia: F. A. Davis Company.

Griffin, S. (1988). Conflicts in professional practice. *Australian Occupational Therapy Journal, 35*(1), 5–12.

Haglund, L. & Kjellberg, A. (1999). A critical analysis of the Model of Human Occupation. *Canadian Journal of Occupational Therapy, 66*(2), 102–108.

Hardy, M. E. (1985). *Theory development and evaluation.* Kingston: University of Rhode Island College of Nursing.

Harvey, D. (1989). *The condition of postmodernity: An enquiry into the origins of cultural change.* Oxford: Basil Blackwell.

Henderson, A. (1988). Occupational therapy knowledge: From practice to theory. 1988 Eleanor Clarke Slagle Lecture. *American Journal of Occupational Therapy, 42*(9), 567–576.

Higgs, J. & Jones, M. (2000). *Clinical reasoning in the health professions* (2nd ed.). Oxford: Butterworth-Heinemann.

Javetz, R. & Katz, N. (1989). Knowledgeability of theories of occupational therapy practitioners in Israel. *American Journal of Occupational Therapy, 43*(10), 664–675.

Keating, D. & Hertzman, C. (Eds). (1999). *Developmental health and the wealth of nations: Social, Biological, and Educational Dynamics.* New York: The Guilford Press.

Kielhofner, G. (1992). *Conceptual foundations of occupational therapy.* Philadelphia: F. A. Davis Company.

Keilhofner, G. (1995). *A model of human occupation: Theory and application* (2nd ed.). Baltimore: Williams & Wilkins.

Kielhofner, G. & Burke, J. (1977). Occupational therapy after 60 years: An account of changing identity and knowledge. *American Journal of Occupational Therapy, 31,* 675–689.

Laukran, V. H. (1977). Toward a model of occupational therapy for community health. *American Journal of Occupational Therapy, 31,* 71.

Law, M. (1991). *Canadian occupational performance measure.* Toronto: Canadian Association of Occupational Therapists.

Law, M. (Ed.). (1998). *Client-centred occupational therapy.* Thorofare: Slack Inc.

Law, M., Cooper, B., Strong, S., Stewart, S., Rigby, P. & Letts, L (1996). The person-environment-occupational model: A transactive approach to occupational performance. *Canadian Journal of Occupational Therapy, 63,* 9–23.

Law, M. & McColl, M. A. (1989). Knowledge and use of theory among occupational therapists: A Canadian survey. *Canadian Journal of Occupational Therapy, 56*(4), 198–204.

Leutz, W. N. (1999). Five laws for integrating medical and social services: Lessons from the United States and United Kingdom. *The Millbank Quarterly, 77*(1), 77–110.

Licht, S. (1947). The objectives of occupational therapy. *Occupational Therapy Rehabilitation, 28,* 17–22.

Losardo, A. & Notari-Syverson, A. (2001). *Alternative approaches to assessing young children.*

Manstead, A. S. R. & Hewstone, M. (Eds). (1995). *The Blackwell encylopaedia of social psychology.* Boston: Blackwell Reference.

Mattingly, C. & Fleming, M. H. (1994). *Clinical reasoning: Forms of inquiry in a therapeutic practice.* Philadelphia: F. A. Davis Company.

Meleis, H. I. (1991). *Theoretical nursing: Development and progress.* Philadelphia: JB Lippincott.

Mental Health Coordinating Council. (1999). *Submission to the welfare reform reference group.* From http://www.facs.gov.au/internet/facsinternet.nsf/aboutfacs/ welfaresubmissions3.htm

Meyer, A. (1922). The philosophy of occupational therapy. *Archives of Occupational Therapy, 1,* 1–10.

Moore, J. (1975). Behaviour, bias and the limbic system. The 1975 Eleanor Clarke Slagle Lecture. *American Journal of Occupational Therapy, 30*(1), 11–19.

Morse, J. M. & O'Brien, B. (1995). Preserving self: From victim, to patient, to disabled person. *Journal of Advanced Nursing, 21,* 886–896.

Mosey, A. C. (1985). Eleanor Clarke Slagle Lecture, 1985: A monistic or a pluralistic approach to professional identify? *American Journal of Occupational Therapy, 39,* 504–509.

Mosey, A. C. (1986). *Psychosocial components of occupational therapy.* New York, NY: Raven Press.

Mosey, A. C. (1996). *Applied scientific inquiry in the health professions: An epistemological orientation* (2nd ed.). Bethesda, MD: AOTA Inc.

National Health and Medical Research Council. (2000). *How to use the evidence: Assessment and application of scientific evidence.* Australia: NHMRC Publications.

National Ethnic Disability Alliance, (1999). *Welfare reform.* From http://www.facs.gov.au/internet/facsinternet.nsf/aboutfacs/welfaresubmissions3.htm

Norris, C. (1992). *Uncritical theory: postmodernism, intellectuals and the Gulf War.* London: Verso.

Oliver, M. (1996). *Understanding disability: From theory to practice.* London: Macmillan.

Oliver, M. & Barnes, C. (1998). *Disabled people and social policy.* London: Longman.

Patel, V. L. & Fredreiksen, C. H. (1984). Cognitive processes in comprehension and knowledge acquisition by medical students and physicians. In H. G. Schmidt & M. L. De Volder (Eds), *Tutorials in problem based learning,* pp 143–157. Holland: van Gorcum.

Peters, S. (2000). Is there a disability culture? A syncretisation of three possible work views. *Disability and Society, 15*(4), 583–601.

Petersen, A. R. (1994). *In a critical condition: Health and power relations in Australia.* Sydney: Allen & Unwin.

Radomski, M. V. (2002). Assessing abilities and capacities: Cognition. In C. A. Trombly & M. V. Radomski (Eds), *Occupational therapy for physical dysfunction,* pp 213–234. Philadelphia: Lippincott Williams & Wilkins.

Ramsden, P., Whelan, G. & Cooper, D. (1989). Some phenomena of medical students' diagnostic problem solving. *Medical Education, 23,* 108–117.

Ranka, J. (1997). Developing postmodern occupational therapy curriculum model using the structure and operations of occupational performance. In C. Chapparo & J. Ranka (Eds), *Occupational Performance Model (Australia): Monograph 1.* Lidcome, Australia: University of Sydney.

Reilly, M. (1962). 1961 Eleanor Clarke Slagle Lecture: Occupational therapy can be one of the great ideas of 20th century medicine. *American Journal of Occupational Therapy, 16,* 1–9.

Reilly, M. (1969). The education process. *American Journal of Occupational Therapy, 23,* 299–307.

Reilly, M. (1974). *Play as exploratory learning.* Beverly Hills: Sage Publications Inc.

Riggar, T. F., Crimando, W., Bordieri, J., Hanley-Maxwell, C., Benshoff, J. J. & Calzaretta, W. A. (1989). Managing organisational change: A review of the literature. *Journal of Rehabilitation Administration. 13,* 134–140.

Rose, N. (1989). *Governing the soul: The shaping of the private self.* London: Routledge.

Royeen, C. B. (2003). Chaotic occupational therapy: Collective wisdom for a complex profession. *American Journal of Occupational Therapy, 57*(6), 609–624.

Schön, D. (1983). *The reflective practitioner.* New York: Basic Books.

Schorr, L. B. (1991). Children, families and the cycle of disadvantage. *Canadian Journal of Psychiatry, 36*(6), 437–441.

Schkade, J. K. & Schultz, S. (1992). Occupational adaptation: Toward a holistic approach for contemporary practice, Part 1. *American Journal of Occupational Therapy, 46,* 829–837.

Seedhouse, D. (1986). Theories of health. In D. Seedhouse, *Health: The foundations for achievement,* pp 26–56. Chichester: John Wiley & Sons.

Shakespeare, T., Gillespie-Sells, K. & Davies, D. (1996). *The sexual politics of disability.* London: Cassell.

Shannon, P. (1977). The derailment of occupational therapy. *American Journal of Occupational Therapy, 31,* 229–234.

Sherry, M. (2002). Welfare reform and disability policy in Australia. *Just Policy, 28,* 3–11.

Sibthorpe, B. & Dixon, J. (2001). Rethinking evaluation for policy action on the social origins of health and well-being. In R. Exkersley, J. Dixon & B. Douglas (Eds), *The social origins of health and well-being.* Cambridge, UK: Cambridge University Press.

Sieg, K. (1988). Theory analysis: In B. Miller, K. Seig, F. Ludwig, S. Shortbridge & J. Van Duesen. *Six perspectives on theory for the practice of occupational therapy.* Rockville, MD: Aspen Publications.

Solet, J. M. (2002). Optimizing personal and social adaptation. In C. A. Trombly & M. V. Radomski (Eds), *Occupational therapy for physical dysfunction,* pp 761–781. Philadelphia: Lippincott Williams & Wilkins.

Spackman, C. (1968). A history of the practice of occupational therapy for restoration of physical function: 1917–1967. *American Journal of Occupational Therapy, 22,* 67–76.

Swain, J. & French, S. (2000). Towards an affirmation model of disability. *Disability and Society, 15*(4), 569–582.

Swales, J. (2000). Inequalities: A challenge to science and politics. *New Zealand Medical Journal, 11*(August), 324–325.

Trombly, C. A. & Radomski, M. V. (Eds). (2002). *Occupational therapy for physical dysfunction* (5th ed.). Philadelphia: Lippincott Williams & Wilkins.

Van Duesen, J. (1988). Mary Reilly. In B. Miller, K. Seig, F. Ludwig, S. Shortbridge & J. Van Duesen. *Six perspectives on theory for the practice of occupational therapy.* Rockville, MD: Aspen Publications.

Veatch, R. M. (1990). Justice in health care: The contribution of Edmund Pellegrino. *The Journal of Medicine and Philosophy, 15,* 269–287.

Vickers, M. (2001). *Work and unseen chronic illness: Silent voices.* London: Routledge.

Waters, B. (1986). Ministry and the university in a post-modern world. *Religion and Intellectual Life, 4*(1), 113–122.

Wilcock, A. (1998). *An occupational perspective of health.* Thorofare: Slack.

Willis, E. (1983). *Medical dominance, the division of labour in Australian health care.* Sydney, Australia: George Allen & Unwin.

Winter, I. (Ed.). (2000). *Social capital and public policy in Australia.* Melbourne, VIC: Australian Institute of Family Studies.

Zemke, R. & Clark, F. (1996). *Occupational science: The evolving discipline.* Philadelphia: F. A. Davis Company.

CHAPTER FIVE

Professional Education in Context

Clare Hocking

Nils Erik Ness

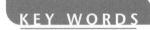

KEY WORDS

Higher education
Local health needs
Educational relevance
Health promotion

Chapter Profile

Doctors, nurses, podiatrists, physiotherapists, audiologists, dentists and other health professionals know what their profession involves, and what members of their profession can do. This shared understanding of the unique role and purpose of their profession crosses international boundaries and medical specialties. Accordingly, we expect to be able to recognise fellow professionals by the work they do, how they do it and what they believe. We imagine that this will hold true regardless of whether they are working in a high-tech medical setting in the United States of America, or developing a primary health-care initiative in a remote location. What's more, we draw comfort from the fact that despite qualifying in countries with different demographic, climatic and socio-economic characteristics, we can tell who is and who is not part of our profession. Whatever the setting, we believe, nursing is still nursing, doctoring is still doctoring, and the same holds for the other health professions. Moreover, because there is a common understanding of what a nurse, speech-language therapist or pharmacist is, there is a perception that the focus and standard of practice is, or should be, comparable between countries.

Concerns expressed over the last 25 years, however, strike at the heart of the consistencies in practice that health professionals value. Nonetheless, they are worthy of our attention because they bring into question the effectiveness of delivering health care in the ways we do. Therefore, the purpose of this chapter is to explore some of the pressures being exerted on the health professions, and the implications of these demands for health-profession education. The specific objectives of the chapter are to examine key documents and consider their implications for the education of health professionals, explore the way one health profession responded to the contextual demands and to offer some reflections on the way forward. To contextualise the discussion, the chapter begins by outlining the contributions educational curricula have made to consistencies in practice. Historical and professional reasons for this consistency are advanced.

Educating for consistency

Underpinning the consistency that characterises each profession, there are commonalities in how practitioners are educated. That is, within each profession there is a "standard" educational curriculum that prescribes the knowledge, skills and attitudes that are traditionally taught. Some programs deviate from this curriculum, yet even they are likely to preserve core concepts of the profession. For perhaps a majority of educational programs, however, similarities in curricula may extend to what is learned and in what sequence. For example, doctors trained in Western medicine typically study physiology and anatomy, and are required to dissect cadavers in order to build up knowledge considered foundational to understanding medical and surgical conditions. While sharing much of the same knowledge, physiotherapists as a rule develop skill in palpating muscles and reducing inflammation in soft tissues, and occupational therapists learn to analyse, adapt and grade the occupations of daily life. Indeed, some aspects of our educational experiences have been so stereotypical as to become part of the professional identity, such as the sea grass stools and cane baskets constructed by occupational therapy students internationally. The global similarities in educational experience extend to the texts students read, with some, such as *Gray's Anatomy of the Human Body*, Brunner and Suddarth's *Textbook of Medical-Surgical Nursing* (Smeltzer & Bare, 2003) or *Willard and Spackman's Occupational Therapy* (Crepeau, Cohn & Schell, 2003), becoming institutions in themselves and appearing in multiple editions over decades.

As well as students of each profession being taught much the same things, regardless of their location, some of the ways students are taught appear to be common to most health professions. Perhaps the best example is the practice of placing students in health-care settings for periods of time, in order to promote the application of academic knowledge to the real world of health care. Despite being called different things, occurring at different points in the educational program and being of varying duration, this is essentially an apprenticeship model. That is, novices are placed under the supervision of more experienced members of the profession to learn their trade. Moreover, a good proportion of this experience is likely to be in a hospital setting, even in countries where community-based services are well established.

The high level of consistency in both educational curricula and professional identity that is evident can, in part, be attributed to history. In general terms, the present day health professions associated with Western medicine arose in Britain, Europe and North America. From there, they diffused into Eastern, Middle Eastern, African, South American and Pacific nations (Hocking, 2003). This history of radiation out from a common source, often in conjunction with broader processes of colonisation, has contributed to a general expectation that the pinnacle of practice is located in the countries of origin. This orientation back towards the United States, the United Kingdom and Europe continues, with professional literature, higher-level qualifications and research endeavours located there being generally highly regarded. Accordingly, practice in other places has tended to mirror developments in those countries rather than developing ways of practising tailored to the culture and climate in which it is embedded.

As well as this common history, the professions themselves have, to a greater or lesser extent, actively maintained a high level of consistency. Two mechanisms by which this has come about are apparent. The first is that at some point in their development, many health professions established an international body. Examples are the International Council of Nurses, the World Federation of Occupational Therapists and the World Federation of Medical Education. These bodies have supported the development of their profession in countries where it had not previously existed. By sharing expertise, advice, and resources, they have explicitly or implicitly moulded practice and educational models in their own image.

A second mechanism by which consistency in practice has been fostered is the process of professionalisation. The health professions have sought recognition as autonomous, self-governing groups within society; a key part of this is determining what members of the profession should know and be able to do. Because of the increased status accorded to groups recognised as professions, scholarly and research effort has focused on the development of a unique body of knowledge to inform each profession. In general, such efforts have been driven by the concerns of the profession itself and in response to the needs of the health system within which it operates, rather than to the broader social context of practice. While such advances have stimulated changes in educational curricula over time, these changes have tended to extend or support existing modes of practice as opposed to fostering localised variations. For example, substantial theory development has taken place in occupational therapy over the last three decades, and occupational therapists in Japan, Thailand and Australia have been taught successive versions of the Model of Human Occupation (Kielhofner, 1985, 1995, 2002). However because it has largely been developed in the United States, concepts of identity, independence and gender relations that reflect American values and perspectives are embedded in the theory (Hocking, 1999; Haglund & Kjellberg, 1999; Iwama, in press, a). Despite the misfit of assumptions, efforts to develop explanations of occupational performance relevant to their own countries have only recently been initiated and are only now beginning to be taught (Chapparo & Ranka, 1993, 1997; Iwama,

2003a, 2003b, in press, b; Iwama, Hatsutori & Okuda, 2002; P. Jananya, personal communication, 16 March 2003).

Against this background of historical development and contemporary educational practice, concerns have been raised about whether the professions' valuing of international consistency best serves the health needs of all people. Most vocal in this regard are two international bodies, the United Nations Educational, Scientific and Cultural Organization (UNESCO) and the World Health Organization (WHO). Together, they have identified a range of educational, health and welfare issues facing people in different regions of the world and the radically different resources they can access to address those health threats. The WHO initiatives, which call for major reform in the ways health professionals are educated, are the subject of the next section of discussion.

Health for all

The strategies WHO has advocated to address the unique health requirements of people in different regions of the world have a long history, and bring into question the actual contribution health professionals make to population health. Two documents are particularly germane to this discussion. The first is the 1978 *Declaration of Alma-Ata*, which contains the WHO's much publicised call for "Health for all by the year 2000". While acknowledging the importance of environmental measures, and curative and rehabilitative health care, the Declaration proposed a radical new approach to population health. Arguing that keeping people well is fundamentally important, the Declaration emphasised the need for preventive programs. Achieving this, it envisioned, would require a major reorientation of the health professions towards illness prevention.

The second, more recent document relevant here is the *Ottawa Charter* (1986). It arose from a conference on health promotion that was sponsored by the WHO and convened in Ottawa in November 1986. The 212 invited participants came from 38 countries, and brought together laymen and health professionals, administrators, and academics from governmental, voluntary and community organisations. The Charter they drew up pronounced that "health is created and lived by people within the settings of their everyday life; where they learn, work, play, and love" (p 8). Intended to stimulate action towards achieving the goal of Health for All, the Charter called on people from all walks of life to join forces with government, non-government and voluntary organisations to advocate for health promotion.

Five focuses of action were identified. One repeated the call to reorient the health services, stating "the role of the health sector must move increasingly in a health promotion direction, beyond its responsibility for providing clinical and curative services" (Ottawa Charter, 1986, p 4). Achieving this would require the majority of health professionals to incorporate a societal perspective on health, rather than an individually-focused, medical view of ill health. Furthermore, to act at a societal level would require health professionals to be skilled in building healthy communities. They would need to be able to take a developmental approach to health and welfare issues, and to support people to develop the capacity to make healthy life choices. It was recognised that altering health professionals' mode of working in this way would require fundamental changes in their education. These changes were identified as imperative. Despite the best intentions of the authors of the visions forged in Alma-Ata and Ottawa, however, "prevention did not become, and still is not, a priority in health service offerings" (Wilcock, 2003, p 33).

Perspectives on health

The notion of Health for All marks a move away from medical perspectives of health to acknowledge the social and psychological dimensions of wellbeing. Another perspective on health that has been promoted by the United Nations is that health is something all people should be able to achieve regardless of race, sex, colour, language, political orientation or other personal factors. From this perspective, health is viewed as a fundamental human right. Initiatives of this kind include the 1982 *World Program of Action Concerning Disabled Persons* and the 1993 *Resolution on Standard Rules of the Equalisation of Opportunities for Persons with Disabilities*. Protecting the rights of people with a disability is both a community development and a health promotion issue, and strategies to enable people with a disability to participate in all aspects of social and economic life have been proposed. The 1989 United Nations *Convention on the Rights of the Child* was updated in 2002 to bring children's rights into focus in relation to issues such as the sale of children, child prostitution and child pornography, and children's involvement in armed conflict. Children caught up in such activities are likely to experience poor health outcomes, in the short or longer term, and to require special health and social supports. Again, this support is likely to be most effective if it takes a socially orientated approach.

Mirroring the United Nations move towards a focus on individual's rights, the WHO was also involved in a radical re-conceptualisation of health and how it might be measured. This rethink involved a major review of the *International Classification of Impairment, Disability and Handicap* (ICIDH; 1980), which had described the consequences of health conditions in terms of the disabilities and handicaps individuals might experience. The revised version, the *International Classification of Functioning, Disability and Health* (ICF) was finalised in 2001. It incorporated feedback from people with a disability who demanded, in place of the ICIDH's focus on deficits and limitations, acknowledgement of what they can do (Gillette, 2000). Accordingly, the ICF classifies the outcomes of health as participation in the personal, domestic, vocational, educational, leisure, social and civic occupations that make up daily life. It also catalogues aspects of the physical and attitudinal environment that, by supporting or inhibiting participation, may enhance or undermine wellbeing. Clearly, this rethinking of how health is experienced and how the environment influences health also have implications for the education of health professionals.

Health professional education

Even before the ICF was finalised, a WHO Study Group met in Geneva to consider the improvements required in health care systems to "ensure equal access to all who seek health care, as well as optimal protection against avoidable causes of suffering and death" (p 1). Their specific brief was to address the education of health professionals. In a report titled *Increasing the Relevance of Education for Health Professionals* (1993), the Group emphasised that educational programs need to:

- be relevant to social and community concerns, as well as the prevailing health needs and priorities, and
- increasingly advocate for healthy behaviour in the population.

Achieving this, they suggested, would involve a four-step process. The first step is to define the population that will be the recipients of health services. This might involve, for example, researching the demographic, cultural and educational characteristics of the population since these things influence people's attitudes towards health care, and their beliefs about the nature, cause, course and prevention of illness, as well as what should be done to care for people with a health condition. Defining the population also implies investigating and acknowledging the diversity that exists within each population. The second step is to determine what their health-related problems are. This includes identifying the incidence of both health conditions and exposure to health risks, in order to establish health priorities. Clearly, the nature of the predominant health issues will vary according to local factors such as the climate, population demographics, the means by which people earn their livelihood (because that influences the kinds of illnesses and injuries they might sustain) and the political situation and socio-economic factors influencing the general standard of the available housing, education and health care. The third step identified by the Study Group is to ensure that existing and new educational programs respond to the identified problems, which is an acknowledgement that although the directions promoted in this report are not new, programs have so far failed to respond adequately. The final step is to monitor how effective graduates of educational programs are in addressing health priorities. The intention of this step is that by seeking and responding to information about graduate effectiveness, programs would become increasingly effective at producing graduates with relevant skills.

In accepting these recommendations, the WHO is suggesting that qualified health professionals may not currently be targeting the most important health needs. At least in part, that failing is considered to be an outcome of educational programs not adequately preparing them to do so. In light of the previous discussion, the WHO is signalling that the very consistency of education and practice that the professions value may be inconsistent with the goal of delivering health services that best meet the needs of local populations. Increasing the relevance of health professional education, it would seem, demands increased diversity in educational curricula. Furthermore, this diversity would seem to encompass both what students are taught and the ways they are taught to work. That is, for graduates to be effective, there needs to be good match between their skills and the prevalent health conditions. In addition, their mode of delivering health care must reflect both the available resources and the numbers of health professionals in relation to the size of the population. To give an extreme example, an educational curricula designed to produce health practitioners skilled in ameliorating the chronic diseases of old age would have limited relevance to a population with a low life expectancy. Equally, health professionals skilled in working one-to-one with patients may be less effective in implementing health promotion programs aimed at changing the population's health behaviours or supporting community-based rehabilitation initiatives.

To support and ensure the refocusing of health professionals' education, the WHO report makes two other important recommendations. The first is that representatives from the community be involved in identifying the problems health professionals should address, and evaluating their effectiveness in addressing them. This would include determining how satisfied recipients are with the health care they receive. Fully implementing this recommendation might again pull educational curricula away from the assumed wisdom of curricula developed in Britain or the United States in that the point of reference would be local conditions rather than professional traditions or ideals.

The final recommendation in the WHO report is that the outcome required of educational programs is to produce graduates skilled in retaining, applying, searching for and managing information. In addition, according to the WHO, graduates should have enhanced critical reasoning skills and the ability to promote teamwork. These generic skills reflect contemporary understandings of what is required to deliver effective health care. Two assumptions are evident. The first is that health knowledge is both rapidly changing and voluminous, which means that in order to remain competent, health professionals need to be skilled in constantly updating their knowledge. The second assumption is that health care is complex. This means that health professionals need to be able to make judgements about the trustworthiness of the available information, so that they can make well-founded decisions about what to do, as well as being able to work effectively alongside professionals attending to other aspects of people's health care.

Perspectives on higher education

As described above, concerns have been expressed at a global level about how effective health professionals are in improving people's health status. In part, these concerns are aligned with a more general anxiety about whether higher education fulfils its intended function of improving general social and economic conditions. UNESCO has framed this concern in terms of the social responsibilities of graduates of higher education, and questioned the extent to which individuals fulfil those responsibilities.

Higher education, in the sense in which UNESCO uses the term, refers to those formal educational processes that prepare individuals to fulfil professional roles in society, regardless of whether the academic award gained is a Diploma, or at a Bachelor's, Master's or Doctoral level. While it is acknowledged that different countries and regions have their own educational systems and preferred teaching strategies, increasing concern has been expressed about the quality and variability of higher education offered internationally. These issues are brought together in the 1995 UNESCO publication, *Policy Paper for Change and Development in Higher Education*. As the title suggests, the focus of this document is on improving the outcomes of higher education. The strategies by which this might come about are encapsulated in three watchwords for higher education — relevance, quality and internationalisation. That is, UNESCO has strongly advocated that all higher education be made more relevant to the context in which it takes place, so that graduates are able to work effectively in that environment. All education should also be of the highest possible quality, which means that systems for ongoing review and continuous updating must be designed and implemented. Finally, while it must be locally contextualised, all higher education must also draw from global knowledge developments.

Following on from this initiative, UNESCO issued a document titled *World Declaration on Higher Education for the Twenty-First Century: Vision and Action* (1998). This document raises four key concerns relevant to this discussion. The first is equality of access to higher education. Of prime concern are people who may be disadvantaged in society, including indigenous peoples, members of cultural and linguistic minorities and groups that are often the target of discrimination such as people with a disability or those living under the rule of an occupying force. The importance of actively assisting members of these special target groups to participate in higher education is stressed.

The 1998 Declaration also places emphasis on the social responsibilities that graduates of higher education programs must acknowledge and accept. The rationale advanced by UNESCO is that providing higher educational opportunities requires a substantial economic commitment that is borne by the society as a whole. Furthermore, rather than being the preserve of individuals, the knowledge and expertise conferred by higher education represents an accumulation of wisdom built up over centuries. On this basis, UNESCO proposes that recipients of such knowledge have a responsibility to use what they have learned for the betterment of society, rather than merely using it for personal gain. A third point highlighted in the 1998 Declaration is the need for transferability of skills, meaning that it is not enough for graduates to be taught skills that will enable them to function within known parameters of present day practice. Rather, professionals must be equipped to apply their skills to novel situations and to critique and update their knowledge constantly. The final point relevant here is that recipients of higher education, including health professionals, must respect diversity and difference. This implies that they will provide a skilled and competent service to everyone who needs it, without prejudice.

As this discussion has shown, there is a long-standing and intensifying call for reform in the ways that all professionals, and health professionals in particular, are prepared for practice. The key messages stressed by UNESCO and the WHO are that change is urgently required, and that the direction of that change must be towards ensuring that health graduates:

1. represent all groups within the community;

2. address their nations' prevailing health needs and community concerns;

3. actively promote health;

4. seek, appraise and apply up-to-date information;

5. view health as a universal right;

6. respect diversity and difference; and

7. evaluate their success in terms of the activities in which recipients of health care participate.

The health sector response to the WHO proposals has, in the main, been less than impressive (Wilcock, 2003). Educational curricula have not been radically revised. However, there are signs that change may be on the way. In the next section, one profession's response to UNESCO and the WHO imperatives is briefly presented.

CASE STUDY

Occupational Therapy's Minimum Standards

As previously identified, many health professions have an international body that exists to promote the profession's interests and to assist it to spread into new countries. The World Federation of Occupational Therapists (WFOT), founded in 1952, is one such organisation. WFOT is chosen as a case study for discussion here because it has been particularly active in promoting international consistency of educational practice. To achieve this end, WFOT published a set of Minimum Standards for the Education of Occupational Therapists in 1958. Over the years, these standards have been reviewed and revised to reflect changes in the profession's knowledge base and relationship with medicine, and advancements in educational theory. The most recent revision, completed in 2002, explicitly acknowledges the concerns expressed by the WHO and UNESCO. The description that follows provides an overview of the ways in which those concerns were incorporated into the WFOT *Revised Minimum Standards for the Education of Occupational Therapists* (Hocking & Ness, 2002).

An early decision was to adopt the language of the ICF. Accordingly, key ICF concepts such as health conditions, body structures and functions, activity, participation and environment are used throughout the document. In addition, the focus of the profession is described in ICF terms as:

1. the relationship between health and wellbeing and people's participation in self-care and domestic activities; interpersonal interactions and relationships; major life areas including education, work and leisure; and in community, social and civic occupations; and

Occupational Therapy's Minimum Standards — *continued*

2. the environmental factors that support or impede participation in those occupations (Hocking & Ness, 2002, p 4).

Important differences in perspective between the ICF and occupational therapy were also noted, in respect of personal factors affecting people's experience of health and welfare issues, occupational therapy's concern with consumers' subjective experience of occupation, and its concern with factors in addition to health conditions that may influence an individual's participation in activities of everyday life.

Several structural features of the Revised Minimum Standards were also informed by the concerns of the WHO and UNESCO (see Figure 5.1). First, occupational therapy educational programs are depicted as embedded in an international context in which particular health, welfare and educational perspectives have been advanced. This influence takes practical effect in specifications for the design of the educational program. For example, one specification for program curricula is that they draw from international research findings and expectations of practice. Another is that students are exposed to inclusive practices, whereby services are provided to all people without prejudice, in the course of their fieldwork. A further specification is that the educators themselves be able to demonstrate links with international perspectives, whether through visiting lecturers, international conferences or via the professional literature.

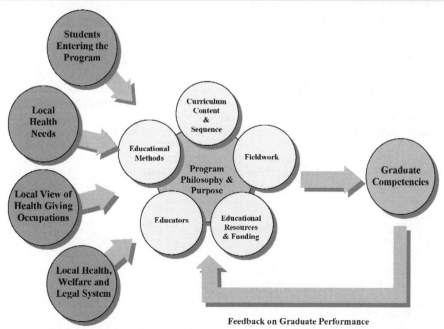

Figure 5.1 Context and components of an occupational therapy education program

Occupational Therapy's Minimum Standards — *continued*

Another strong feature of the Standards is that curricula should be founded on knowledge of the local health and welfare needs, as well as the local legislation and systems that address health, welfare and disability issues. The intent of this feature is that all educational programs for occupational therapists should be designed in response to national health priorities rather than established health practices, as well as being informed about local housing and employment conditions, educational opportunities, the arts and cultural sectors of society, the justice system and so on. Readers will recognise these as factors identified in the Ottawa Charter as influencing health. The intent of both the Charter and the Declaration of Alma-Ata is also captured in a further specification that programs be specifically informed about local health promotion and community development funding.

Two further aspects of the local context that are singled out in the WFOT Minimum Standards are relevant here. One is that the program should incorporate knowledge of local beliefs and values about the ways occupation contributes to people's health, as well as the ways it may undermine it. This knowledge is seen to inform the selection of occupations to be taught within the program, and the understandings students should gain about the therapeutic use of occupation. It also underpins occupational therapists' valuing of participation in a range of occupations that make up daily life as a health outcome. The second feature of the local context to note relates to students entering the program. Here, UNESCO's plea that higher education be open to disadvantaged groups is reflected in specifications that the student group reflect the demographics of the local population, and that discrimination on racial, gender, religious, disability or other grounds is unacceptable.

Two further WHO imperatives arising from its report on increasing the relevance of health professionals' education are also structured into the WFOT Minimum Standards. The notion of collecting feedback on graduates' performance so that the program can be continually improved is clearly evident in the diagram. In addition, the program is required to address the knowledge and skills occupational therapists need to work effectively as members of health-care teams. A final specification relevant here is that the program develop students' ability to locate, understand, evaluate and apply information to practice and that they recognise the need to update their knowledge, skills and attitudes continually throughout their professional lives.

Whether the WFOT Minimum Standards will prove effective in moving occupational therapy towards the outcomes promoted by the WHO is as yet untested. As the authors of the revised standards, our hope is that they stimulate new ways of thinking, legitimise changes that the previous Standards seemed to constrain, and create opportunities to produce different kinds of occupational therapists than the more traditional programs have allowed.

Reflections on the future

It is reasonable to assume that each health profession will determine its own response to the issues raised by UNESCO and the WHO, and do so at its own pace. The means occupational therapists have adopted may not be feasible or desirable to other professions, and may or may not be effective in bringing about the sorts of changes the WHO and UNESCO have envisaged. Nevertheless, it may be possible to foresee some of the opportunities and challenges the professions might encounter as they move forward into a future shaped by expectations that health will be measured in terms of participation in everyday life despite impairments, that health promotion will be given substantially increased attention and that health care services will be tailored to local health priorities.

In developed countries, particularly those with a Western heritage, the path to this future may appear smoother. First, since the professions themselves have a long history in those places, there is a natural goodness of fit. Secondly, health professionals and educators in those countries have ready access to vast arrays of health and welfare data with which to determine social and community needs. Moreover, their governments are likely to have already determined health priorities. Having a wealth of data, however, carries an implicit risk of information overload, such that making sense of the data in relation to a specific profession's domain of concern may represent a substantial challenge. In addition, the data may not be entirely helpful if it cannot be broken down to give a picture of the concerns of minority groups within the population. Finally, it cannot be assumed that official data has captured the right information. For example, it is likely that the health statistics reflect biomedical concerns, rather than broader understandings of the factors that influence health. New Zealand Māori, for example, identify spiritual, family and tribally-based aspects of health that are not represented in official health statistics. In failing to address implicit understandings of health, health promotion programs may fail to achieve the intended outcomes with such groups.

In countries with less comprehensive or less accurate health information, programs may need to develop and test their own strategies to build up knowledge of the range and incidence of health needs and risk factors. Involving students enrolled in the program in surveying the incidence of health conditions and their impact on participation might, for example, serve to generate this knowledge at a local level and simultaneously orient students to the purpose of the profession they will become part of. Certainly, actions directed towards ensuring graduates' skills are directly applicable to local health needs might enhance their sense of competence and the level of responsibility they feel towards practising in their own country. Designing health education curricula in response to contextual issues and cultural understandings might also create an opportunity to embed health practices within local perspectives of health rather than taking a strictly biomedical stance. This might, for example, include perceived relationships between health and the land, or between health and the spiritual world. It may also encompass communal rather than individual decision-making about health matters.

The challenge for the professions themselves is how to maintain a sense of fellowship across national and regional borders, in the face of increasingly diverse practice born of locally-tailored educational curricula. The essence of this challenge is how we might recognise and articulate the commonalities that unite the profession, as knowledge, skills and modes of practice diverge. One approach suggested by occupational therapy's example is that rather than a sense of unity based on familiarity with the same texts, theories and educational experiences, occupational therapists will share a vision of enabling people's participation in daily life. That is, despite differences in everyday practice, requiring each educational curriculum to articulate its philosophies about occupation and the outcomes of participating in occupation, may bring to light similarities in the outcomes the profession works towards and it guiding assumptions.

A further challenge that may emerge from increasing diversity of educational curricula internationally is in relation to the international transportability of qualifications. Here, perhaps more than in other aspects of professional life, there has been an assumption that health professionals educated in one locality will have the credentials to practice in another. The transportability of qualifications has benefits and drawbacks. The benefits to individuals wishing to relocate are self-evident. The disadvantages are perhaps most evident in poorer countries, which have been victim to relatively wealthy countries recruiting locally trained health professionals. Notwithstanding the rights or wrongs of this situation, getting one's qualifications recognised in other places may be more complex as educational programs diverge. This is because existing systems to evaluate foreigners' competence to practice have tended to focus on their knowledge and clinical reasoning. In the future, these systems may need to be redeveloped to evaluate professionals' skill in accessing, comprehending, evaluating and applying knowledge and in recognising the limits to their competence.

Finally, increased diversity of health professionals' educational curricula may make it more difficult to establish the health professions in countries where they do not yet exist. This possibility relates to the increased difficulty in comprehending the role and function of a particular profession if it manifests differently in different places. Conversely, the essence of each of the health professions may be more clearly evident if variations on practice can be viewed, each in their own context. In addition, the applicability of a health profession to a new setting may be more apparent if its unique contribution to people's health within similar contexts, rather than the standardised practice of old, could be investigated.

Conclusion

While the future cannot be foretold with any accuracy, the WHO and UNESCO have clearly charted their preferred future. Although the health professions have been slow to adopt their message, the authors are optimistic that the pace of change is quickening. This optimism is based on two discrete things. First, the challenge to make health services more effective is compelling and, as the WHO has recognised, people's most pressing health need is to retain their health. Equally persuasive is the fact that health comprises different things in different places, because the health threats people face and the occupations they need to participate in vary with the geographical and socio-economic context. Where context is so influential to health, it makes sense that context must also shape health practice. Secondly, occupational therapy's response to both the educational and health practice changes that have been advocated will provide a working example of some of the ways change might be implemented. While this profession's response is in no way held up as perfect in itself, nor directly applicable to other professions, it may nonetheless stimulate others to explore new ways of achieving a goal shared by the health professions and the WHO alike — of protecting and promoting people's health and wellbeing.

References

Crepeau, E. B., Cohn, E. S. & Schell, B. A. B. (Eds). (2003). *Willard and Spackman's occupational therapy* (10th ed.). Philadelphia: Lippincott Williams & Wilkins.

Chapparo, C. J. & Ranka, J. L. (1993). *Identification of information processing deficits through the use of the perceive, recall, plan and perform subsystem (The PRPP system).* Paper presented at the Australian Association of Occupational Therapists 17th National Conference, Occupational therapy: A unique profession, Darwin, Australia.

Chapparo, C. & Ranka, J. (1997). *Attention and perception: New ways to identify problems during task performance.* Proceedings of the Occupational Therapy Australia 19th National Conference, Perth, Australia, 87–91.

Declaration of Alma-Ata. (1978). Retrieved 15 February 2004, from http://www.who.int/hpr/archive/docs/almaata.html

Gillette, N. P. (2000). Practice shapes research agenda for the profession. *Occupational Therapy Practice, January 31,* 29–30.

Haglund, L. & Kjellberg, A. (1999). A critical analysis of the model of human occupation. *Canadian Journal of Occupation, 66*(2), 102–108.

Hocking, C. (1999, September). *The cultural nature of occupation: A model of human occupation perspective.* Paper presented at the 2nd Asia-Pacific Occupational Therapy Congress, Taipei.

Hocking, C. (2003). *The relationship between objects and identity in occupational therapy: A dynamic balance of rationalism and romanticism.* Unpublished doctoral dissertation, Auckland University of Technology, Auckland, New Zealand.

Hocking, C. & Ness, N.-E. (2002). *Revised minimum standards for the education of occupational therapists.* Perth: World Federation of Occupational Therapists.

Iwama, M. (2003a). Illusions of universality: The importance of cultural context in Japanese occupational therapy. *The Japanese Journal of Occupational Therapy, 37*(4), 319–323.

Iwama, M. (2003b). The issue is ... toward culturally relevant epistemologies in occupational therapy. *American Journal of Occupational Therapy, 57*(5), 217–223.

Iwama, M. (in press, a). Situated meaning: An issue of culture, inclusion and occupational therapy. In F. Kronenberg, S. Simo Algado & N. Pollard (Eds), *Occupational therapy without borders: Learning from the spirit of survivors.* Edinburgh: Churchill Livingstone.

Iwama, M. (in press, b). The Kawa (River) model: Nature, life flow and the power of culturally relevant occupational therapy. In F. Kronenberg, S. Simo Algado & N. Pollard (Eds), *Occupational therapy without borders: Learning from the spirit of survivors.* Edinburgh: Churchill Livingstone.

Iwama, M., Hatsutori, T. & Okuda, M. (2002, September). *Emerging a culturally and clinically relevant conceptual model of Japanese occupational therapy.* Paper presented at the 13th International Congress of the World Federation of Occupational Therapists, Stockholm, Sweden.

Kielhofner, G. (1985). *A model of human occupation: Theory and application.* Baltimore: Williams & Wilkins.

Kielhofner, G. (1995). *A model of human occupation: Theory and application* (2nd ed.). Baltimore: Williams & Wilkins.

Kielhofner, G. (2002). *A model of human occupation: Theory and application* (3rd ed.). Baltimore: Williams & Wilkins.

Smeltzer, S. C. & Bare, B. G. (2003). *Textbook of medical-surgical nursing* (10th ed.). Philadelphia: Lippincott.

United Nations. (1982). *World programme of action concerning disabled persons.* New York: Division of Economic and Social Information for the Centre of Social Development and Humanitarian Affairs. Retrieved 15 February 2004, from http://www.un.org/esa/socdev/enable/diswpa00.htm

United Nations Development Programme. (1993). *United Nations standard rules on the equalization of opportunities for persons with disabilities.* Vienna: United Nations. Retrieved 15 February 2004, from http://www.un.org/esa/socdev/enable/dissre00.htm

United Nations. (1989). *Convention on the rights of the child.* Office of the High Commissioner for Human Rights. Retrieved 15 February 2004, from http://www.unhchr.ch/html/menu2/6/crc/treaties/crc.htm

United Nations. (2002). *Convention on the rights of the child.* Office of the High Commissioner for Human Rights. Retrieved 15 February 2004, from http://www.un.org/Depts/dhl/pathfind/frame/start.htm

UNESCO. (1995). *Policy paper for change and development in higher education.* Paris: UNESCO.

UNESCO. (1998). *World declaration on higher education for the twenty-first century: Vision and action.* Retrieved 15 February 2004, from http://www.unesco.org/educprog/wche/declartion_eng.htm

Wilcock, A. A. (2003). Population interventions focused on health for all. In E. B. Crepeau, E. S. Cohn & B. A. B. Schell (Eds), *Willard and Spackman's occupational therapy* (10th ed.), pp 30–45. Philadelphia: Lippincott Williams & Wilkins.

World Health Organization. (1980). *International classification of impairment, disability and handicap (ICIDH).* Geneva: WHO.

World Health Organization. (1993). *Increasing the relevance of education for health professionals: Report of a WHO study group on problem-solving education for the health professions.* Geneva: WHO.

World Health Organization. (1994). *Declaration on occupational health for all.* Geneva: WHO.

World Health Organization. (2001). *International classification of functioning, disability and health.* Geneva: WHO.

World Health Organization, Health and Welfare Canada, & Canadian Public Health Association. (1986). *Ottawa charter for health promotion.* Ottawa: WHO.

CHAPTER SIX

Professionalism and Accountability: Accreditation Examined

Rebecca Allen

Lin Oke

Carol McKinstry

Michelle Courtney

KEY WORDS

Professional accreditation

Continuing professional development

Competence

Professional standards

Chapter Profile

In previous chapters, consideration has been given to issues relating to the knowledge base of practitioners and their utilisation of theory in practice. In this chapter, the focus is on how practitioners maintain the currency of their knowledge base and their competency levels over time, and how this can be monitored at a professional level through accreditation processes. Programs of professional accreditation seek to assure external groups, such as governments and service consumers, that professional practice is of a high standard. This chapter discusses some of the current political and professional issues that have shaped accreditation, through presenting the profession of occupational therapy's new accreditation program in Australia as a case study. Central to this specific accreditation program is the philosophy that professionals who actively engage in continuing professional development activities are maintaining and improving their levels of knowledge and skills so that they practise competently and safely. The chapter details some of the elements of the accreditation program which aims to influence practitioners positively to participate in ongoing professional development. The program also aims to assist consumers, governments and other external groups readily identify and seek out practitioners who are accredited. The chapter concludes with reflections on future directions for the profession of occupational therapy and other health professions in their collective pursuit of excellence in practice.

Introduction

There are increasing demands for professional groups to improve their level of accountability to external bodies such as consumers, governments and other purchasers of services. "Accreditation" is the term broadly used to refer to a process of external approval for performance in a particular field, and the terms "licensing", "certification" and "regulating" may be used for similar purposes (Scrivens, 1995). This chapter describes the broad political and professional imperatives for developing programs for accrediting health professionals. The development of an Accredited Occupational Therapist program in Australia will be presented as a case example, highlighting the response of the occupational therapy profession to these imperatives.

The amount and type of external scrutiny and internal regulation of professional practice varies greatly between professions, and there may be different levels of regulation within a profession (Brown, Esdaile & Ryan, 2003). Accordingly, professional groups have traditionally assumed a major responsibility for determining practitioner standards. However, the service environment is such that professional practice is increasingly regulated through external means. A variety of mechanisms such as practice and legislative guidelines are being used both to prescribe and proscribe practitioner activities in order to reduce risks (Fish & Coles, 1998). Such regulation has not necessarily required practitioners to participate in ongoing professional education; however this is increasingly becoming an integral component of such programs for health and other human services professionals. Continuing professional development is often a requirement of professional accreditation programs.

OT AUSTRALIA's accreditation program was established by the professional association with the intention of positively influencing the standards of practice within the Australian occupational therapy profession. A major objective of the program was to acknowledge those occupational therapists who maintain the currency of their knowledge and skill through ongoing professional development. The program also aimed to assist consumers and purchasers of occupational therapy services to identify therapists committed to ongoing learning. The program was developed to enable both the external scrutiny of practitioner activity as well as satisfy the profession's need for self-determination.

The chapter begins with a discussion of the professional and political pressures that influenced the structure of the accreditation program, in particular the current concern with safety and quality practice in the health-care system. It will then consider the meaning of professional competence and the process of maintaining it, prior to describing the accredited occupational therapist program as a case illustration of these broader issues.

Background

Higher demand for services coupled with increasing consumer expectations and environments where resources are either static or reducing place human service systems under immense pressure. This is particularly evident in health care.

Although there is an increasing diversity, complexity and variety of services in our health-care systems, more continues to be expected of them. Governments, insurance companies and consumers expect a higher quality of health care including its safer delivery (Commonwealth of Australia, 2001). The past two decades have witnessed a major focus on developing quality-improvement systems in organisations. However, despite the progress achieved with quality-improvement activities in countries such as the United Kingdom, the United States of America, Canada and Australia, there has been a growing awareness that health professionals are human and do make mistakes. Accordingly, there has been an increased demand for systems to be established to minimise mistakes, thereby protecting patients and consumers (Saltman, Figueras & Sakellarides, 1998; Grbich, 1996; Hogg, 1999).

A number of high-profile inquiries and reports have highlighted the need for mechanisms to ensure health professionals maintain and update their skills, with clinical services ensuring that staff have the appropriate credentials to practice. The Inquiry into the Bristol Royal Infirmary 1984–1995 (Kennedy, Jarman, Howard & Maclean, 2001), for example, investigated the adverse events associated with paediatric cardiac surgery and made over 200 recommendations for corrective action. These recommendations included the need for health professionals to undertake continuing professional development as well as regular performance appraisal of clinical staff. The *Bristol Report* also promoted the revalidation of fitness to practice as necessary. The development of appropriate mechanisms to deal with misconduct and poor performance, as well as mechanisms for appropriate supervision and training to ensure ongoing competence, were also highlighted (Kennedy et al). The inquiry into the deaths of twelve children who had open heart surgery at Winnipeg Health Sciences Centre in Manitoba, Canada, also reinforced the need for such mechanisms. This inquiry recommended that recruitment, professional development and performance management systems need to be adequate to ensure that health professionals' skills and expertise match their specific position requirements (Sinclair, 2000).

In Australia, there have been two similar inquiries. The first was into the King Edward Memorial Hospital's obstetric and gynaecological services 1990–2000 where there had been a high rate of stillbirths, maternal deaths and deaths following gynaecological procedures (Australian Council for Safety and Quality in Healthcare, 2002). The second inquiry investigated serious allegations involving two nursing staff members at the Royal Melbourne Hospital (Wilson, 2002). Both of these inquiries highlighted serious system failures relating to the professional standards of the health professionals involved. Recommendations were made to improve post-graduate learning and ongoing training while compliance with standards, policies and procedures was also found to be in question. In addition, the credentialing program was also strongly criticised in the King Edward Memorial Hospital Inquiry.

In light of these investigations, the clinical governance movement in Britain started to address "deep public and professional concern" that "threatened to undermine confidence in the National Health System" (Halligan & Donaldson, 2001). Clinical governance has been described as "an umbrella term" that provides a single framework for a range of quality control concepts (Warne, 2002). It includes new approaches for effective leadership, staff and process management, consumer involvement and strategic planning to improve quality within health service organisations. Learning from complaints and other forms of consumer feedback as well as effectively using information and data to enhance policy decisions and processes are some of the key elements of clinical governance. With the emergence of the clinical governance movement, there is a greater focus on reassuring the general public that health systems are safe and accountable. A strategy to reduce clinical risk involves the implementation of credentialing systems in which health professionals are required to provide evidence of their competency. At the health service organisation level, professional bodies need to examine their systems to ensure the quality of the services meet industry and consumer expectations. Colleges or associations of health professionals are expected to have established Codes of Ethics with which members need to abide, or face deregulation or disciplinary procedures. While professional Codes of Ethics formulate the expectation of professional competency, there is an increasing emphasis on participation in continuing professional development to increase competence in practice. In many instances, sufficient participation in continuing professional development activity is becoming a mandatory requirement of health professionals' membership of their college or professional association as consumers, health authorities and governments require regulation and reassurance.

Clinical governance has developed within the context of the broader consumer movement in which consumers expect health-care services to be designed to enable them to participate in the decision-making involving their care. Clinical governance promotes patient or client-centred services. Consumers want access to information to enable them to be fully informed and more in control of their own health choices. According to Hogg (1999), "consumers need unbiased information with which to make choices about services and treatment and who should provide them. This requires open access to information about the effectiveness and outcome of treatments and the performance, qualifications and experience of providers" (p 170). Consumers require access to relevant information to enable them to seek out and receive safe, high-quality services and allow them to participate more actively in their own health care. Health-care consumers, like other service consumers, currently expect regulatory bodies and individual institutions to ensure that the best possible care is provided, to protect them from adverse events and under-performing practitioners.

Professionalism considered

While consumers and governments may be seeking external checks of practitioner activity, self-regulation has been a traditional identifier for a profession. According to Bosser, Kernaghan, Hodgins, Merla, O'Connor & Van Kessel (1999) a "profession is autonomous, self-directing and embodies trustworthiness through adherence to ethics and knowledgeable skill" (p 117). While there is no agreement on the specific criteria which define a profession, those identified in the literature often draw on criteria developed by Schein (1972) which include that it:

- is founded on intellectual activity;
- has definite and practical purpose;
- has techniques that can be communicated;
- is effectively self-organising;
- has a highly developed Code of Ethics; and
- assumes a lifelong commitment.

Traditional notions of professionalism suggest that a profession controls its own work and assesses the performance of its practitioners. The profession as a collective determines what is right or wrong and enshrines these principles within its Code of Ethics. The profession sets professional standards with the implicit understanding that individual practitioners will strive to maintain their competence and comply with the Code of Ethics, thus protecting those using the profession's service. The profession determines the level of education or skill required for entrance into it. In this context, external regulatory bodies primarily protect the public from substandard or poor practice and do not necessarily determine what is required in order to maintain good practice. Professionalism has more recently been constructed as a context-bound concept (Ford, 1999). That is, given that society is increasingly diverse and complex, social attitudes and the settings in which professionals work are changing the criteria that define a profession. Consequently, many conceptualisations of professionalism have been criticised as failing to acknowledge the mounting influence of the public and the consumer demand for transparency and accountability by professional groups (Youngstrom, 1998).

In comparison to other occupational groups, it is assumed that professionals have high incomes, enviable status and significant power within the community (Irvine & Graham, 1994). Although in today's society, these assumptions are not always borne out in fact, they continue to imply common "rights" for the professions, comprising status and power. Concurrently, the implication is for common "responsibilities" that increasingly include accountability for the continuing development and improvement of professional practice. Significantly, the concept of professionalism has implications for both collective and individual continuing development and improvement. The power and status of the professions hinge on the prominent theme of demonstrating individual and collective continuing professional development. Thus, within today's cultural and economic milieu, matters relating to professional competence are seen as a means by which professional status can be galvanised (Curry Wergin & Associates, 1993).

Professional knowledge

Professionalism involves commitment to a specific body of knowledge and skill as well as a systematic process to reserve, refine and elaborate on that knowledge and skill to serve the community (Harris, 1993). Professions are considered to be based on intellectual activity; primarily knowledge and learning. Professional knowledge is characterised by applied theory. Health professionals have a responsibility not only to expand and critique their own knowledge continually, but also to contribute to the development of their profession's knowledge base (Higgs & Titchen, 2000). The amount and rate of cultural and technological change in the latter half of the twentieth century has drastically altered the nature of professional knowledge. There are significant challenges to professions maintaining valid knowledge, including the rapid growth rate of new knowledge, the increasing complexity of that knowledge, the hastened obsolescence of knowledge and enormous technological change and innovation (Dubin, 1990). Given these changes, even if currency of knowledge is achieved, it is transitory, requiring constant updating. Therefore, an initial licence to practice gained through entry level education is not considered enough to maintain professional knowledge in the longer term.

One of the challenges to making professional groups more accountable is that while the routine elements of professional practice may be easily scrutinised externally by employing organisations and regulatory bodies, not all elements of professional practice are so easily defined (Fish & Coles, 1998). There is little argument that professional groups must be open to scrutiny. The professional literature abounds with statements supporting this, exhorting practitioners to continue to advance their knowledge. However, professional groups consider that the expectation that all aspects of professional intervention can be monitored is unrealistic. This is a significant issue, as in attempting to ensure professional practices are open to external scrutiny and monitoring, regulation of professional activity can at times appear to be reducing professional knowledge and decision-making to only those features that are measurable. The clinical governance movement has developed in what O'Neill (2002) has called "a climate of distrust", in which health professionals and others in positions of authority are increasingly "regarded with suspicion". O'Neill believes that "the pursuit of ever more perfect accountability provides citizens and consumers, patients and parents with more information, more comparisons, more complaint systems; but it also builds a culture of suspicion, low morale, and may ultimately lead to professional cynicism" (p 57). In this climate, attempts to reduce risk by developing documented procedures, and ensuring that professional intervention conforms to these procedures, abound. Unfortunately, in many instances, the focus has been on "performance indicators chosen for ease of measurement and control rather than because they provide an accurate measure of quality" (O'Neill, p 55). This view conveys well the discomfort many professionals feel with some of the account-ability systems being established. Brown et al (2003) note that "there is a delicate balance between public accountability and professional self regulation and control" (p 9) and this balance is highlighted in the current environment of clinical governance. Given these issues, it remains crucial that professional associations take a leading role in establishing monitoring or accountability systems that satisfy the profession as well as assuring external groups that practice is based on sound processes.

The broad scope for interpretation of professional knowledge implied by "knowing how" can never be refined into a list of procedures, being learned most effectively through practice and systematic reflection on practice (Schön, 1983). Reflection in professional practice is a means by which the increasing limitations of professional knowledge can be addressed, and there has been a move toward conceptualising professionalism emphasising reflective practice (Harris, 1993). The goal of the reflective practitioner is wise judgement and action constituting professional practice in all situations (Parham, 1987). Current views of professionalism highlight the responsibility not only for valid, specialised knowledge but also for a tradition of deliberation (Keilhofner, 1997). This new concept of professionalism for both the collective and the individual involves the integrated and complementary use of a specialised body of knowledge, including evidence of best practice and reflective practice. However, notions of reflective practice and professional views about what constitutes valid evidence can be at odds with the approach that aims to scrutinise and control professional action so as to reduce risk.

Reflective professional practice emphasises responsibility for action directed toward developing and improving professional practice, which ultimately protects the right to status and power within the professions. The individual and collective responsibility to be accountable to the profession can be used as a means of ensuring the standards of practice and conduct implied by the concept of profess-ional competence (Youngstrom, 1998). Thus, the advantages of professionalism to occupational therapy are seen to impact both on the group's external relations and on its internal structure. A profession can initiate activities including accreditation, collectively and individually, as a means not only of meeting responsibilities but also of guarding the rights implied by the label of professional. The following section explores how these issues, and those covered earlier with respect to knowledge generation and transference, have been addressed through the development of a profession-specific accreditation program.

Continued competence: Occupational therapy as a professional case example

The Australian Association of Occupational Therapists (1994) defines a competent professional as:

> [One] having the relevant knowledge, skills and attributes necessary for job performance to the appropriate standard …[professional competence] is a complex interaction and integration of knowledge, judgement, higher-order reasoning, personal qualities, skills, values and beliefs. In their everyday work competent professionals will recall and apply facts and skills, evaluate evidence, create explanations from available facts, formulate hypothesis, and synthesise information from a rich and highly organised knowledge base.
>
> (p 2)

A further dimension of professional competence is how well the occupational therapist copes with the service environment. Levels of competence may fluctuate depending on career development, how knowledge and skills are updated and the various roles and functions assumed in day-to-day practice (Evert, 1993). The literature emphasises the power and responsibility of both the individual and the collective to establish, maintain and measure professional competence (Thomson, Lieberman, Murphy, Wendt & Poole, 1997).

In a study of occupational therapy practitioner perceptions in the United States, Fawcett and Strickland (1998) frequently heard the statement: "I know a competent practitioner when I see one, but I cannot describe this for you" (p 741). While competency must be a demonstrable component of any profession, the occupational therapy literature concurs with the broader professional view that competence, being multifaceted and dynamic, is difficult to define (Youngstrom, 1998). One proposal is that practitioner autonomy can be used as an indicator of competence (Fawcett & Strickland). Other authors suggest that different models of practice and health service environments require different competencies (Ford et al, 1999). No profession has succeeded in defining or measuring competency cost effectively or using a method that ensures competence beyond a single point in time. For occupational therapy and other professions dealing with these themes, there is growing attention and concern about the valid assessment of competence.

Research among practising occupational therapists has concluded that more years of experience did differentiate higher skill level (Nordholm, Adamson & Heard, 1994) and a more sophisticated level of clinical reasoning (Burke & DePoy, 1991). However, mindful of the imperative among professionals for currency of knowledge, years of experience alone will not translate into professional competence. Indeed, the more years of experience, the larger the potential for discrepancy between the knowledge taught during initial education and the knowledge that should be appropriate for current use as a basis for practice (Stancliff, 1996). Given that professional competence is multifactorial and dynamic, the currency of knowledge and skill alone is not directly predictive of competence. Nevertheless, a competent practitioner must be an up-to-date practitioner.

The literature outlines a range of approaches to assessing, planning for, maintaining and documenting professional competence for individual occupational therapists. Youngstrom (1998) reinforces the integrative, diverse and complex nature of the issue for the occupational therapy profession by suggesting that fully developed competence goes beyond the checklists and tests that are often used to assess competence. For individual occupational therapists, the key to assuring competence is the self-perpetuating attitude of lifelong learning, reflective practice and professional development. For example, the more actively occupational therapists update and improve their knowledge and skills, the less satisfied they are with their foundational information for practice and the more actively they seek to improve and update their knowledge and skills further. This basic philosophy of lifelong learning and professional development provides the framework for OT AUSTRALIA's accreditation program.

Competence is not just maintaining knowledge and skills, but also updating and improving them. Thus, competence in professional practice is continuous. Foto (1998) suggests that to be valued by the user community in the future, the collective group and the individual members of the occupational therapy profession must be committed to assuring continuing competency as individuals and as a profession. Continuing professional development can encompass all post entry-level activities directed toward lifelong learning. Stancliff (1996) has described continuing professional development as "a vehicle; it's not an outcome" (p 51). Accordingly, the "outcome" is centred on assuring continuing competence. For the occupational therapy profession, continuing professional development is not viewed as optional for the individual practitioner (Brockett & Bauer, 1998). The path one takes, however, to achieve and maintain professional competence is a personal decision with continuing professional development being viewed as a combination of advanced skills, education and socialisation (Evert, 1993). It requires an organised and systematic approach to continuing professional development (Cusick & McCluskey, 2000). Youngstrom (1998) suggests that learning how to undertake effective continuing professional development is a competency in itself and that this improves with practice. According to Thomson et al (1997), the requirement to demonstrate that one is undertaking continuing professional development has been proven to be better for assuring competency than no formal requirements.

The model of continuing professional development most recommended in the occupational therapy literature, and on which the Australian accreditation program is based, involves habitual needs' assessment. Each occupational therapist must identify his or her individual learning needs and use various tools for self-assessment of continuing competence. This involves an assessment of his or her current level of competence, a determination of what needs to be enhanced and the method to be used to gain such knowledge or skill. Participation in activities aimed at continuing competence is voluntary with responsibility for continued learning resting with the individual.

There are no short cuts in continuing professional development and it does not simply involve continuing education. Continuing education does not necessarily change practice and, in isolation, continuing education will not necessarily ensure continuing competence. Given that continuing competence is ongoing and developmental, it requires a variety of learning methods (Thomson et al, 1997). Continuing professional development encompasses all activities undertaken to maintain and update competency. The occupational therapy literature includes reference to a variety of methods including independent study, academic coursework, continuing education, teaching, presentations, publications, research, professional certification, accreditation, participation in supervision/mentor relationships, peer review, on-the-job training and experience. Significantly, it is often suggested that pursuing various avenues for professional socialisation is imperative to continuing professional development, as a competent health practitioner cannot work in isolation from other members of their profession (Hocking, Levack & Chester, 2002). Incorporating Grossman's (1992) view that professional excellence is modelled, participation in the process of mentoring or supervision has long been seen as valuable within the occupational therapy profession (Schemm & Bross, 1995). More recently, Burke (1998) reinforced the value of contact with occupational therapy colleagues for participation in discussion using the language of occupation. The accreditation program reinforces the value of positive relationships within the profession.

The professional association's role in relation to professional competence

Establishing the framework

> The professional associations provide a framework for members to pursue common interests, set requirements for entry into the profession, and establish mechanisms to monitor and regulate standards of practice.
>
> (Cusick, 1999, p 70)

Additionally, the professional association's role is to provide opportunities for growth in clinical practice, education and research to its members (Brockett & Bauer, 1998). Through these activities, the collective profession, represented by the professional association, can promote professional competence in individual members. By addressing accountability through demonstrations of competence, the professional associations will encourage and enhance development of critical behaviours for professionalism (Fidler, 1996).

As the peak body representing occupational therapists in Australia, OT AUSTRALIA, the Australian Association of Occupational Therapists has had a central role in establishing and maintaining practice standards for the profession. OT AUSTRALIA promotes the competency of its members through providing continuing professional development programs, a code of ethics, entry and specialist level competency standards, accreditation of entry level education programs, incentives for research, policies to guide practice and, most prominently, the Accredited Occupational Therapist (AccOT) Program. The development of the AccOT Program is indicative of the integration of the current concepts of professional competence into the occupational therapy culture in Australia. Moreover, it is an example of the vital role of the professional association in establishing and maintaining standards of professional behaviour and responsibility for individual occupational therapists.

In Australia, a number of medical colleges and allied health associations require their members to undertake a level of continuing professional education as do other professional bodies such as the Australian Institute of Architecture and the Society of Certified Practising Accountants. At the time the occupational therapy accreditation program was being developed, the Dieticians Association of Australia had introduced its Accredited Practising Dietician program in response to the closure of state registration boards for dietetics. In New Zealand, the OT Association introduced the Cornerstone Program in which members could demonstrate that they were pursuing professional learning. The National Certification Board for Occupational Therapy in USA was also developing a re-certification process to replace a one-off examination.

The common feature of all these programs was the requirement for members to demonstrate that they had been participating in professional education or development activities. There are a variety of ways in which the education or development activities are defined, categorised or weighted for achieving the required level for entry or renewal. The re-submitting cycle varies from one year with membership renewal, through to a five-year cycle in the Cornerstone Program. They are all member-exclusive programs. Most of these programs involve members collecting a minimum number of points per annum or over a two or three-year period usually based on the hours spent in participating in continuing professional education activities. Only a minority of accreditation programs award points based on the level of participation or assessment requirements as most are based on the length of time spent in the activity.

To reward therapists who undertook activities that involved assessment of their knowledge and skills adequately, it was decided that the model designed by OT AUSTRALIA would use the concept of weighted points. More points are awarded for activities that required assessment or for formal courses such as postgraduate certificates, diplomas or degrees. Assessed programs can provide some assurance that participants have gained some measurable level of learning. In a study of Victorian occupational therapists' involvement in continuing professional education, McKinstry (1995) reported that therapists had low participation rates in activities that involved assessment. They also preferred to undertake activities with a direct relationship to the enhancement of intervention skills that could be incorporated into their practice. In the Accredited Occupational Therapist program, points are also awarded for activities that contributed to the profession such as convening a special interest group, holding office within OT AUSTRALIA or supervising entry-level students on fieldwork placements. The latter also recognises the contribution to the learning of others and, in turn, the learning of other professional knowledge and skills.

To reflect the diverse range of workplace settings and positions in which occupational therapists are employed, including generic health-care positions, the activities that qualify for points also vary greatly. This feature is considered vital if the program is to meet the needs of all occupational therapists and continue to be relevant in the future. The program was designed to ensure that some groups of occupational therapists such as rural therapists are not disadvantaged. Points can be obtained through private study activities such as reading journals, undertaking database searches or researching literature to develop an assessment tool within the workplace. To encourage therapists to use a variety of learning methods, a maximum is placed on the number of points that can be obtained in certain categories such as private study. Rural therapists, however, have a higher point maximum for private study than metropolitan therapists who do not have the same problems accessing continuing professional education activities. The design of the program acknowledges that occupational therapists have varied learning needs and preferences in styles of learning, thus aiming to empower occupational therapists to be self-directed in determining their own learning needs and strategies to meet those needs. The process of implementing and reviewing the program is detailed below.

The professional association's role in relation to professional competence

Implementing the program

After the development of the initial table of activities and allocation of points, the program was piloted with 400 occupational therapists across Australia. Some rural and part-time therapists were concerned that they would be disadvantaged and requested that they should not have to acquire as many points in total as metropolitan or full-time therapists. In reality, almost all of the pilot study therapists achieved the required number of points for accreditation. The program sets a minimum standard benchmark. This benchmark is the amount of professional development activity that the profession as a collective expects of an individual occupational therapist to maintain currency of skill and knowledge. Hence, every participating therapist has to achieve the same minimum number of points regardless of geographical location or working status.

The Accredited Occupational Therapist program has several features not always present in other professional accreditation programs. One such feature is the requirement for the newly graduated to gain up to half of their accreditation points from supervision and mentoring. Newly-graduated therapists, particularly those in generic positions, are at a crucial stage of their professional identity and need the guidance and support of positive role models (McKinstry, 2003). Supervision or peer review is also a strategy to enhance professional development and safety in the individual professional. As part of the development of the program, best practice standards for supervision and mentoring were developed and the professional association has increasingly developed its role in facilitating access to mentors and supervisors for therapists. The program has also been made available to all occupational therapists in Australia, not just members of the professional association, as OT AUSTRALIA wants to influence the practice of the whole profession.

The program recommends that participants document and submit to OT AUSTRALIA a continuing professional development (CPD) plan and a record of their CPD activities when they renew their membership of the program (OT AUSTRALIA, 2001). Random audits of CPD records are undertaken to maintain integrity of reporting. The CPD plan can assist in facilitating reflection to identify the individual's learning needs. Rather than haphazardly participate in continuing professional development activities, therapists are encouraged to examine their current and future learning needs. OT AUSTRALIA also uses the CPD plans to gather information to assist with the planning of educational activities. The program has a manager who can assist practitioners with their plans and determine whether a continuing professional development activity did result in new learning.

During the development of the program and prior to its launch, the AccOT Program was extensively marketed to the profession. It was, and continues to be, marketed to employers of occupational therapists, to organisations using the services of occupational therapists, to general practitioners and allied health professionals who often refer clients to occupational therapists and to consumers.

The external marketing strategies promote the benefits of choosing an AccOT and also assist external groups to identify accredited therapists. Central to the accreditation program is the philosophy that professionals who actively engage in continuing professional development activities are maintaining and improving their levels of knowledge and skills so that they practise competently and safely.

As with all programs that measure participation, there is an underpinning assumption that participation has an impact on practice. Accreditation facilitates competence by setting expectations and standards for participation in CPD (Courtney & Farnworth, 2003). While participation does not equate with competence, having such standards is better than having no expectation (Thompson et al, 1997). As noted previously, the expectation of professionals is that they engage in lifelong learning as one way to demonstrate competence to practise (Alsop, 2000). The AccOT program aims to facilitate a culture of ongoing learning and enquiry within the profession, along with a willingness to have that activity scrutinised and measured. Hence, it aims to create a culture that becoming accredited is part of a process of continuous professional development rather than "an act of compliance" (Cross, 1998, p 531). By taking the lead, OT AUSTRALIA aimed to develop a program that would satisfy governments, regulatory bodies and individual therapists at the same time, while maintaining self-determination for the profession.

Over 75 per cent of OT AUSTRALIA's members joined the inaugural cycle of AccOT, along with a small number of non-member occupational therapists, indicating successful marketing and appeal to members of the Australian occupational therapy profession. As well as the higher than expected number of occupational therapists joining the program, there was strong support from the Commonwealth Government and a number of health-care bodies. Congratulatory letters were received from the Division of Health Industry and Investment in the Commonwealth Government's Department of Health and Aged Care and the Safety and Quality in Health Care Council of Australia. These acknowledged the program's contribution to improving the safety of the health-care system by ensuring that people working in health care are well trained and actively engaged in continuous professional development. Many workplaces now include a preference for occupational therapists who have satisfied accreditation requirements in position advertisements. Government agencies and health insurance companies have also indicated a preference for engaging accredited occupational therapists as it is recognised as the Australian benchmark.

The Accredited Occupational Therapist Program's promise of "assuring professional excellence" required the development of a process to assist accredited occupational therapists when there were concerns about their practice. In Australia, Registration Boards where they exist, state government statutory bodies such as the Health Complaints Commission or the state occupational therapy association manage issues relating to substandard practice by occupational therapists. The accreditation program does not have any statutory powers and does not compete with or replace the role of the Registration Boards or other regulatory processes. OT AUSTRALIA's philosophy and aim is to embed a positive culture of ongoing professional development. Hence, a remedial approach has been developed when problems are identified with the practices of an accredited occupational therapist. This is particularly important in Australia as there are some states with registration and some without. For those states without registration, the only role of OT AUSTRALIA is to assist with providing opportunities for remediation.

OT AUSTRALIA recognises that customer feedback, whether it is from consumers, referees, employers or others, is an extremely valuable source of information, providing an opportunity for improving the quality of a service. The AccOT Manual (OT AUSTRALIA, 2001) outlines a best practice approach to managing consumer expressions of concern. Accredited Occupational Therapists are encouraged to respond to any expressions of concern as an opportunity to review and enhance their standards of practice. With such an approach, it is assumed that consumer concerns are most likely to be resolved and not lead to complaints being made. However, to meet its assurance of quality services from AccOTs fully, OT AUSTRALIA has introduced a national system for managing concerns about the standards of practice of AccOTs, wherever this may assist Registration Boards and Health Complaints Commissioners.

The AccOT Program: Future development and directions

While the AccOT program has provided Australian occupational therapists with a framework for maintaining and developing competence and demonstrating a degree of accountability, the requirements of the program are only minimal. As the first cycle of accreditation was completed in August 2003, a review of the activities and points occurred to ensure continued relevance for the profession. It is anticipated that regular reviews of the program will be necessary to reflect the ongoing needs of both participants and the key stakeholders of the program.

Advanced knowledge and skills of experienced practitioners who have chosen to specialise is currently not recognised in the AccOT program. During the development of the program, some sectors of the health industry expressed a desire to be readily able to recognise occupational therapists with the particular knowledge and skill required in their service delivery area. Given the diversity of occupational therapy practice, it is important that the purchasers or consumers of occupational therapy services can easily identify therapists with specialist knowledge, skill and competence. This identified need gave rise to a project to develop specialist levels of the accreditation program. The project has specified the purpose of these specialist levels of accreditation as follows: first, to ensure quality occupational therapy practice in specialty areas to meet the needs of consumers and purchasers of occupational therapy services; secondly, to enable consumers and purchasers of occupational therapy services and also members of the occupational therapy profession to identify readily occupational therapists with expert knowledge and skills in specialty areas; and thirdly, to protect and enhance the reputation of occupational therapy by continuing to promote the value of occupational therapy services and thus increase the profile of the profession.

Conclusion

Professional accountability is achieved through ongoing development of competence throughout a practitioner's career (Fawcett & Strickland, 1998). Consumers need a mechanism not only to identify competent professionals, but also to be reassured that there is quality and safety in the service they are receiving or paying for. Continuing professional development activities are viewed positively in enhancing professional competence. Involvement in these activities also often promotes the exchange and dialogue important in professional socialisation.

The Accredited Occupational Therapy Program is an example of an Australian professional response to these increased demands that has gained wide acceptance from the majority of practitioners and employers. The program was developed by the profession and its implementation welcomed as symbolising the importance of professional development activity to professional practice. It is a program that accommodates therapists working in a diverse range of workplaces and allows them to be self-directed learners, rewarding those who meet minimum participation requirements in continuing professional development. AccOT status has also given some therapists additional leverage to seek support from workplaces to implement supervision or support for professional development activities. New practitioners, for example, are able to be more assertive in seeking formal supervision because supervision is a requirement of accreditation status.

The benefits are not just for the practitioners, however. Consumers and employers can access the national list of accredited occupational therapists and identify practitioners who are working to maintain their knowledge and skill though ongoing professional development. OT AUSTRALIA now has evidence that practitioners are engaging in ongoing professional development which can be used to promote the practice of occupational therapy and to tailor educational activities towards the learning needs of practitioners.

The question of whether accreditation programs actually ensure professional competence remains. However, the profession of occupational therapy, through the implementation of its AccOT program, can demonstrate that it has a reliable system in place to encourage and monitor professional development activities. With increasing regulation of practice likely, more focus will be directed towards such systems. This represents a real and pressing challenge for all professional groups as we move toward an uncertain yet demanding future.

References

Alsop, A. (2000). *Continuing professional development. A guide for therapists.* Oxford: Blackwell Science.

American Association of Occupational Therapists (1999). Standards for continuing competence. *American Journal of Occupational Therapy, 53,* 599–600.

Anderson, L. T. (2001). Occupational therapy practitioners' perceptions of the impact of continuing education activities on continuing competency. *American Journal of Occupational Therapy, 55,* 449–454.

Australian Association of Occupational Therapists. (1994). *Australian Competency Standards for Entry-Level Occupational Therapists.* Melbourne: Australian Association of Occupational Therapists.

Australian Council for Quality and Safety in Health Care (2002). *Lessons from the Inquiry in Obstetrics and Gynaecological Services at King Edward Memorial Hospital 1990–2000*, July.

Bosser, A. M., Kernaghan, J., Hodgins, L., Merla, L., O'Connor, C. & Van Kessel, M. (1999). Defining and developing professionalism. *Canadian Journal of Occupational Therapy, 66,* 116–121.

Brockett, M. & Bauer, M. (1998). Continuing professional education: Responsibilities and possibilities. *Journal of Continuing Education in the Health Professions 18,* 235–243.

Brown, G, Esdaile, S. & Ryan, S. (2003). *Becoming an advanced healthcare practitioner.* Edinburgh: Butterworth-Heinemann.

Burke, J. P. (1998). Clinical interpretation of 'Health and the human spirit for occupation'. *American Journal of Occupational Therapy, 52,* 419–422.

Burke, J. P. & DePoy, E. (1991). An emerging view of mastery, excellence, and leadership in occupational therapy practice. *American Journal of Occupational Therapy, 45,* 1027–1032.

Courtney, M. & Farnworth, L. (2003). Professional competence for private practitioners in occupational therapy. *Australian Occupational Therapy Journal, 50,* 234–243.

Commonwealth of Australia (2001) *Consumer Participation in Accreditation. Resource Guide.* Melbourne: National Resource Centre for Consumer Participation in Health.

Crist, P., Wilcox, B. L. & McCarron, K. (1998). Transitional portfolios: Orchestrating our professional competence. *American Journal of Occupational Therapy, 52,* 729–735.

Cross, V. (1998). Framing experience. Towards a model of CPD outcomes. *Physiotherapy, 84,* 53–54.

Curry, L., Wergin, J. F. & Associates. (1993). *Educating professionals: Responding to new expectations for competence and accountability.* San Francisco: Jossey-Bass.

Cusick, A. (1999). Accreditation of occupational therapy educational programmes in Australia: Time we did it our way? *Australian Occupational Therapy Journal, 46,* 69–74.

Cusick, A. & McCluskey, A. (2000). Becoming an evidence-based practitioner through professional development. *Australian Occupational Therapy Journal, 47,* 159–170.

Dubin, S. S. (1990). Maintaining competence through updating. In S. L. Willis & S. S. Dubin (Eds), *Maintaining professional competence: Approaches to career enhancement, vitality, and success throughout a worklife,* pp 9–43. San Francisco: Jossey-Bass.

Evert, M. M. (1993). Nationally speaking: Competency: Ethical issues and dilemmas. *American Journal of Occupational Therapy, 47,* 487–489.

Fawcett, L. C. & Strickland, L. R. (1998). Accountability and competence: occupational therapy practitioner perceptions. *American Journal of Occupational Therapy, 52,* 737–743.

Fidler, G. S. (1996). Developing a repertoire of professional behaviors. *American Journal of Occupational Therapy, 50,* 583–587.

Fish D. & Coles, C. (1998). *Developing professional judgement in health care.* Oxford: Butterworth-Heinemann.

Ford, L. (1999, April). *Quality and competency: Underpinning of the OT AUSTRALIA Accreditation Program.* Paper presented at the Australian Occupational Therapy Conference, Canberra.

Ford, L., Dorries, V., Fossey, E., do Rozario, L., Mullavey-O'Byrne, C., Shuey, H. et al (1999). *Australian competency standards for occupational therapists in mental health.* Fitzroy: OT AUSTRALIA Australian Association of Occupational Therapists Inc.

Foto, M. (1996). Nationally speaking: Delineating skilled versus nonskilled services: A defining point in our professional evolution. *American Journal of Occupational Therapy, 50,* 168–170.

Grbich, C. (Ed.). (1996). *Health in Australia. Sociological concepts and issues.* Sydney: Prentice Hall.

Grossman, J. (1992). Commentary: Professionalism in occupational therapy. *Occupational Therapy Practice, 7*–10.

Halligan, A. & Donaldson, L. (2001) Implementing clinical governance: turning vision into reality. *British Medical Journal, 322,* 1413–1417.

Harris, I. B. (1993). New expectations for professional competence. In L. Curry (Ed.), *Educating professionals: Responding to new expectations for competence and accountability,* pp 17–52. San Francisco: Jossey Bass.

Higgs, J. & Titchen, A. (2000). Knowledge and reasoning. In J. Higgs & M. Jones (Eds), *Clinical Reasoning in the health professions* (2nd ed.), pp 23–32. Oxford: Butterworth-Heinemann.

Hocking, C., Levack, H. & Chester, M. (2002). The professional competence context in New Zealand. *WFOT Bulletin, 45*, 12–16.

Hogg, C. (1999). *Patients, Power & Politics. From Patients to Citizens.* London: Sage Publications.

Irvine, R. & Graham, J. (1994). Deconstructing the concept of profession: A prerequisite to carving a niche in a changing world. *Australian Occupational Therapy Journal, 41*, 9–18.

Kennedy I., Jarman, B., Howard, R. & Maclean, M. (2001) The Inquiry into the Management of Care of Children Receiving Complex Heart Surgery at the Bristol Royal Infirmary — Final Report, July.

Kielhofner, G. (1997). Professional identity and competence. *Conceptual foundations of occupational therapy* (2nd ed.), pp 303–319. Philadelphia: F. A. Davis Company.

McKinstry, C. (1995). *Continuing Professional Education in the Victorian Occupational Therapy Profession. Unpublished Master's thesis*, La Trobe University, Bendigo, Australia.

McKinstry, C. (2003, April). *Enhancing workplaces to maximise learning for newly graduated occupational therapists.* Paper presented at the OT AUSTRALIA 22nd National Conference, Melbourne.

Nordholm, L. A., Adamson, B. J. & Heard, R. (1994). Australian physiotherapists' and occupational therapists' views on professional practice. *Journal of Allied Health, 24*, 267–282.

O'Neill, O. (2002). *A question of trust. The BBC Reith Lectures 2002.* Cambridge: Cambridge University Press.

OT AUSTRALIA. (2001). *Accredited occupational therapist program manual.* Melbourne: OT AUSTRALIA, Australian Association of Occupational Therapists Inc.

Parham, D. (1987). Nationally speaking: The reflective practitioner. *American Journal of Occupational Therapy, 41*, 555–561.

Saltman, R. B., Figueras, J. & Sakellarides, C. (Eds). (1998). *Critical Challenges for Health Care Reform in Europe.* Buckingham: Open University Press.

Schein, E. A. (1972). *Professional education.* New York: McGraw-Hill.

Schemm, R. L. & Bross, T. (1995). Mentorship experiences in a group of occupational therapy leaders. *American Journal of Occupational Therapy, 49*, 32–37.

Schön, D. A. (1983). *The reflective practitioner: How professionals think in action.* New York: Basic Books.

Scrivens, E. (1995). *Accreditation: Protecting the professional or the consumer?* Bristol: Open University Press.

Sinclair, M. (2000) The Report of the Manitoba Pediatric Cardiac Surgery Inquest — an Inquiry into Twelve Deaths at the Winnipeg Health Sciences Center in 1994.

Stancliff, B. L. (1996). Demonstrating continued competency. *OT Practice, 1*(9), 49–52.

Thomson, L., Lieberman, D., Murphy, R., Wendt, E. & Poole, J. (1997). Developing, maintaining and updating competency in occupational therapy: A guide to self appraisal. *OT Week*, 28–34.

Warne, C. (2002). Keeping in shape: Achieving fitness to practice. *British Journal of Occupational Therapy, 65*, 219–223.

Wilson, B. (2002, August) Royal Melbourne Hospital Inquiry — August 2002. Retrieved from http://www.health.vic.gov.au/hsc/rmh.report0802.

Youngstrom, M. J. (1998). Evolving competence in the practitioner role. *American Journal of Occupational Therapy, 52*, 716–720.

CHAPTER SEVEN

World Connected: The International Context of Professional Practice

Kit Sinclair

KEY WORDS

Human rights
Consumer empowerment
and technology
Practice trends
Globalisation
Education

Chapter Profile

This chapter investigates the present context of health-care practice from a global perspective and explores the major international trends that impact health-care practice including globalisation, social justice imperatives, education, technological advances and the mobility of human resources. The impact on people with disabilities is discussed where relevant. These trends are interpreted as they relate to traditional and emerging fields of health practice. In addition, the responses that health care professionals, and occupational therapists in particular, are making to these challenges and trends are considered. This chapter explores the traditional, present and future trends in health-care practice. Finally, the role of international, professional organisations in promoting practice worldwide is considered.

Introduction

In this market driven, interconnected world, major international trends are impacting on health-care practice. Challenges to traditional health-care systems and approaches include the continuing population growth in some countries, globalisation, re-emergence of communicable diseases and epidemics, increasing proportions of elder populations and the concomitant burden of chronic diseases, privatisation of health care, requirements for improving quality of care, a focus on poverty and deprivation and increasing marginalisation of peoples in developed and developing countries (Haines & Antezana, 1997; Hall & Taylor, 2003; Islam & Tahir, 2002; Rafei, 2000). For example, human immunodeficiency virus/acquired immunodeficiency syndrome (HIV/AIDS) has become a global epidemic. Severe acute respiratory syndrome (SARS) and other communicable diseases are challenging health systems. Both are having a direct impact at all levels from the World Health Organization (WHO) to national governments to health-care workers to families and communities.

Within this context, health services in developed countries are facing major health-care reforms, as well as cutbacks in hospital funding (Atkinson, 1993; Cortinois, Downey, Closson, & Jadad, 2003; Davidhizar, 1996). There is an increasing emphasis on client-oriented, community-based practice and health promotion (Baum, 1991; Chilton, 1995; Gage, 1995; Heitkamp, 1998; Nelson, 1997), evidence based practice and continuing educational development for individual practitioners (Shim, 2002). In developing countries, there is a struggle to develop services and meet basic needs in light of the lack of trained professionals as a consequence of migration and the "brain drain" (Collins, 1994; Marchal & Kegals, 2003; United Nations Economic Forum, 1956).

Technological advances, consumer awareness, human rights and factors related to the global mobility of human resources are also changing the face of health care (McChesney, 2000). Though global issues can be categorised in a number of ways and addressed from a number of perspectives, I have chosen to address issues related to globalisation, technological advances and the mobility of human resources to illustrate the challenges and opportunities for health-care practitioners.

Globalisation

Globalisation is a complex and multidimensional phenomenon that broadly covers macroeconomic, social and environmental factors affecting our world today. It has impacted on the international context of practice through economic growth and the dissemination of technologies. It is shaping the patterns of global health and challenging our health systems (Frenk, Gomez-Dantes, Macguinness & Knaul, 1997; Martens, 2002; Ugalde & Jackson, 1995). Positive impact occurs in the globalisation of knowledge and practice (Leggat & Tse, 2003) through the internet and by the knowledge transfer and extension of specific health-care interventions internationally and particularly to developing countries (Cortinois, Downey, Closson & Jadad, 2003). This should ultimately contribute to improvement in access and delivery of modern and effective health services (Ellis, 2003).

On the downside, globalisation has effected greater differences between the rich and the poor. In some instances, globalisation has also led to socioeconomic inequalities and political instability. Two years after the historic "call for action" by the United Nations, the World Health Organization published its annual health report, *Reducing risks, promoting healthy life* (WHO, 2002). It stated the obvious. It reiterated the close and self-evident links between poverty and disease. It added that disease often meant people could not work which in turn led to a lack of food on family tables with the inevitable results; malnutrition and other health issues. Global statistics tell the stark facts. More than half of the world's people suffer from malnutrition and have access to substandard health care (Smith, 2002). The wealth that has been created is being shared by few in the world (International Labour Organization, 2004).

Health sector reforms

As a consequence of global economic adjustments, the health sector in many countries has undergone major reforms (Islam & Tahir, 2002; Mercer et al, 2002). Health-care organisations in developed countries have experienced major changes to their structure, procedures and personnel in response to the need to increase clinical accountability, efficiency and become more cost-effective (Lloyd & King, 2002). They have been impacted upon by new government policies, new information, new technology, public expectations and changing health needs of the population (Collis, 2003; Cortinois, Downey, Closson & Jadad, 2003). Among aspects of recent health-care reform are the decentralisation of health systems, increased consumer choice, emphases on clinical effectiveness and health outcomes, the development of the private sector and the introduction of new delivery systems such as managed care (Bassett & Lloyd, 2000).

The provision of services is also affected by the mobility of the global population. On the positive side, this can promote and enhance cultural understanding and international learning. On the negative side, it creates disparity both in the provision of services to poorer or disadvantaged populations and between education for health professionals and the ability of governments to meet health-care needs and services. Such mobility also generates concerns over the appropriate distribution of government funding for long-term support and the stability of services for the total population (Kim, Millen, Irwin & Gershman, 2000; Mercer et al, 2002). (See Box 1 for a case example illustrating these phenomena.) Distribution of services is affected by political action, traditions, values and pressure strategies used by existing governmental and non-governmental stakeholders (Walsh, 2000). Disabled Peoples International for instance, with one peak organisation to represent each country, now has standing at the United Nations thus wielding power to influence governments internationally.

Policy makers and practitioners are faced with the demands of considering the value of dignity, equity and ethical dimensions for successful health reform, diverse opportunities for educating health professionals and issues such as international deployment of resources. Evidence based policy options, technical support and co-operation among agencies ought to be incorporated into all aspects of practice (The International Forum on Globalisation, 2002). Educational programs should

CASE STUDY

Nigerian occupational therapy brain drain

In 2002, statistics for Nigeria showed the poorest doctor to patient ratio in Africa at 1:3500. In 1998, only 2.5 per cent of the government budget was spent on health. According to Yesufu (2000), local health-care manpower is enticed to advanced countries through higher remuneration and greater opportunities for professional specialisation, whereas Nigeria has shrinking opportunities, deficit facilities and oppressive governance.

There are 22 educational degree programs for medical doctors, five educational degree programs for physiotherapist and one program for occupational therapy assistants. There are no degree courses presently available for occupational therapists. Occupational therapy in Nigeria is recorded for leprosy patients as early as 1944. Of 48 occupational therapists trained primarily in Britain for Nigeria, 20 have emigrated (between 1986–1996), 8 were expatriate, 8 have retired, 3 passed away and 8 are presently practising in Nigeria. Of those now practising, five have been pulled out of retirement to teach at a new school for occupational therapy assistants set up by the Psychiatric Hospital Management Board in 2002. All are city hospital based but are attempting to provide grassroots therapy. No trained staff are available to take up faculty positions for a degree program that has been accredited at the University (Coker, 2003).

be established of a minimum standard, culturally relevant and available to all countries (Hocking & Ness, 2002).

Technological advances

Ease of access to information through the internet, media and travel have influenced the process of globalisation in our increasingly mobile society. Health-care information and knowledge in the public domain is empowering for populations and for individuals who take advantage of this medium to understand their own health-care issues (Ellis, 2003; Kari & Michels, 1991; Labonte, 1989). For example, in 2003, the Australian government purchased access to the Cochrane Library database for all Australians. As a consequence, the gate-keeping role of health professionals to high levels of information about treatment effectiveness no longer exists.

Technology empowers people with disabilities

The widespread adoption of email and internet services is facilitating information exchange for people with disabilities (Carlson, Ehrlich, Berland & Bailey, 2002) and new technology is at the forefront, including interactive communications and enhanced equipment for people with a range of sensory impairments. It provides a foundation for greater connectedness (see Box 2).

The technology that supports advancement in communication improves efficiency but also increases the demand for greater individual involvement and productivity. The challenges and opportunities afforded by new technology lie in the ability to harness it for the benefits of the individual and the community without creating an untenable stress of too much demand. New techniques and assistive technology have opened new opportunities that should empower people by facilitating access and inclusion for improved health and wellbeing (Kari & Michels, 1991). Prior to the major breakthrough in microcomputer technology in the early 1990s, Kaiser (1987) described the impact of technical aids and switches, environmental controls, powered mobility, computer interfacing and communication as new specialty areas for occupational therapy in Canada and noted issues of therapists having to deal with their own "technophobia". Oke and French (1987) wrote of the developing use of microcomputers as an adjunct in special education in Australia.

A decade and a half later, people with mobility challenges are heading into their communities using electric scooters, electric shopping carts, power wheelchairs, ramps, lifts, adapted bicycles and go-karts. Travellers can now rent accessible vans and cars with hand controls. Automatic doors make more buildings, stores, trains and even ships accessible. Telecommunication devices are found in airports, hotel stores, universities and libraries. Recreational technology facilitates the enjoyment of hiking, camping, boating and running. Audio books are sold in bookstores. Information is published in Braille, large print and on cassette tapes for banks, stores, restaurants and the travel industry. Voice activated telephones access the web or assist people with disabilities to call friends. Students with disabilities can use assistive technology at all levels of education (Gitlow, 2002; Shim, 2002). All of this advanced technology provides for a more inclusive society.

However, not all people, even in the developed world, have access to this technology or can afford it, if they know about it. Teachers, health-care professionals and the population at large need a better understanding of its use and potential (Barney, 2002; Williams, 2003). In less developed countries, the impact of technology has depended on access to and affordability of this new technology. For example, 80 per cent of the population living in developing countries represents less than 10 per cent of internet users (Frenk & Gomez-Dantes, 2002).

A shift in philosophy

With the move from an industrial to knowledge-base society in many countries over the last two decades, there has been a change in emphasis from a welfare-based system to an equity and empowerment philosophy focused on enabling everyone to participate in all aspects of the community (Fox, 2001; Labonte, 1989). As a result, effecting a "cure" through remedial activities has gradually given way to dealing with real life issues through occupations and alterations to environmental barriers, redefining independence on the basis of experience and insights about quality of life to gain control over one's own life and activities, irrespective of dependency on others to complete tasks (Bontje, 1998; Law, 1998).

CASE STUDY

Impact of the internet on community participation

A survey reported by Rehabilitation Engineering and Assistive Technology Society of North America (RESNA) (Carlson, Ehrlich, Berland & Bailey, 2002) noted that approximately 64 per cent of persons with disabilities in the United States aged 18 and over used some form of assistive or information technologies in 2002. This estimate was based on a prevalence rate of disability among adults in the United States of America (USA) of 16 per cent. Put differently, 10 per cent of adults in the USA, or nearly 21 million people not counting persons under age 18, used some type of assistive technology to help them with their daily lives and activities. The internet has had a significant impact on community participation and quality of life for people with and without disabilities. According to a report giving highlights from the 2000 National Organization on Disabilities/Harris Survey on community participation (Williams, 2003), the internet appears to be effective in overcoming social isolation and helping people with disabilities become better informed about the world around them. For this study, 535 adults (aged 18 and over) with disabilities and 614 adults (aged 18 and over) without disabilities were interviewed online. A respondent was included in the sample of adults with disabilities if he or she had a health problem, disability or handicap that kept him or her from participating fully in work, school, housework or other activities. On average, people with disabilities spent 30 hours per week online. In contrast, people without disabilities spent significantly less time online, an average of 18 hours per week.

Impact of the internet on quality of life

Nearly half (48 per cent) of the respondents with disabilities said that the internet had significantly improved their quality of life. Only 27 per cent of people without disabilities said the same.

Be better informed about the world

Fifty-two per cent of those with disabilities said the internet had significantly improved their ability to be better informed about the world surrounding them, while only 39 per cent of those without disabilities said the same.

Reach out to people with similar interests and/or experiences

The Internet also was effective in helping people with less severe disabilities to reach out to other people with similar interests and/or experiences. Fifty-two per cent of disabled respondents said that the internet had significantly enhanced their ability to do this whereas only 30 per cent of people without disabilities and 34 per cent of people with severe disabilities said the same.

Finding a common language

The World Health Organization (2001) has focused attention on the participation perspective with the development of the International Classification of Functioning, Disability and Health (ICF) previously known as the ICIDH. This framework, which has a foundation in the philosophy of occupational therapy (Law, 2002), provides a common language to describe how people live with a health condition. It highlights the international concern about health-care outcomes and proposes a shift in emphasis away from viewing a person in terms of impairment and handicap and towards the perspective of a person as a human being —functioning in daily tasks, undertaking a variety of roles and being a member of society (Brintnell, 2002). It also provides a positive terminology of accessibility in terms of transport, public areas, equipment and communications (Stewart, 2002). The term "accessible" is taking over from the term "disabled facilities" in many developed countries (Fox, 2001).

The ICF defines participation as involvement in a life situation and uses the domains of learning and applying knowledge, general task and demands, communication, mobility, self-care, domestic life, interpersonal interactions and relationships, major life areas such as work, or school, community and social and civic life (Brintnell, 2002). It implies being involved, making choices and taking risks. It also implies that issues of access gain greater consideration. Access developments can be easily measured in high-technology urban areas, but in the majority of the world, priorities of hunger, shelter and health care often make participation and access priorities difficult to achieve (Fox, 2002).

The implications of this major WHO document for health-care practitioners lie in reinforcing the client-oriented and community approaches already being implemented in many aspects of practice. From the practitioners' view, now reinforced by this document, the focus is on people's occupations within the natural environment and on occupational routine for quality of life (Law, 1998). Occupation-focused services, therefore, centre on people's opportunity to make choices, set goals and better control circumstances to make life more meaningful (Menon, 2002).

Historical perspective of human rights and inclusiveness

Globalisation of ethical and judicial standards was initiated with the UN Convention on Human Rights in 1966. As can be seen in Table 7.1, the international community has experienced a paradigm shift in thinking from the idea that people with disabilities are objects of care and services to the paradigm of equal rights and opportunities for all. Some of the outcomes of this shift include the International Year of Disabled Persons (IYDP) in 1981, which outlined and encouraged adherence to a plan of action at the national, regional and international levels, with an emphasis on equalisation of opportunities, rehabilitation and prevention of disabilities. This was followed by the Decade of Disabled Persons (1983–1992), and subsequently, in the adoption by the UN General Assembly of

1948	United Nations Convention on Human rights promulgated from the draft international bill of Rights of the League of Nations started in 1945.
1966	The International Covenant on Economic, Social and Cultural Rights and the International Covenant on Civil and Political Rights were adopted by the United Nations General Assembly.
1978	United Nations Declaration of Alma Ata stating the Fundamentals of human rights.
1981	International Year of Disabled Persons.
1983–1992	Decade of Disabled Persons declared by United Nations.
1983	International Labour Organization (ILO) Vocational Rehabilitation and Employment (Disabled Persons) Convention.
1987	Global meeting of experts to review experience gained from UN Decade of Disabled Persons: – no consensus on convention for rights of persons with disability; – standard rules elaborated equalisation of opportunities for people with disabilities; and – led to development of ICIDH and subsequently the ICF.
1993	World Conference on Human Rights. Vienna Declaration and World Plan for Action. UN Standard rules on Equalization of Opportunities cover all aspects of a disabled person's life and show how governments can make social, political and legal changes to ensure full participation of disabled people as equal citizens of their countries. It identified 22 policy/program areas for the development of persons with disabilities.

Table 7.1 Some historical examples of international development of human rights perspectives for people with disabilities

1995	Copenhagen Declaration. Promoted "social" model of disability, focusing on the constraints arising from social, political, economic and cultural factors, as well as barriers in the built environment, and on solutions through measures to remove these constraints and barriers.
1993–2002	Asian and Pacific Decade of Disabled Persons declared by the Economic and Social Commission for Asia and the Pacific (ESCAP) in response to the UN decades of Disabled Persons 1983–1992, in which equal opportunities for full participation could not be achieved for the disabled persons especially in the developing countries of Asia Pacific Region where approximately two-thirds of the World's disabled persons live.
2000	UN Millennium Development Goals with aims to eradicate extreme poverty and hunger, achieve universal primary education, promote gender equality and empower women, reduce child mortality, improve maternal health, combat HIV/AIDS, malaria, and other diseases, ensure environmental sustainability, develop a global partnership for development.
2002	Post-Decade United Nations ESCAP high level Inter-governmental Meeting to conclude the Asian and Pacific Decade of Disabled Persons 1993–2002 on 25–28 October 2002 held in Shiga, Japan. Seven priority areas for action identified: – Strengthening self-help organisations for persons with disabilities and related family and parent associations; – Development of women with disabilities; – Early detection, early intervention and education; – Training and employment, including self-employment; – Access to build environments and public transport; – Access to information and communications, including information, communications and assistive technologies; and – Poverty alleviation through capacity building, social security and sustainable livelihood programs.

Table 7.1 Some historical examples of international development of human rights perspectives for people with disabilities — *continued*

2002	Change of WHO international classification of disability (ICIDH) to incorporate affirmative terminology of activity and participation (ICF).
2003	European Year of People with Disabilities. Events throughout the year highlight challenges and potential for people with disabilities in European countries.

Table 7.1 Some historical examples of international development of human rights perspectives for people with disabilities — *continued*

the *Standard Rules on the Equalization of Opportunities for Persons with Disabilities* in 1993. The *World Programme of Action concerning Disabled Persons* is summarised in 22 Standard Rules that serve as an instrument for policy-making and as a basis for technical and economic co-operation. They represent a strong moral and political commitment to promote effective measures for prevention of disability, rehabilitation and the realisation of the goals of full participation of disabled persons in social life and development, and of equality. Full participation means opportunities equal to those of the whole population and an equal share in the improvement in living conditions resulting from social and economic development. These concepts should apply with the same scope and with the same urgency to all countries, regardless of their level of development, according to the Standard Rules. As we move forward in this millennium, health-care practice must be based on the belief that all people have the right to respect, care, comfort, meaningful occupations and a place in society. According to Lindquist (2002), one way that we can have a global effect is to form local and international partnerships and mobilise for the development of a Convention on the Rights of People with Disabilities. That is one avenue of many.

Legal backup for human rights initiatives

With the enactment of statutes such as the *Americans with Disabilities Act* in the USA, the *Disability Discrimination Act* in Australia in 1992 and the *Disability Discrimination Ordinance* in Hong Kong in 1995, discrimination on the grounds of disability has been made illegal (Fox, 2001). This access and equity movement has had an impact on developed countries such as Australia, New Zealand, Japan, Hong Kong, Canada, Northern Europe, United Kingdom and the United States of America but has still left about 80 per cent of the world's population unable to share the significant benefits of a rights-based approach (Fox, 2002). The Standard

Rules on The Equalization of Opportunities for Persons with Disabilities state that governments should ensure the provision of rehabilitation services for persons with disabilities in order for them to reach and sustain their optimum level of independence and functioning (Eagle, 2003). Though not directly stated in the Standard Rules, this should include the removal of barriers and limitations that prevent people with disabilities from full participation in community life (Townsend, 1999).

Human resources for health care

Development and sustainability of human resources

A positive global effort is embodied in the Millennium Development Goals (MDG) established by the United Nations in 2000. It aims to eradicate extreme poverty and hunger, achieve universal primary education, promote gender equality and empower women, reduce child mortality, improve maternal health, combat HIV/AIDS, malaria, and other diseases, ensure environmental sustainability and develop a global partnership for development (United Nations, 2003). The Millennium Development Goals are being implemented to promote health and wellness for all people worldwide. The lack of human resources is, however, a constraint to the achievement of the Goals.

The health sector is a major employer in all countries with 35 million persons currently employed worldwide (Mercer et al, 2002). Human resource development and sustainability require education and job availability. At the local level, individual practitioners may be affected by problems such as insecurity of employment or inadequate pay. On a larger scale, the health services in many countries are affected by migration and poor distribution of health professionals. Incentives need to be established to keep personnel where they are needed. Governments need to address the ethical recruitment and distribution of skilled health-care workers and promote sound national policies and strategies for the training and management of human resources for health (Bryde, 1989).

Positive and negative aspects of mobility

As the global marketplace expands, so does the cross-border movement of health practitioners. The World Trade Organization (WTO) requires reciprocity of services and this has also pushed the need for greater reciprocal access to education at both the undergraduate and postgraduate level (Larsen, 2002). This emphasis on international mobility has its positive side in the sharing of skills and development of new services (Westcott &Whitcombe, 2003). However, a question is raised about the role of examination and gate-keeping strategies to limit access to people from other countries. The WTO demands that there be no differential gate-keeping rules for the movement of professional people of different countries (WTO, 1998). Following this rule, if all locally and internationally trained practitioners must pass the same exam, it is not discrimination. Discrimination occurs, however, if a written exam is demanded only of non-resident and overseas practitioners.

Overseas recruitment thwarts government planning

Health-care workers tend to prefer to work in cities rather than rural areas as well as using their skills to migrate to more affluent countries for work or higher education (Mercer et al, 2002). In order to meet the health-care needs of a country's population, governments must consider planning for appropriate levels of training, creation of jobs and services as well as quality of services (Segall, 2000). It is important to understand the education and training perspective and its inherent relation to often competing political interests. Too often this planning is thwarted by the migration of therapists from rural to urban settings and from developing to more developed countries. Recruitment companies in developed countries respond to the expressed market requirement of certain countries for more staff by actively advertising in less developed countries. The issue then arises of considering what is ethical in recruitment. Personal choice of jobs is one issue, but active international recruitment by companies in developed countries depletes the human resources in developing countries to the extent that the service may no longer be viable (Simo-Algado & Kronenberg, in press; Whiteford, 1997) An example lies in the recruitment of 11 of the 14 occupational therapists from a large Nairobi hospital in the early 1990s which devastated that hospital's rehabilitation services for many years (F Amalia, personal communication, 28 March 1996).

In the case of occupational therapy, personal choice and individual opportunities for migration may be held up in some countries by the national approval system for education programs (Stohs, Rene, Coppard & Royeen, 2002). Also, in spite of the World Federation of Occupational Therapists' introduction of minimum education standards, differences in national standards of occupational therapy education make global mobility more difficult (Brockett, 1988). Though

---

CASE STUDY

Migration opportunities drain country's services

In the Philippines, many occupational therapists trained at university level in the 1980s were immediately recruited to work in the United States. The Philippines' rehabilitation services suffered for many years from this recruitment and migration. In response to the recruitment companies' major marketing campaigns in the Philippines in the mid-nineties, the number of private occupational therapy programs increased sharply, almost overwhelming the national association's education program approval process (Patrinos, 2002; Sinclair, 1999). In 1999, the national professional association had approved three schools while 31 were awaiting approval.

Now that jobs are more difficult to find in the United States and recruitment from the USA has almost totally ceased, the occupational therapy services in the Philippines are benefiting from the increased graduate output and rapidly expanding services (Sinclair, 2000).

codes of conduct for international recruitment have been produced by various international and governmental agencies over the last several years, recruitment still affects the level of local services in many parts of the world.

Emerging fields of practice in occupational therapy

Practitioners are positively influencing health, welfare, education, social financial, legal/justice and political issues for individuals and groups at local, national and international levels (Baum & Law, 1998; Grady, 1994; Townsend, 1999). Through the proactive nature of the profession, practitioners have a valuable contribution to make to occupational performance as it affects the health and wellbeing of people globally (Shackleton & Gage, 1995; Wilcock, 1998; Wood, 1998).

Emerging fields of occupational therapy are responding to changing needs (see Table 7.2). There are trends toward community-based rehabilitation (CBR), working with marginalised people and working from a human rights and social justice perspective (Kronenberg, 2003; Townsend, 1992; Townsend, 1999; Whiteford, 2000). Such programs are being developed to facilitate individual and group survival and coping, as well as community reintegration (Somers, 2001).

An area where occupational therapists have been very effective in promoting these opportunities has been in the community (Carswell-Opzoomer, 1990; McColl, 1998) and in CBR (Kronenberg, 2003). CBR is a strategy within general community development for rehabilitation, equalisation of opportunities and social inclusion of all children and adults with disabilities (Deepak & Sharma, 2001). Occupational therapists in particular are able to facilitate the process of establishing CBR program development at both government and community levels (Menon, 2002; Thibeault, 2002). Occupational therapists are capable of providing and passing on to community workers and disabled persons relevant knowledge and skills to enable them more actively to participate in and take control of their lives and the lives of others within the community. CBR and CBR principles are an important way of empowering people with a disability in under-serviced and disadvantaged communities (Labonte, 1989). The World Federation of Occupational Therapists (WFOT) supports the international community in the development of CBR as a strategy to develop civil society, to create healthy and accessible communities for all members (specifically those with disabilities) and to extend equal opportunities for education, transportation, housing and employment for all members of the community (Bontje, 1998; Kronenberg).

Practitioners are working with policy makers at government and community levels to improve access for all people using innovative solutions (Townsend, 1992). For example, not only are they working with individuals on basic community participation skills like crossing a street safely, but with city planners to create safer pedestrian crossings. Not only are they working with individuals to cope with climbing stairs at home, but with architects to create apartment buildings that do not cause barriers to participation. It is the breadth, depth and scope of intervention and influence at many levels that will allow practitioners to make a positive change within communities, countries and internationally.

Country	Emerging Fields of Practice
Argentina	Work rehabilitation, community service, sheltered workshop
Australia	Access
Belgium	Private practice, palliative care, technical aids, home adaptation
Bermuda	Home care
Brazil	Social problems
Canada	Community-based practice, self employment
Finland	Project work
Germany	Paediatrics (new born), vocational therapy, increasing numbers private practice
Greece	Community health centres, school system, ergonomic consultants
Hong Kong	Community rehabilitation, elderly care, home care
Iceland	Community health sector, school system, ergonomic consultants, private practice
Japan	Private practice, CBR, home care
Luxembourg	Private practice, hospital sector, primary schools, OT at home, "assurance dependence" – dependency insurance
Malaysia	Home care, palliative care, cardiac rehab, community and forensic psychiatry, community rehabilitation, occupational health and safety
Malta	Community, psycho-geriatrics, paediatrics
Netherlands	Home care

Table 7.2 Emerging Fields of Practice in WFOT Member Countries
Ref: van-Bodegom, Knutsson &Valentin, 2000

Country	Emerging Fields of Practice
New Zealand	Private practice, injury prevention programs, occupation therapists working in schools
Norway	Rehabilitation in local communities, adjusting labour situations for disabled adults and children; community-based occupational therapy
Philippines	Private practice, school system, paediatrics, community-based occupational therapy; adolescent programs, mental health, health maintenance org.
Portugal	Community
Taiwan	School-based occupational therapy, home care, occupational therapy in long term care, occupational therapy in early intervention
Singapore	Community-based occupational therapy, geriatric care, work rehabilitation, private practice
Spain	Community occupational therapy, geriatrics, social services occupational therapy
Sri Lanka	Rehabilitation for physical handicap, mental health
Sweden	Public health, working life, allergy; in preventive and in emergency care
Switzerland	Private practice
United Kingdom	Primary care, pain management, working in accident and emergency department, forensic psychiatry, health promotion, work rehabilitation, insurance industry
USA	Ergonomics, public health community, architectural environment, industrial sites, private practice

Table 7.2 Emerging Fields of Practice in WFOT Member Countries
Ref: van-Bodegom, Knutsson &Valentin, 2000 — *continued*

Many human rights initiatives have been undertaken by occupational therapists throughout the world (Lindstrom & Ohlsson, 2001). Refugees and victims of torture who seek asylum in other countries are not only traumatised by their experience but are also unable to utilise the life skills they have, for lack of cultural skills (Connor-Schisler, 2002; Somers, 2001; Wilson, 2004). Occupational therapists work with marginalised people to promote occupational justice (Whiteford, 2000). The challenge of HIV/AIDS is being taken up by therapists working at all levels of care, from treatment for individuals to working with communities in developed and developing countries. Such initiatives can make a difference in a different tomorrow. Staying with traditional roles will lead to diminished influence in a changing world. Funding and government decisions are not tied to improving the life of individuals; they are about having the greatest impact on the most people with the least resources. This has to be a principle by which we operate in the future in order to truly create change.

Education to support best practice

Access for all to "best practice" via the worldwide web has meant that consumers have increased access to knowledge and evidence, thus challenging the once-held secure authority and exclusive knowledge of health and best practice by professionals. Practitioners cannot be complacent, but must be informed and must increase the use of evidence and research (Eakin, 1997).

Foundations through education and continuing competence

The WFOT's revised Minimum Standards of Education provide a good example of a response to globalisation and de-medicalisation (Hocking & Ness, 2002). The previous standards were written in the 1950s, based on the Western medical model of the time. Over the last five years, the Federation has reviewed and revised the WFOT Minimum Standards of Education for Occupational Therapists in response to feedback from occupational therapists around the world to be in line with the changes that have taken place in social thinking. The Standards now reflect this shift. The revision of the standards is a positive response to the challenges of breaking down international barriers, supporting reciprocity and promoting quality and vision for occupational therapy. As an internationally approved set of Standards, this document can thus be used as tool to influence governments and policy development.

The increased emphasis in the Minimum Standards for students to understand people as occupational beings, and to improve their experience of health and well-being, has far reaching implications. They provide guidelines which incorporate the occupational basis of the profession, providing countries with developmental, mentoring and review/monitoring processes. They promote learning through innovative approaches, facilitating students to acquire professional competences in clinical reasoning, skills and attitudes so they function successfully in specific situations (Palmadottir, 1996). Educational programs must retain a strong cultural component and be relevant to local needs, an example being the innovative use of students' own village life experience illustrated in Box 4.

CASE STUDY

Innovative application of culturally appropriate competency development

The undergraduate program in Uganda is an example of how one country developed a culturally-appropriate occupational therapy program to meet local needs. In a country that had no occupational therapist previously, there were 18 students in this program. A competency-based curriculum was devised to help qualifying therapists to be able to face the enormous levels of disability. Relevant issues were that students should they start learning about the needs of their communities, in particular the many people who had suffered the effects of cerebral malaria or meningitis, the absence of services for people with psychiatric problems, the AIDS epidemic and the fact that a repressive regime had left the country devastated. Students learned activities particularly suited to the local needs such as to cook in the traditional way or design an accessible outdoor shower using local reed and available materials. Others demonstrated their use of paper technology by making chairs for children with disabilities using the very strong glue made from local cassava root. Before reporting for studies, the students were required to visit three disabled or mentally disturbed friends or neighbours in their home village and chat with them about their lives. These observations were used to help students identify knowledge, skills and attitudes they would like to acquire in order to be able to help in each situation thus ensuring the integration of theory with grassroots practice (Smyth, 1997).

Learners need to be highly motivated, critical and analytical thinkers, adaptable and willing to work in teams. They need the scientific and technological literacy to respond to the challenges posed by the knowledge economy and the promotion of lifelong learning. In the United Kingdom's Hospital Trusts for example, there is an active Continuous Professional Development (CPD) program which includes regular professional supervision for all staff, dedicated CPD time, peer review within service areas, a critical appraisal scheme, development group, a support worker's group, fieldwork education and research projects. These are measures to sustain service quality and lifelong learning.

Education and research are the foundation for the development of services and evolution of best practice throughout the world. Best practice cannot happen without the creation of new knowledge. Educational institutes that limit their core business to teaching are doing a disservice to the profession. In order to provide the evidence that is needed across so many areas of specialty, support for quality research that is accepted as trustworthy in the health and social service arena is needed. Practitioners cannot produce this level of research without education and training in research design and methods. Academic-practice partnerships ought to be established and the "town-gown" distance bridged to enable health practitioners to provide best practice in their response to the global challenges (T Packer, personal communication, 2 March 2004).

Expanding options for providing and improving educational opportunities are seen in online education as well as the assistance of second country providers, partnering with international organisations, to supplement national systems of higher education. The European community has addressed cross-border issues by focusing on comparable degrees and joint degrees. For example, the European Network of Occupational Therapy in Higher Education (ENOTHE) was founded in 1995, within the framework of the European Union, on the initiative of the Committee of Occupational Therapists for European Communities (COTEC), the European regional group of occupational therapists. With financial support from the European Union, ENOTHE aims to unite European occupational therapy programs in order to advance education and occupational therapy's body of knowledge in Europe. The aim includes the integration of European dimensions within curriculum content and inter-institutional co-operation with integrated programs of study, training and research. Another emphasis of this group has been the development of Problem Based Learning in Occupational Therapy.

ENOTHE approaches governments in the European region to support service development and provides education modules to assist local health-care personnel to upgrade qualifications. A major thrust of higher education in health care in the European region is to make all education programs available at university level. International support for educational and service development often comes through neighbouring countries, for example Swedish Association and St Petersburg education, Australia and Singapore, Japan Association and Beijing, China. In the African region, the Occupational Therapy Africa Regional Group (OTARG)

CASE STUDY

WFOT leads the trends of occupational therapy

The World Federation of Occupational Therapists incorporates the rich cultural diversity of occupational therapy worldwide. As a dynamic and accessible world body, it impacts occupational therapy at all levels. The global role of the World Federation lies in being responsive to the professional needs, issues and requirements of its membership of national occupational therapy associations by providing a strong unified leadership through the WFOT Council. The World Federation of Occupational Therapists directly links 57 countries across the world. Its mission is to support the development, use and practice of occupational therapy worldwide, demonstrating the relevance and contribution to society. WFOT has an individual membership of over 6000 and a national membership that represents over 130,000 occupational therapists worldwide. The national membership is increasing with the regional support and mentoring of neighbouring countries in many part of the world.

acts as a co-ordinating body working together for Africa to meet felt needs, identify continental strategies and prepare a plan of action. In Asia, therapists are finding their roots in Eastern philosophy and drawing on empirical experience, establishing and articulating this in an emerging model for practice (Iwama, 2003). WFOT acts as a disseminator of information and support at all levels of international action through the networking activities of the website and OTION, through the promotion of education and setting of minimum educational standards and, most recently, through the emerging development of an international competence model.

The new practice world

Globalisation will continue to shape the world. Faced with the increasing global challenges posed by migration, poverty and changing labour markets, health practitioners can help people and communities flourish through enabling individuals and groups to establish and participate in meaningful, culturally-relevant occupations. Occupation-focused practice can help counter the negative effects of globalisation by facilitating people and supporting communities to find sustainable solutions to problems of living (Law, 2002; Townsend, 1993). New services which involve consumers in service planning and delivery (Chilton, 1996) for the creation of environments which support people's healthy lifestyle choices and ways that enable them to age successfully within a changing world must continue to emerge (Jackson, Carlson, Mandel, Zemke & Clark, 1998; Jackson, Mandel, Zemke & Clark, 2001).

New health-care paradigms have impacted the design of services (Gage, 1995). Continuous planning and management of human resources and the education and training of health service providers must develop to support service delivery at all levels (Chilton, 1995). Social and economic equity, empowerment and community practice are all relevant and emerging aspects of occupation-focused practice (Carswell-Opzoomer, 1990). According to Nelson (1997), the profession will flourish because occupation is fundamental to human health.

In many underdeveloped areas, the difficulties with public health promotion and personal health and rehabilitation services have a lot to do with general economic issues. With widespread poverty, insufficient infrastructure, poor education and a total absence of democratic structures, the outlook is grim for practitioners seeking to improve the life and health of their clients and the community. Occupation-focused practitioners, as facilitators, can help highlight and make public the problems faced by the disabled and disadvantaged. They can challenge invisibility, discrimination and poverty. They can facilitate people with disabilities to develop their full potential and enable those on the fringe of society to take part in different spheres and activities. The future trend in professional education must include a strong component on enablement, advocacy and social reform (Freire, 1985; Higgs & Edwards, 2002).

Conclusion

Practitioners in the new world must be flexible and resourceful in order to promote effective partnerships focused on developing relevant services and changing methods of service delivery to meet the health needs of communities and societies. This means being involved with consumer groups and organisations at local, national and international levels. It means taking up grassroots, public awareness initiatives. Practitioners will be faced with the challenge of identifying and developing new ways of working with people in communities to meet the new social demands. Their roles as agents of social change and social justice will be aimed at taking health practice to a new level, one that focuses on enabling participation at a community level. To become effective agents of change, the way in which practitioners are educated must come under sweeping review. Practitioner competencies related to enablement, advocacy and social reform will become the cornerstone of health professional education.

References

Atkinson, K. (1993). Reprofiling and skill mix: Our next challenge. *British Journal of Occupational Therapy, 56*(2), 67–69.

Bassett, J. & Lloyd, C. (2000). New challenges and opportunities for service delivery. *British Journal of Therapy and Rehabilitation, 7*(10), 424–427.

Barney, K. (2002). *Survey research: Using the brave new WWW.* 13th World Congress of Occupational Therapists, Stockholm, Sweden, WFOT.

Baum, C. (1991). Professional issues in a changing environment. In C. Christiansen & C. Baum, (Eds), *Occupational therapy: Overcoming performance deficits*, pp 805–817. Thorofare: Slack.

Baum, C. & Law, M. (1998). Community health: A responsibility, an opportunity, and a fit for occupational therapy. *American Journal of Occupational Therapy, 52*, 7–10.

Bontje, P. (1998). Trends in occupational therapy: A worldwide perspective. *WFOT Bulletin, 37,* 43–50.

Brintnell, E. S. (2002). WHO-International classification of functioning, disability and health-development and Canadian content. *WFOT Bulletin, 45*, 33–37.

Brockett, M. (1988). Occupational therapy resources worldwide. *WFOT Bulletin, 17*, 8–11.

Bryde, G. (1989). Ethics and occupational therapy. *WFOT Bulletin, 19*, 34–37.

Carlson, D., Ehrlich, N., Berland, J. & Bailey, N. (2002). *Highlights from the NIDRR/RESNA/University of Michigan survey of assistive technology and information technology use and need by personals with disabilities in the United States.* NIDRR/RESNA/University of Michigan.

Carswell-Opzoomer, A. (1990). Occupational therapy: Our time has come. *Canadian Journal of Occupational Therapy, 57*, 197–203.

Chilton, H. (1995). Partners in practice: Riding the waves of change. *Canadian Journal of Occupational Therapy, 62*, 183–187.

Chilton, H. (1996). Challenges and opportunities: Meeting the competitive edge. *Canadian Journal of Occupational Therapy, 63*, 155–161.

Coker, O. (2003). *Surviving challenge beyond challenge.* 3rd International Congress: Occupational Therapy Africa Regional Group, Mombasa, Kenya.

Collins, C. & Green, A. (1994). Decentralization and primary health care: Some negative implications in developing countries. *International Journal of Health Service, 24*(3), 459–475.

Collis, T. (2003). Globalisation, global health, and access to healthcare. *International Journal of Health Planning Management, 18*(2), 97–104.

Connor-Schisler, A. M. (2002). The individual as mediator of the person– occupation–environment interaction: Learning from the experiences of refugees. *Journal of Occupational Science, 9*(2), 82–92.

Cortinois, A., Downey, S., Closson, T. & Jadad, A. R. (2003). Hospitals in a globalized world: A view from Canada. *Healthcare Papers, 4*(2), 14–32.

Davidhizar, R. (1996). Surviving organizational change. *Health Care Supervisor*, 14(4), 19–24.

Deepak, S. & Sharma, M. (2001). Volunteers and community-based rehabilitation. *Asia Pacific disability rehabilitation*, 12(2), 141–148.

Dillard, M., Andonian, L., Flores, O., Lai, L., MacRae, A. & Shakir, M. (1992). Culturally competent occupational therapy in a diversely populated mental health setting. *American Journal of Occupational Therapy*, 46, 721–726.

Eagle, M. (2003). Challenging society's perception of disability. *British Journal of Occupational Therapy*, 66(4), 35.

Economic & Social Commission for Asia and the Pacific (ESCAP) (2003). *Policy paper on disability — Nepal 2004*. Retrieved from http://www.disability.dk/images/docpics/1043663724_Final_disability_policy_paper_22jan2003.doc

Ellis, P. (2003). Globalisation of healthcare: A UK perspective. *Healthcare Papers*, 4(2), 14–32.

Foto, M. (1995). New president's address: Challenges, choices, and changes. *American Journal of Occupational Therapy*, 49, 955–959.

Fox, M. (2001). *Impact of the Access Movement in Australia: Rehabilitation International.* International Commission on Technology and Accessibility (ICTA).

Fox, M. (2002). *International access and equity perspectives: From catalyst to mainstream.* Australia Council of Rehabilitation of the Disabled (ACROD) NSW conference, Sydney, Australia.

Freire (1985). *The politics of education: Culture, power and liberation.* South Hadley, MA: Bergin & Garvey Publishers.

Frenk, J., Gomez-Dantes. O., McGuinness, M. J. & Knaul, F. (1997). The future of world health: The new world order and international health. *British Medical Journal*, 314(7091), 1404–1407.

Frenk, J. & Gomez-Dantes, O. (2002). Globalisation and the challenges to health systems. *British Medical Journal*, 325(7355), 95–97.

Gage, M. (1995). Re-engineering of health care: Opportunity or threat for occupational therapists? *Canadian Journal of Occupational Therapy*, 62, 197–207.

Gitlow, L. (2002). *Research investigating global occupational therapists' preferences for assistive technology education.* 13th World Congress of Occupational Therapists, Stockholm, Sweden, WFOT.

Grady, A. (1994). *Building inclusive communities: A challenge for occupational therapy.* 1994 Annual Conference, Boston, USA, American Occupational Therapy Association.

Haines, A. & Antezana, F. S. (1997). Future of international health. *British Medical Journal 315*, 1163–1164.

Hall, J. J. & Taylor, R. (2003). Health for all beyond 2000: The demise of the Alma-Ata Declaration and primary health care in developing countries. *Medical Journal of Australia*, 178(1), 17–20.

Harris, R. (1992). *Second Chronicle of the World Federation of Occupational Therapists, 1982–1992.* Perth, World Federation of Occupational Therapists.

Heitkamp, P. (1998). Promoting People's Health: Challenges and Opportunities. *Health Millions*, 24(4), 3–5.

Higgs, J. & Edwards, H. (2002). Challenges facing health professional education in the changing context of university education. *British Journal of Occupational Therapy* 65(7), 315–320.

Hinojosa, J. & Kramer, P. (1994). Defining multiculturalism for occupational therapy. *WFOT Bulletin*, 30, 9–10.

Hocking, C. & Ness, N. E. (2002). Introduction to the Revised Minimum Standards for the Education of Occupational Therapists. *WFOT Bulletin*, 46, 30–33.

International Labour Organization. (2004). *World commission says globalization can and must change, calls for urgent rethink of global governance.* International Labour Organization press release. Retrieved 24 February 2004, from http://wwwilo.org/public/english/bureau/inf/pr/2004/7.htm

Islam, A. & Tahir, M. (2002). Health Sector reform in South Asia: New challenges and constraints. *Health Policy*, 60(2), 151–169.

Iwama, M. (2003). Towards culturally relevant epistemologies in occupational therapy. *American Journal of Occupational Therapy*, 57, 582–588.

Jackson, J., Carlson, M., Mandel, D., Zemke, R. & Clark, F. (1998). Occupation in lifestyle design: The well elderly study occupational therapy program. *American Journal of Occupational Therapy*, 52, 326–336.

Jackson, J., Mandel, D. R., Zemke, R. & Clark, F. A. (2001). Promoting quality of life in elders: An occupation-based occupational therapy program. *WFOT Bulletin*, 43, 5–12.

Kaiser, P. (1987). The effect of modern technology on the practice of occupational therapy. *WFOT Bulletin*, 15, 12–14.

Kari, N. & Michels, P. (1991). The Lazarus project: The politics of empowerment. *American Journal of Occupational Therapy, 45*, 719–725.

Kim, J. Y., Millen, J., Irwin, A. & Gershman, J. (2000). *Dying for growth: Global inequality and the health of the poor.* Monroe, Maine: Common Courage Press.

Kronenberg, F. (2003). *WFOT Draft Position Paper on Community based Rehabilitation.* Perth, Australia: World Federation of Occupational Therapists.

Labonte, R. (1989). Community empowerment: The need for political analysis. *Canadian Journal of Public Health, 80*, 87–88.

Law, M. (1998). *Client centred occupational therapy.* Thorofare: Slack.

Law, M. (2002). Participation in the occupations of everyday life. *American Journal of Occupational Therapy, 56*, 640–649.

Leggat, S. G. & Tse, N. (2003). The role of teaching and research hospitals in improving global health (in a globalized world). *Healthcare Papers, 4*(2), 34–38.

Lindquist, B. (2002). *All means all.* Rehabilitation International Congress, Osaka, Japan, Rehabilitation International.

Lindstrom, I. & Ohlsson, J. (2001). Occupational therapy — what's it worth to society. *WFOT Bulletin, 44*, 23–25.

Lloyd, C. & King, R. (2002). Organizational change and occupational therapy. *British Journal of Occupational Therapy, 65*(12), 536–542.

Marchal, B. & Kegals, G. (2003). Health workforce imbalances in times of globalization: Braindrain or professional mobility? *International Journal of Health Planning Management, 18* (Supplement 1), S89–101.

Martens, P. (2002). Health transitions in a globalizing world: Towards more disease or sustained health? *Futures, 34*(7), 635–648.

McChesney, A. (2000). *Promoting and defending economic, social and cultural rights: A handbook.* Washington, DC: American Association for the Advancement of Science.

McColl, M. (1998). What do we need to know to practice occupational therapy in the community? *American Journal of Occupational Therapy, 52*, 11–18.

Menon, S. (2002). Toward a model of psychological health empowerment: Implications for health care in multicultural communities. *Nurse Education Today, 22*, 28–39.

Mercer, H., Dal Poz, M., Adams, O., Stilwell, J., Dreesch, N., Zurn, P. & Beaglehole, R. (2002). *Human resources for health: Developing policy options for change.* Geneva, World Health Organization, 1–26.

Nelson, D. (1997). Why the profession of occupational therapy will flourish in the 21st century. *American Journal of Occupational Therapy, 51*, 11–24.

Newton, E. (2002). OTION: The occupational therapy international outreach network. *WFOT Bulletin, 45*, p 39.

Oke, L. & French, M. (1987). Occupational therapy's role in the development of the use of microcomputers by people with severe disabilities. *WFOT Bulletin, 15*, 15–17.

Palmadottir, G. (1996). Occupational therapy education program in Iceland: Needs and development. *WFOT Bulletin, 33*, 19–23.

Patrinos, H. (2002). *The role of the private sector in the global market for education.* Washington, DC: World Bank.

Rafei, U. (2000). Public health in the new millennium. *Health Millions, 26*(2), 8–10.

Segall, M. (2000). From cooperation to competition in national health systems and back?: Impact on professional ethics and quality of care. *International Journal of Health Planning and Management, 14*(1), 61–79.

Shackleton, T. & Gage, M. (1995). Strategic planning: Positioning occupational therapy to be proactive in the new health care paradigm. *Canadian Journal of Occupational Therapy, 62*, 188–196.

Shim, M. (2002). *Exploring the use of technology in continuing education for occupational therapists.* 13th World Congress of Occupational Therapists, Stockholm, Sweden, WFOT.

Simo-Algado, S. & Kronenberg, F. (in press). *Occupational therapy without borders: Spirit of survivors.* Oxford: Elsevier Science.

Sinclair, K. (1999). *Report of informal meeting between WFOT and OTAP.* Taipei, World Federation of Occupational Therapists.

Sinclair, K. (2000). Assessment of the profession: An historical perspective. *WFOT Bulletin, 42*, 29–30.

Smith, D. J. (2002). *If the world were a village: A book about the world's people*. Canada: Kids Can Press.

Smyth, J. (1997). News from national associations: Uganda. *WFOT Bulletin, 35,* 43–44.

Somers, A. (2001). The human rights initiative. *Advance for Occupational Therapy Practitioners,* (11 June 2001).

Stewart, D. (2002). *The new ICF and occupational therapy: Potential uses in practice, research, education and management.* 13th World Congress of Occupational Therapists, Stockholm, Sweden, WFOT.

Stohs, S. J., Rene, P., Coppard, B. & Royeen, C. (2002). *Entry level and post-professional clinical doctoral programmes in occupational therapy.* 13th World Congress of Occupational Therapists, Stockholm, Sweden, WFOT.

The International Forum on Globalization. (2002). *Alternatives to economic globalization: A better world is possible.* San Francisco: Berrett-Koehler Publishers.

Thibeault, R. (2002). Occupation and the rebuilding of civil society: Notes from the war zone. *Journal of Occupational Science, 9*(1), 38–47.

Townsend, E. (1992). Institutional ethnography: Explicating the social organization of professional health practices intending client empowerment. *Canadian Journal of Public Health, 83*(supplement 1), S58–S61.

Townsend, E. (1993). Occupational therapy's social vision. *Canadian Journal of Occupational Therapy, 60*(4), 174–184.

Townsend, E. (1999). Enabling occupation in the 21st century: Making good intentions a reality. *Australian Occupational Therapy Journal, 46,* 147–159.

Ugalde, A. & Jackson, J. T. (1995). The World Bank and international health policy: A critical review. *Journal of International Development, 7*(3), 525–541.

United Nations Economic Forum (UNECF). (1956). Measures to facilitate the return and reintegration of highly skilled migrants into African countries. *The International Migration Review, 24*(1), 197–212.

United Nations. (2000). *United Nations Millennium Development Goals.* New York, United Nations.

United Nations. (2003). *Biwako millennium framework for action toward an inclusive, barrier-free and rights-based society for persons with disabilities in Asia and the Pacific.* Otsu City, Shiga, Japan, United Nations Economic and Social Council.

U.S. Government. (2002). *A Nation Online: How Americans are expending their use of the Internet.* Washington, DC, US Department of Commerce, Economics and Statistics Administration.

van Bodegom, B., Knutsson, H. & Valentin, C. (2000). The professional practice questionnaire: A worthwhile project? *WFOT Bulletin, 42,* 30–33.

Walsh, J. (2000). The impact of globalisation upon prospects for peace and cooperation: Evidence from Southeast Asia. *International Journal of Humanities and Peace, 16*(1), 16–18.

Wescott, L. & Whitcombe, S. (2003). Globalisation and occupational therapy: Poles apart? *British Journal of Occupational Therapy, 66*(7), 328–330.

Whiteford, G. (1997). Occupational deprivation and incarceration. *Journal of Occupational Science, 4*(3), 126–130.

Whiteford, G. (2000). Occupational deprivation: Global challenge in the new millennium. *British Journal of Occupational Therapy, 63*(5), 200–204.

Wilcock, A. (1998). *An occupational perspective on health.* Thorofare: Slack.

Williams, J. (2003). *Assistive technology is creating a more inclusive America.* National Organization on Disability. Retrieved 28 February 2004, from http://www.nod.org/content.cfm?id=1441

Wilson, C. (2004). *Occupational opportunities for asylum seekers: Newsletter.* Brisbane.

Wood, W. (1998). It is jump time for occupational therapy. *American Journal of Occupational Therapy, 52,* 403–411.

World Health Organization. (2001). *International Classification of Functioning Disability and Health.* Geneva: World Health Organization.

World Health Organization. (2002). *The World Health Report 2002: Reducing risks, promoting healthy life.* Geneva: World Health Organization.

World Trade Organization. (1998). *Trade in Services* Annex I-IV S/L/64, 17 December 1998, 98-5140.

Yesufu, T. M. (2000). *The human factor in national development: Nigeria.* Lagos: University of Benin Press and Spectrum Books Ltd.

The Organisational Context of Practice

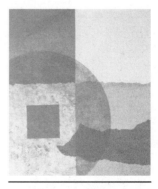

From Graduate to Practitioner: Rethinking Organisational Support and Professional Development

Carol McInstry

KEY WORDS

New graduates
Continuing professional development
Supervision
Workplace learning
Situated learning theory
Communities of practice

Chapter Profile

In this section of the book, we reflect on a context of practice that has increasingly become the focus of inquiry: the organisational context. This chapter considers the role, and indeed the responsibility, of organisations in supporting the transition of newly graduated professionals into practice. Specifically, data from research undertaken by the author on newly graduated occupational therapists is presented and discussed, highlighting the importance of active learning through reflective practice and workplace interaction. The theoretical framework of situated learning is utilised within the chapter, examining how the features of the community of practice influence processes of knowledge acquisition and transference for new graduates. The importance of understanding the culture, customs and values of the community of practice is also explored. The chapter concludes with a series of recommendations for educators, supervisors and managers.

Introduction

While the transition from student to new graduate in the health professions has recently received more diverse attention from researchers, previous research tended to focus narrowly on the psychological/emotional stresses that newly graduated professionals' experience (Atkinson & Steward, 1997; Hummell & Koelmeyer, 1999; Leonard & Corr, 1998; Parker, 1991; Rugg, 1996; Rugg, 1999; Tryssenaar, 1999). Methodologically, this research largely involved use of survey instruments (Atkinson & Steward; Cracknell, 1981; Hummell & Koelmeyer; Parker, 1991; Rugg, 1999) and, while this research has been useful in identifying major issues, it has been of limited use. Specifically, it has failed to provide rich data to illuminate the learning needs and learning processes of new graduates in the workplace.

In occupational therapy, many of the previous researchers were based in undergraduate professional schools (Atkinson & Steward, 1997; Parker, 1991; Rugg, 1999). Understandably, these researchers were oriented towards following-up final year students after graduation to evaluate the effectiveness of their under-graduate programs.

Apart from exploring program effectiveness, however, Rugg (1999) also sought to explain some of the ongoing recruitment and retention problems experienced by the occupational therapy profession in the United Kingdom. In contrast, Canadian and Australian authors directed their research towards identifying strategies to assist the newly graduated therapist in overcoming transitional problems in the workplace (Hummell & Koelmeyer, 1999; Sutton & Griffin, 2000; Tryssenaar, 1999). Additional themes in the literature include the influencing factors in choosing the first position for an occupational therapist, the job satisfaction for newly graduated therapists and the major problems encountered (Atkinson & Steward, 1997; Hummell & Koelmeyer; Parker 1991; Rugg, 1999; Tryssenaar & Perkins, 1999). Peer support and supervision required by junior therapists has also been highlighted (Hummell & Koelmeyer, 1999; Rugg, 1996; Parker).

While there has been a focus on the reasons why newly graduated therapists have chosen to work in a particular setting or location, health professionals such as occupational therapists are increasingly moving into more diverse roles and positions. There are now increased employment opportunities in areas such as community-based health services, occupational rehabilitation and private practice. Despite this more diverse range of options, however, it seems there is still a trend for new graduates to commence employment in traditional settings. Indeed, newly graduated occupational therapists surveyed during their first year of practice (Britain, Atkinson & Steward, 1997) reported choosing to commence their careers in the public health system. One factor that apparently influences newly graduated therapists' preference for the public hospital system is that the majority of undergraduate clinical fieldwork is undertaken there. Experience in undergraduate clinical placements is a major factor in determining where newly graduated therapists commence their career (Adamson, Harris & Hummel, 1998; Cracknell, 1981; Toulouse & Williams, 1984). The other characteristic that appealed to junior therapists was the rotational aspect of these positions. Junior therapists prefer rotational positions as they offer experience in a variety of clinical areas, thus increasing the range of learning opportunities (Ryrie, Williams, Wamsley & Dwyer, 2000; Lansdowne, 1989).

Newly graduated therapists in Australia have also been attracted to the public hospital system (Hummell & Koelmeyer, 1999; Sutton & Griffin, 2000). While this has been a well-established trend, there is evidence that this may be changing. Hitch (1998) believes that there are more newly graduated therapists now seeking employment outside the public hospital system. These newly graduated occupational therapists may still be the minority. However more are being employed in generic positions such as case managers, mental health workers or occupational health consultants.

With an increasing diversity in the initial positions in which newly graduated therapists are working, providing adequate support for them is becoming more complex. Access to supervision and support is reported as a major problem in many countries (Hummell & Koelmeyer, 1999; Lee & Mackenzie, 2003; Rugg, 1999; Parker 1991; Tryssenaar, 1999). Difficulties gaining access to regular supervision within the workplace increased the stress experienced by beginning therapists and the quality of supervision is also questioned (Copeland, 1998; Sweeney, Webley & Treacher, 2001b).

Copeland (1998) focuses on the benefits of supervision in assisting the transition between student and therapist. Finding time to provide regular supervision is reported as the greatest barrier to effective supervision for both the newly graduated therapist and the senior therapist. According to Copeland, supervision for newly graduated therapists is important in developing confidence, role identity and for professional development. Newly graduated therapists require feedback, support and opportunities for personal reflection, which can be provided in supervision sessions. To gain the maximum benefits from supervision, it is recommended that supervision be regular, for a set duration, and with clearly defined goals negotiated by both parties.

Sweeney, Webley & Treacher (2001b) report that junior occupational therapists are often dissatisfied with the quality of their supervision. Some junior therapists being supervised believed that their supervisors had insufficient clinical and management skills and experience. They reported that supervision sessions often lacked clearly defined objectives and guidelines. Junior therapists prefer autocratic supervisors, as they want structure and direction, while many senior therapists feel uncomfortable taking on this type of style (Sweeney et al, 2001a, b). Supervisors also report high levels of dissatisfaction, feeling inadequate to fulfill this role due to limited knowledge of the supervision process and understanding of their role. Line supervisors often provide the supervision, affecting the level of trust and openness experienced in supervision sessions (Sweeney et al, 2001b).

Many researchers also suggest that the stress and dissatisfaction experienced by newly graduated therapists is due to their high or unrealistic expectations. In research undertaken by a number of authors in this area, there was found to be discrepancies between what new therapists expected and what they experienced in practice, in particular, in regard to amounts of direct supervision. Some newly graduated therapists apparently also reported that they expected to receive more respect and support from colleagues including senior therapists (Leonard & Corr, 1998; Rugg, 1999; Sutton & Griffin, 2000).

Other challenges facing newly graduated therapists include time management, workload issues and completion of administrative tasks (Leonard & Corr, 1998; Tryssenaar & Perkins, 1999; Rugg, 1996; Sutton & Griffin, 2000). These issues may also result from unrealistic expectations originating from their experiences as undergraduate students on clinical placement. Hummell and Koelmeyer (1999) recommend that workplaces be structured to enable newly graduated therapists to have adequate supervision, continuing professional development opportunities and support from their colleagues. Parker (1991) also recommends that undergraduate students need better preparation for their transition into their roles as beginning therapists.

Workplace learning: A qualitative study of the transitional journeys of five newly graduated therapists

Previous research into newly graduated therapists has focused on the individual therapist and how they have coped with the transition. As a result, there have been lost opportunities to enhance learning through greater understanding of the workplace context. This situation, coupled with a long-standing interest in the topic, was the motivation behind a research project undertaken by the author to investigate effective workplace learning (McKinstry, 2003). The major part of this qualitative study involved following five newly graduated therapists from their last days as final year students through eighteen months post graduation in their new workplaces.

Initially, a pilot study was conducted to ascertain issues relating to the transition of students to therapists. This preliminary study explored the experiences of four occupational therapists working for twelve months in varying workplaces and two occupational therapy managers regularly employing newly graduated occupational therapists. Following data analysis, the themes identified were further explored in three focus groups. Participants in the focus groups were final year occupational therapy students from two universities and occupational therapy managers. The focus groups identified a number of major issues that influenced the experiences of newly graduated therapists that warranted further exploration. From the two focus groups of final year occupational therapy students, five were purposely selected and invited to continue in the study. Selection was based on workplace features such as location, services offered, model of service delivery, existence or size of occupational therapy department and the position title.

Two new graduates worked in rural settings and three therapists worked in mental health. Three therapists were based in hospitals while the other two new graduates were working in community-based settings. One newly graduated therapist had two part-time positions at the same organisation, while another therapist worked in multiple teams at her hospital — community, outpatients, hospital inpatients and nursing home. One therapist worked as a generic mental health worker while the other community-based therapist worked in a specialised head injury unit. Two of the newly graduated therapists were sole occupational therapists in their workplaces, relying heavily upon colleagues of other health professions to pass on their knowledge and skills. Three therapists worked for government-funded health agencies while the other two therapists worked for private, not-for-profit health organisations. Four newly graduated therapists were working in positions specified for occupational therapists and one therapist was working in a generic position.

Semi-structured interviews with the newly graduated therapists were conducted at six, twelve and eighteen month intervals at the workplace following graduation. Interviews were also conducted with the supervisors of these newly graduated therapists to seek their perceptions of the newly graduated therapists' experiences. Data analysis consisted of line-by-line coding, category coding and then thematic coding (Strauss & Corbin, 1998).

Theoretical basis of the study

To guide the analysis of the data, the theory of situated learning was utilised as the theoretical framework for this research study. Situated learning is a useful theory to explain the importance of workplace features for continued learning of newly graduated professionals. Similar to the dynamic systems theory, situated learning theory focuses on understanding the context of learning rather than the individual's learning style. Previously, Jenkins and Brotherton (1995a, b) have utilised the theory of situated learning to examine occupational therapists' acquisitions in practice situations.

Figure 8.1: Situated Learning Theory: Core concepts

The situated learning theory approach is based on the belief that knowledge and skills are learned in contexts that reflect how the knowledge is obtained and applied in authentic situations. Learning is about creating meaning from everyday activities and is grounded in the engagement of practice. As knowledge is situational, it can only be transferred to similar contexts (Lave & Wenger, 1991).

With learning being viewed as a social process, it incorporates thinking, perceiving and problem solving. Knowledge is created through the social interactions of the learners with others and also the environment. A learner observes a more experienced colleague perform the task and then engages in the task or is guided through the task by a colleague with more expertise. Through ongoing practice, the acquired knowledge and skills are refined and perfected by the novice. Working with others and participating in the work tasks needed to achieve the desired results, meaning is generated for all involved (Billett, 1994).

Situated learning theory originated in the early 1900s from the social development theory of Dewey (1938) and then Vygotsky (1978). The basic premise of situated learning is that all learning is socially based and grounded in practice. The researchers were interested in practices that enabled learning and helped to frame a curriculum of learning. The social learning theory was further refined for workplace learning by Lave and Wenger (1991) who developed the framework of situated cognition. As part of the situated theory, learning takes place within communities of practice, which are defined as "a set of relations among person, activity and world over time and in relation with other tangential and overlapping communities of practice" (Lave & Wenger, p 98). Workers with the same goals are often drawn together regardless of the organisational structure and management cannot artificially put communities of practice together as they will occur with minimal input (Wenger, 1998).

Situated learning has four basic components: community, context, access and language. Lave and Wenger (1991) also describe the process of belonging to a community of practice as legitimate peripheral participation. This concept defines how learners move from peripheral participation within a community of practice to full participation or membership. As learners become full participants, their identities and sense of belonging increases in addition to understanding the language of the community of practice. The person is accepted as a full member, taking on responsibility to then share the knowledge with other newcomers to the community of practice. Sharing of knowledge with newcomers also involves ensuring that they understand the customs, values and main objectives of the workplace.

As with all theories, there are limitations to their practical implementation. Critics such as Greeno, Moore and Smith (1993) and Tennant (2000) have drawn attention to possible conceptual and practical concerns. One such concern is the notion that if learning is context specific, how similar does another situation need to be for the learner to utilise skills and knowledge acquired in another setting or situation? The ability to transfer learning from one context to another may be limited. However Billett (1999) believes that this claim is negated if a combination of workplace learning tools is utilised in the social learning process. While the transfer of learning is a valid issue, according to Greeno et al, the important thing is that the goal of situated learning is to learn from interacting with others and things within the environment.

Vygosky (1978) also developed the concept of the zone of proximal development, describing successive learning opportunities for the learner (Davis & Polatako, 2004). While his original intention was to enable children to maximise their learning through engagement in practice or activities that were within their learning capacity, this is also a useful concept for the further learning of newly graduated therapists. Where newly graduated therapists are given too many challenges within their workplace, they can be pushed outside their "zone". Billet (2000) suggests that learning is maximised when the learner within the community of practice is given routine tasks to develop their level of competence and mastery. More novel or complex tasks are then provided to the learner to increase their repertoire of skills and knowledge from engaging in different practices, activities and tasks.

Findings of the study: Understanding newly graduated therapists' learning within diverse workplaces

In the profession of occupational therapy, new graduates are not considered novices when they enter the workforce or communities of practice as they have had some engagement in practice through undergraduate clinical placements. There are, however, considerable differences between undertaking a student placement and commencing work as a therapist. As a student, there is close supervision, regular feedback and assessment and the opportunity to work closely with the supervising therapist. Often there is an emphasis on gaining experience working with patients or clients rather than the tasks that are not directly related to patients. Examples of such tasks are administration, ordering equipment, report writing or participating in team meetings. This may explain why newly graduated therapists report feeling stressed and unsupported as they are basing their expectations on their under-graduate experience.

Experiencing supervision and feedback

The learning tools that were highly valued by newly graduated therapists were tools such as structured supervision, advice from other team members and the opportunity to observe skilled and experienced practitioners in practice. In the transition from student to therapist, they still need the structure and support that supervision provides, which they had relied upon as undergraduates. Supervision provides them with feedback on performance, confirming and reinforcing the aspects of their practice that are progressing well in their development while identifying areas of practice that need further development. As this manager suggests, it has specific foci:

> … yeah, we have formal supervision; weekly to start with, then fortnightly. Going through the therapist's report writing, discovering what happened in team meetings and that.

Supervision is more frequent and intense for an undergraduate occupational therapy student in comparison to that provided to newly graduated therapists. Supervision is a form of guided learning where the newly graduated therapist is provided with feedback and advice relating to his or her therapeutic practice. The supervisor can provide support and identify the need for specific formalised cont-inuing professional development. According to Billett (1998), the supervisor plays a crucial role in assisting the less experienced to reflect on their practice, enabling them to increase their ability to learn and consolidate knowledge and skills. Supervisors can also assist the newcomers to identify learning needs and access formal learning opportunities such as external courses or workshops. Having a supervisor who is also a member of the community of practice to which the newly graduated therapist belongs is a major advantage as the feedback is accurate and perhaps more timely. Availability and approachability also apparently help, as this new graduate reflects:

With the Chief [occupational therapist] being so approachable and open to anything, like if I was ever unsure of what my actual role was or where I should actually take it, I knew I could always pop in and ask her.

The newly graduated therapists viewed supervision from a senior colleague or manager who was also a full member of the community of practice as very relevant and beneficial. Interestingly, though, views of some managers is that supervision serves an almost regulatory function, as this manager suggests:

The supervision structures need to be there ... there is no room for feral behaviour. So there is no just running off doing your own thing and everybody needs to know what is going on. We make no bones about that. It's very structured work.

Where there is limited supervision available, or the supervisor is external or on the periphery to the community of practice the newly graduated therapist strongly identifies with, there is greater reliance upon learning from other team members. Working closely with other interdisciplinary team members provides newly graduated therapists with support and access to more experienced health professions to share their knowledge. Interaction with other experienced team members enables the newly graduated therapist to learn the language of the workplace and the customs or values peculiar to the work setting. Often the newly graduated therapist relies heavily upon colleagues who are not occupational therapists for this learning. Other allied health professionals and nursing managers commonly provided the newly graduated therapists with informal feedback upon their practice. Where this occurred, the newly graduated therapists were very appreciative and would often request this type of feedback when they began to feel a sense of belonging within the community of practice. For example, one of the new graduates working part-time on the medical unit reflected that:

I found it difficult at first to maybe ask the nurses or even the residents [medical officers] as they are sometimes a bit unapproachable ... but I think with my confidence increasing I am feeling more comfortable within myself and just asking has come easier.

With the changing workplace contexts in which newly graduated therapists are now working, often they are the sole occupational therapist or working as a generic health professional. This is increasingly the case for newly graduated occupational therapists working in community-based teams or in mental health services. While they might be receiving supervision and guidance relating to their role within this community of practice, the newly graduated therapists not receiving supervision from an occupational therapist were concerned that their professional identity and specific occupational therapy skills and knowledge may not develop sufficiently. These newly graduated occupational therapists believed that in these situations, having external supervision from an experienced occupational therapist was beneficial and agitated to access it.

Supervisors also have a role to play in determining what tasks or responsibilities the newly graduated therapist can undertake. As the newly graduated therapist becomes more skilled and knowledgeable, he or she can be given more complex patients or tasks. Routine tasks that the newly graduated therapist is easily able to complete successfully are gradually replaced with more novel tasks that require greater knowledge and further developed clinical reasoning. This is also an indication that the newcomer to the community of practice is becoming a full member, assuming responsibility for all practices belonging to the community of practice. This newly graduated therapist considers the movement towards greater depth in their interactions with clients and the feedback experienced from them as they become a more fully engaged member of their community of practice:

> … like the clients who give you hell. [They] have given me feedback both positive and negative, but certainly negative feedback and very strong negative feedback. I mean I work with superficial issues and there are your own frustrations and they are very clear about what they think of you. And that's quite daunting because in one instance you are working with a very strong, serious issue and the person had a lot of stuff about me as a human being and impacted on me quite significantly on reflection. And also to realize that you have to separate out what's the client's stuff and what is true about your performance.

Newly graduated therapists can learn from clients as they often obtain feedback on the quality and effectiveness of their practice. Where the client is encouraged to participate in clinical decision-making with the treating team, he or she could be considered to be a central member of the community of practice. Clients, therefore, could also be viewed as members of the community of practice, though peripheral ones as they often do not fully understand the language used by other members. In this respect, membership of the community of practice is not only restricted to health professionals. Rather, it can incorporate others who experience a sense of understanding and belonging.

Experiencing learning within the organisation

Features of the workplace play a significant part in influencing what and how the newly graduated therapists learn. As all five newly graduated therapists participating in the study commenced their careers in very different communities of practice, the reported learning by the five therapists also differed.

The five therapists described marked variation in their communities of practice. One community of practice had very stable and experienced staff and the newly graduated therapist worked very closely with these therapists and the clients of the unit. Two of the newly graduated therapists had extremely varied caseloads. One worked half-time in an acute psychiatric unit and the other half of the time in a community rehabilitation centre, treating outpatients with a variety of physical conditions. The other therapist worked in a small regional hospital and spent her mornings as a member of the medical unit team. The afternoons for this therapist were spent performing home visits for community patients, assessing and treating paediatric and hand injury outpatients and providing an occupational therapy service to residents of a nursing home. After six months and discussions with her manager/supervisor, a more experienced therapist took over the services to the nursing home. The newly graduated therapist reported that her caseload had been too complex, particularly the associated administration:

> At times [it's] been a bit overwhelming and just getting the paperwork done. That was another part that I got sheltered from in student placements and just having to cope with all the extra paperwork but it's actually got easier.

Learning the language and how to work within a team were frequently reported as being very challenging initially for the newly graduated therapists. To move from being a peripheral member of the multidisciplinary team or community of practice, the newly graduated therapist needed to understand fully the language and the roles of the other team members. The newly graduated therapists working in the rural hospital commented that understanding the language was:

> … a big issue, a big difficulty … even in terms of diagnosis and like all the medical terms, coming to grips with all those things … I got a bit lost, but the nursing staff up on the ward are really helpful.

Mentors and supervisors can also assist new therapists to identify learning opportunities external to their workplace to consolidate and expand their knowledge and skills, as is suggested here:

> I think we have a fairly close working relationship as most places do, with the physiotherapy department in particular here. And the Chief Physio is very supportive and depending upon who is working on the wards, we try and do allied health in-services as well as just occupational therapy in-services … I think I gained a lot of value from interacting with other teams members and actually learning from them as well.

Senior members of the community of practice also have a role in teaching the new members of the team the customs or values of the workplace. An example of this may be the way team meetings are conducted. There may be a certain order in which team members report the progress of their patients or clients, or there may be an allocation of time for discussion of each patient during ward round. Standards of dress, preferences for report writing formats or allocation of car parking may also be covert features of a community of practice so that an outsider would not necessarily be aware of them upon first commencing work.

Learning from practice and participation in everyday work tasks was the most effective method of learning reported by newly graduated therapists. They reported that they had learnt the theory in their undergraduate preparation and then had to learn how to apply this theory when they entered the workforce. One newly graduated therapist remarked that:

... with practice, you get more understanding than you would, say, just reading a textbook, so you get a wider experience than the previous experience that you've had.

Clearly, they no longer wanted to learn from formal tools such as textbooks. Rather, at this stage, they preferred learning from engagement in the community of practice and/or the workplace.

Discussion: Implications for workplace practice and policy

While health professional managers and supervisors may understand the importance of having formal supervision in place, other more informal features of the workplace have not been maximised to enhance learning. One of the major aspects overlooked is the degree of social learning that occurs and how much this is valued by the newly graduated practitioners. Learning from other health professionals is one example of the social learning that is not routinely acknowledged or managed.

Newly graduated practitioners are very aware that they depend greatly upon senior allied health, nursing and medical staff to orientate them to their new communities of practice. Indeed, it is these more senior people who share their knowledge with the new graduate through vehicles such as team meetings, ward rounds, journal clubs and report writing. Through these activities, they introduce the newly graduated therapist to the language, and therefore the culture, of the community of practice. Although other members of a community of practice assist the new practitioner with the transition from being a peripheral member to a central member through such sharing, it is the manager who has the most significant role. While feelings of overwhelmed anxiety are not uncommon for newly graduated practitioners, their supervisor or manager can do a lot to ensure that they are kept within their zone of proximal development.

The novice professional needs to become competent and confident in performing the routine tasks of the community of practice before they are expected to manage the complex tasks that require a high degree of clinical reasoning. The supervisor, therefore, observes the junior practitioner's work and checks with the more central members of the community of practice to determine their competency and success. Based on this information, the supervisor is then able to provide the adequate support, guidance and teaching need by the newly graduated practitioner. As the new therapist learns more from the other members of the community of practice, the support framework from the supervisor and colleagues can be gradually decreased.

Acquisition of supervision skills by senior therapists cannot be assumed. Supervising newly graduated therapists is different from supervising students because the relationship is one of support for another colleague. Both the newly graduated therapist and senior therapist providing the supervision need to understand the importance of regular and high quality supervision. A level of trust and rapport needs to be established to enable the newly graduated therapist to raise concerns and identify areas that require further learning and practice. Further continuing professional development activities focusing on supervision practices would be beneficial for both experienced and inexperienced supervisors.

Reliance upon other health professionals is particularly required when the newly graduated practitioner's supervisor is not a member of their professional community of practice. Indeed, the newly graduated professional may require two supervisors when working in sole or generic positions: one supervisor who is a member of the community of practice and another supervisor who is from their home discipline. What is important to remember is that other health professionals who provide support, learning and feedback to the newly graduated practitioner also need support and acknowledgement of their role in assisting a new member in their transition to the team.

As has been mentioned in the literature, unrealistic expectations of supervisors may arise from the newly graduated therapists expecting the same supervision and support as was afforded to them as students. Undergraduate clinical placements need to be realistic. No aspects of a health professional's role should be overlooked or viewed as unsuitable for a final year student to engage in. Students needed to be supported and supervised in areas where they may not be fully competent; however they need to be fully aware of what is involved in all aspects of practice.

Conclusion

Through greater understanding and awareness of how the workplace can enhance learning, newly graduated practitioners can maximise their learning potential with assistance from their managers, colleagues and team members. Research findings have identified strategies that can be effectively utilised within the workplace to support and ensure newly graduated practitioners such as occupational therapists continue their lifelong learning. Strategies such as utilising feedback and supervision from other members of the community of practice and providing opportunities for the less experienced clinicians to observe senior practitioners that may be from the home or other disciplines are very useful tools of learning. Supporting communities of practice and making known the tools of learning that exist within them, would be beneficial to both newly graduated practitioners and their supervisors or managers.

References

Adamson, B., Harris, L., Heard, R. & Hunt, A. (1996). *University Education and Workplace Requirements. Evaluating the Skills and Attributes of Health Science Graduates.* Lidcombe: The University of Sydney.

Atkinson, K. & Stewart, B. (1997). A Longitudinal Study of Occupational Therapy New Practitioners in their First Years of Professional Practice: Preliminary Findings. *British Journal of Occupational Therapy, 60*(8), 338–342.

Billett, S. (1994). Situated Learning — A Workplace Experience. *Australian Journal of Adult and Community Education, 34,* 112–130.

Billett, S. (1998). Understanding workplace learning: Cognitive and sociocultural perspectives. In D. Boud (Ed.), *Current Issues and New Agendas in Workplace Learning*. Leabrook: National Centre for Vocational Education Research Ltd.

Billett, S. (1999). Experts' ways of knowing. *Australian Vocational Education Review, 6*, 25–36.

Billett, S. (2000). Guided learning at work. *Journal of Workplace Learning, 12*(7), 272–285.

Copeland, K. (1998). Supervision requirements: Perspectives from graduate occupational therapists. *Reflections, Perceptions and Directions. Preparing for Practice in Occupational Therapy and Beyond. A Collection of Papers by Final Year Charles Sturt University Occupational Therapy Students, Charles Sturt University*, Albury.

Cracknell, E. (1981). Clinical Placements and First Appointments. *British Journal of Occupational Therapy, 44*, 149–151.

Davis, J. & Polatajko, H. (2004). Occupational Development. In C. Christiansen and E. Townsend (Eds), *Introduction to Occupation. The Art and Science of Living* (91–101). New Jersey: Pearson Education Inc.

Dewey, J. (1938). *Experience and Education*. New York: The Macmillan Co.

Greeno, J., Moore, J. & Smith, D. (1993). Transfer of situated learning. In D. K. Detterman & R. J. Sternbert (Eds), *Transfer on Trial: Intelligence, Cognition, and Instruction*. Norwood, NJ: Ablex.

Hitch, D. (1998). Stretching the Boundaries of Occupational Therapy: A new graduate experience within a disability environment service. Paper presented at *Victorian Occupational Therapy Conference*, Melbourne.

Hummell, J. & Koelmeyer, L. (1999). New graduates' perceptions of their first occupational therapy position. *British Journal of Occupational Therapy, 62*, 351–358.

Jenkins, M. & Brotherton, C. (1995a). In search of a theoretical framework for practice, Part 1. *British Journal of Occupational Therapy, 58*, 280–285.

Jenkins, M. & Brotherton, C. (1995b). In search of a theoretical framework for practice, Part 2. *British Journal of Occupational Therapy, 58*, 332–336.

Jenkins, M. & Brotherton, C. (1995c). Implications of a theoretical framework for practice. *British Journal of Occupational Therapy, 58*, 392–396.

Landsdowne, J. (1989). To rotate or not to rotate: That is the question. *British Journal of Occupational Therapy, 52*, 4–7.

Lave, J. & Wenger, E. (1991). *Situated learning. Legitimate peripheral participation*. New York: Cambridge University Press.

Lee, S. & Mackenzie, L. (2003). Starting out in rural New South Wales: The experiences of new graduate occupational therapists. *Australian Journal of Rural Health, 11*, 36–43.

Leonard, C. & Corr, S. (1998). Sources of stress and coping strategies in basic grade occupational therapists. *British Journal of Occupational Therapy, 61*, 257–262.

McKinstry, C. (2003) Enhancing workplaces to maximise learning for newly graduated occupational therapists. OT AUSTRALIA 22nd National Conference, Melbourne 6–9, April 2003.

Parker, C. (1991). The needs of newly qualified occupational therapists. *British Journal of Occupational Therapy, 54*, 164–168.

Rugg, S. (1996). The transition of junior occupational therapists to clinical practice: Report of a preliminary study. *British Journal of Occupational Therapy, 59*, 165–168.

Rugg, S. (1999). Factors influencing junior occupational therapists' continuity of employment. A review of the literature. *British Journal of Occupational Therapy, 62*, 151–156.

Ryrie, I., Williams, H., Wamsley, R. & Dwyer, J. (2000). Basic grade occupational therapists: A descriptive evaluation of a community rotation scheme. *British Journal of Occupational Therapy, 63*, 399–404.

Strauss, A. & Corbin, J. (1998). *Basics of qualitative research: Techniques and procedures for developing grounded theory*. Thousand Oaks: SAGE Inc.

Sutton, G. & Griffin, A. (2000). Transition from student to practitioner: The role of expectations, values and personality. *British Journal of Occupational Therapy, 63*, 380–388.

Sweeney, G., Webley, P. & Treacher, A. (2001a). Supervision in occupational therapy, Part 1: The supervisor's anxieties. *British Journal of Occupational Therapy, 64*, 337–345.

Sweeney, G., Webley, P. & Treacher, A. (2001b). Supervision in occupational therapy, Part 2: The supervisee's dilemma. *British Journal of Occupational Therapy, 64*, 380–386.

Tennant, M. (2000). Learning to work, working to learn. In C. Symes & J. McIntyre (Eds), *Working Knowledge. The New Vocationalism and Higher Education.* Buckingham: Open University Press.

Toulouse, J. & Williams, S. (1984). First appointments: A survey of influencing factors. *British Journal of Occupational Therapy, 47,* 111–113.

Tryssenaar, J. (1999). The lived experience of becoming an occupational therapist. *British Journal of Occupational Therapy, 62,* 107–112.

Tryssenaar, J. & Perkins, J. (1999). From student to therapist: Exploring the first year of practice. *The American Journal of Occupational Therapy, 55,* 19–27.

Vygotsky, L. (1978). *Mind in Society: The Development of Higher Psychological Processes.* Cole, M., John-Steiner, V., Scribner, S. & Souberman, E. (Eds). Cambridge MA: Harvard University Press.

Wenger, E. (1998). *Communities of Practice: Learning, Meaning and Identity,* Cambridge: Cambridge University Press.

Wenger, E., McDermott, R. & Snyder, W. (2002). *Cultivating Communities of Practice.* Boston: Harvard Business School Press.

CHAPTER NINE

Challenges of Case Management

Rebecca Allen

KEY WORDS

Service co-ordination

Case management

Organisational context

Management structures

Chapter Profile

In previous chapters, professional issues with respect to knowledge generation, autonomy, utilisation of research and accountability have been explored. This chapter, however, critically analyses case management as a model of professional practice increasingly adopted with health and human service organisations which is founded upon the assumption of a generic skill base amongst professionals in specified settings. Case management is a process of co-ordinating service delivery and the roles associated with it provide numerous challenges to those working within its parameters. This chapter will discuss some of these challenges and will overview current practices and definitions of case management. An outline of some of the professional and consumer concerns about case management are presented before the chapter concludes with a review of key issues now and in the future.

Introduction

Case management is an approach to service delivery that is practised in a wide range of government, non-government and private health and human service organisations internationally. Case management is usually defined as a process of overseeing and co-ordinating the services that a particular client receives, and is generally regarded as a means of improving a client's access to services as well as obtaining and managing the resources required by the client.

While case management is a central feature of many aspects of human service delivery, it is not necessarily well understood. Case management is practised very differently depending on the workplace or service area and the funding arrangements of that workplace. Given the widespread use of case management in health and human services, it is likely that all health-care practitioners will be interacting with or working within case management systems at some stage in their careers. Hence, some understanding of the assumptions and expectations of case management will potentially be of relevance to all practitioners.

This chapter explores some of the challenges of case management. It discusses current practices and definitions of case management with some comment on the way case management operates in different services. The discussion also outlines some of the professional and consumer concerns about case management, and the challenges and criticisms of case management as a process, and gives some consideration throughout to the opportunities, benefits and effective strategies in the practice of case management.

Concept and definitions of case management

Case management is an approach that traditionally involves an identified worker taking responsibility for the co-ordination of services required by a client. However, it is also a term that is used to describe a co-ordinated process of care. The origins of case management are often traced to the work of charitable organisations in the US in the 19th century, where programs for the poor and sick began to establish systems to document need, co-ordinate care and account for resources used (Dill, 2001). Case management became established as an entity in service delivery in the 1970s and 1980s in a number of countries. It appears to have become popular for two main reasons. First, it was recognised that the proliferation and fragmentation of services in the community created barriers to access to services for clients. Case management in mental health, for example, followed the deinstitutionalisation of people with a mental illness. It was particularly important to assist those people who, due to their long periods within institutions, had little experience in negotiating the maze of community services they now needed to survive in the community (Onyett, 1998). Second, the concern about the increasing cost of service delivery and the need for cost containment became evident, particularly in the health-care system, and case management provided a system of managing and containing the interventions a client receives. The case management model of service delivery was described in the 1990s as being somewhat in vogue internationally (Loomis, 1992) and all pervasive (Austin & McClelland, 1996).

Since this time, it has become even more prevalent in a range of human service environments. Case management is the method of service delivery that is chosen by many health, aged care, acute care, rehabilitation, long-term care, disability services, corrections, employment, workers' compensation and insurance services. It has grown exponentially along with the proliferation of human service organisations.

Case management has been described as a process that makes the system work for the client (Rossi, 1999). The case manager has been described as the person who makes the system work, ensuring both the quality of the outcome for the client and containment of the cost of care (Mullahy, 1998a). Case management is also often described as a way of better co-ordinating services for a client who has complex needs. The case management process assumes that clients may have little knowledge of the range of services that are available to them and the process involved to access them. Services can be fragmented and difficult to access because they span administrative or institutional boundaries (Office of the Public Advocate, 1992). However, as case management has become more prevalent, the complexity or otherwise of the clients' needs or the service delivery system are no longer defining features. Case management has simply become the usual way of business for a great many services for all clients, whatever their needs. Case management has become such an accepted modus operandi that it has been suggested that the "preoccupation with case management, and the all encompassing nature of the concept have led to other individualised service delivery approaches being devalued or recategorised to fit a case management label" (Duransky, Harvey & Kennedy, 2003, p 2003). For example, some clinical services have turned their attention from providing therapeutic interventions to case management interventions, and some well functioning models of multidisciplinary service delivery in acute inpatient services are being described as case management. This is probably not surprising given that the rise of case management has occurred in the context of increased managerialism of health and human services. That is, case management has developed at the same time as the increasing demand for efficiency and cost effectiveness of human services, of concern for administrative and accountability systems, for risk management and documented systems of quality improvement and the increased prominence of management control of clinical aspects of service delivery. By definition, case management fits well within this environment.

The key features of case management have been described as "individualised service delivery based on comprehensive assessment that is used to develop a case or service plan. The plan is developed in collaboration with clients and reflects their choices and preferences for the service arrangements being developed. The goal is to empower clients and ensure they are involved in all aspects of the planning and service arrangement in a dynamic way" (Case Management Society of Australia, n.d.). This definition incorporates two key elements that are generally seen in case management descriptions. That is, there is an individualised service plan and this plan is created in collaboration with the client. Case management is generally promoted as being client-centred. It attempts to place clients and their needs central to the decision-making and service provision (Krupa & Clark, 1995).

145

While the focus of case management is described as improving services for the client, there can be tension between client care and fiscal management, and the focus of case management at times appears to be more on cost containment than on client need. The two, of course, are not mutually exclusive. However, what a case manager does, or what the case management process entails, depends very much on the organisation in which it is being practised. For example, the terms "case management" and "managed care" have at times been used interchangeably in the United States (Powell, 2000) and this contributes to the confusion about the intent of case management in some environments. The goal of managed care is to encourage more effective and economical use of health-care resources by consumers (Powell). That is, managed care is explicitly about resources management at a systems level. Case management, however, is focused on client need, being a process of negotiating the various provider systems for the people receiving the service (Powell). In general, case management has had a greater association with the containment of costs in countries such as the US, because of that country's reliance on a user pay system of health, than it has had in other countries, where there are varying levels of national health insurance systems in place. Hence, discussions of case management from the US will necessarily emphasise the management of costs. Wherever it is practised, definitions and discussion of case management retain a determinedly client focus. However, balancing client need with obtaining or containment of resources for care remains a central concern for the person or people operating as case managers.

The practice of case management

Organisations bring to case management their own particular interpretation of the process. Hence, the way case management operates changes according to the organisational brief. It will also change according to the needs of the client, and as will be discussed later, it will change according to the focus of the person providing the case management service. A range of approaches to case management have been documented to describe more specifically the focus of the intervention and the role of the case manager in the case management process. Broadly, case management approaches can be described as those that primarily provide service brokerage and those that primarily provide clinical interventions. Brokerage describes approaches to case management where the case manager's role is a manager or broker of resources to ensure the client has access to needed services. The case manager may determine and co-ordinate the services the client is to receive but not provide any direct services themselves (Clark & Fox, 1993). At the opposite end of the spectrum, clinical case management is an extension of clinical or therapeutic interventions, where the case manager's role is to work directly with the client, providing therapeutic services, as well as assisting the client to access and link to community agencies and services. Some case management approaches also convey a particular philosophy or strategy of care. For example, the "strengths model" (Rapp, 1994) seeks to empower and focus on the strengths of the client, rather than the problems or deficits traditionally the focus of service provider attention. There are increasing descriptions in the literature of the models or approaches as case management evolves and is adapted for various client issues, funding arrangements and service structures (see, for example, Cohen & Costa, 2001; Mullahy, 1998b; Rossi, 1999). Steve Onyett, a key author on mental health case management, suggests that describing case management approaches in detail is important as it allows measurement of outcomes, costing of the approach and facilitates dissemination of the ideas (Onyett, 1998). In order to consider the best practice features of case management, there needs to be a great deal of clarity about what case management is considered to be, and this is particularly so as its practice is so different. Hence, case management needs to be considered carefully before being applied to new environments.

Despite the differences in approaches to case management, there is broad agreement about the central process or steps in case management. The way these steps are carried out will vary enormously.

Intake and assessment

Case managers generally have a "screening" or "gate-keeping" role. That is, the case manager determines a client's eligibility to receive services from the organisation providing the case management service. The case manager also assesses the client's needs by gathering information from the client, family, carers and other service providers. Assessment involves identifying the client's strengths and weakness, problems and skills. This may require case managers seeking formal assessments from a range of service providers, or they may undertake some of these assessments themselves.

Planning

A service plan is developed with the client on the basis of needs assessment which includes short and long-term goals and objectives, locating appropriate service providers and developing time-lines for expected outcomes. Service planning can be considered the crux of case management as it involves the organisation of programs and services that reflect the client's identified needs, preferences and strengths (Raiff & Shore, 1993).

Implementation

Some case managers will provide direct services or "hands on" intervention. Others will "broker" services and resources, that is, identify and ensure other service providers implement the service. Generally, the case manger will provide a counselling and support role to assist clients to make the required links and to support their continuing participation in these services.

Monitoring

The case manager's role in ensuring the client continues to receive effective and optimal intervention is crucial. The case manager will ensure that formal or informal service agreements are in place. He or she will also monitor the appropriateness of services, the effectiveness of the intervention and the client's overall progress and ongoing needs.

Case closure and evaluation

Case management generally operates on the assumption that there will be an end point to the case manager's role. In some systems, case managers will maintain a role in the long term. However, the case management process requires review of outcomes, consideration of the need for future services and determination of action to be taken should the client require services in the future.

The case manager operates as an advocate for the client throughout this process. Advocacy is frequently cited as a core feature of case management and a necessary element throughout (Raiff & Shore, 1993). Advocacy is necessary at a number of levels. Case managers may need to work towards changing processes internal to their own organisation as well as to assist clients to gain access to external facilities and resources (Rothman & Sager, 1998). Advocacy may be required at a systems level whereby gaps in service are identified but it may also be required more broadly by lobbying and negotiating for the general target population (Office of the Public Advocate, 1992).

As previously noted, the way that a case manager carries out the process of case management will vary according to organisational and individual differences. Caseloads vary dramatically and will necessarily influence the level of involvement a case manager has with each client. In addition, services differ in whether or not the case manager has budgetary control, and this impacts on the way the case manager obtains services for the clients. Some case managers will be operating within a pre-determined budget, others will be required to seek out the financial resources necessary for the interventions they agree are needed for their client, while others will be operating within environments where they have no direct access to funding. To illustrate these points, a case manager with 120 clients on the caseload who works for an insurance company may primarily work as a broker of services, emphasising the management and organisation of care, and be required to seek efficient case closure in the short term. Alternatively, a case manager providing intensive outreach work for 10 people experiencing long term mental ill-health may focus on establishing an ongoing supportive therapeutic relationship with the client, locating and fostering community supports and providing long-term monitoring and support for the client.

Each element of the case management process requires the case manager to use a high level of communication and negotiation skills. These advanced skills are needed since case management planning cuts across agency and professional boundaries and case managers need to consider a wide breadth of needs areas. For example, a resource guide for Australian mental health workers (Human Services Victoria, 1998) suggests that case managers should consider the following areas of need in assessment and planning:

- emotional and mental wellbeing;
- dealing with stress;
- personal response to illness;

- personal safety and the safety of others;
- friendships and social relationships;
- work and productive activities;
- leisure;
- education;
- daily living skills;
- the family's response to their relative's illness;
- income;
- physical health;
- housing; and
- rights and advocacy.

Mullahy (1998a) suggested that case managers require broad base knowledge to be effective stating that "they need to be part general practitioner, social worker, psychologist, minister or rabbi" (p 9). A range of additional professional practice areas could be added to this list.

While it is generally assumed that a client will be allocated one case manager in a service to give him or her a central point of contact, a team approach to case management has also been described. A team approach considers that the whole team is responsible for ensuring the client receives a co-ordinated and well-managed service (Clark & Fox, 1993). The team approach is valuable as the client is assured of assistance even when the identified case manager is not available. The team approach assists clinicians to spread the load of working with clients who require a high level of support and input from a case manager and can potentially reduce practitioner burnout (Clark & Fox). Some teams have also successfully included service consumers as "peer specialists" to enhance the case management process. Consumer team members can take significant roles in representing clients' perspectives to the team and have contributed to improved quality of life and consumer outcomes in mental health case management (Felton et al, 1995).

The term case management has also been used to describe a system of care. For example, case management has been used to describe the system of care in acute health and rehabilitation services where critical pathways are established to determine practitioner input, client length of stay and anticipated outcomes. This process has been associated with improved outcomes from team members' perspectives, an increase in the consistency and timeliness of care as well as reduced cost (Latini, 1998). Perhaps one of the key advantages of using a case management process in this environment is that usual clinical service delivery is overlaid with a system of management that attempts to ensure that all interventions are co-ordinated and provided in timely sequence. The client receives the interventions when they are considered to be most effective and the process ensures that necessary elements of intervention are not missed.

The process of case management has also been used by some professional groups to describe the core organisational elements of their intervention. For example, Hagedorn (1995) describes case management as integral to an occupational therapist's practice. Hagedorn uses the term case management to replace the term "occupational therapy process" when describing the core treatment planning process. This process is not unique to one profession as it is basically a problem-solving or analytical process that is used by most health-care practitioners (Hagedorn). Mayer (1998) suggests that case management has a practical use as a philosophic "mindset" of patient care delivery that has relevance for all patients in all environments.

Challenges of case management

The client or consumer experience of being "case managed" is one that is under-explored. However, what is well documented is that the somewhat bureaucratic assumptions in the language of case management have not been considered to be all that palatable by some consumers and service providers. Service consumers have reacted to the objectification implied in the use of the term "case". The term has been described as being "redolent of outdated attitudes ... no-one likes to be thought of as a case, and most people do not want to be managed" (McDonald, 1989, p 39). Some of the greatest criticism of the term has come from the mental health sector, where there is ongoing discussion about the appropriate terminology for people who make use of the mental health system. A range of alternative terms have been used to describe case management. For example "care co-ordinator", "keyworker" and "service co-ordinator" are more acceptable in some areas of practice. Some disability support workers in Australia have likened the case management role to being a "navigator" of services, and refer to themselves in these terms. "Care management" has been preferred in the UK because the term case was considered offensive to those using services (Burns, 1997).

While case management approaches are philosophically client-centred, like other areas of health practice, it is only in recent years that this claim has been tested with clients. For example, a study by Crane-Ross, Roth and Lauber (2000) of mental health case management indicated that case managers and clients had very different views about how well client needs were being met by case management. These authors suggested that service providers may be overestimating the effectiveness of their services and that attempts to increase consensus could be enhanced by changing the philosophy in services so that clients are seen as "treatment team leaders" rather than "treatment recipients".

Another example of the unequal relationship between case manager and client is that clients usually do not choose their case manager, nor usually given the opportunity to review case managers' expertise in the detail that they are reviewed by the case manager. A service may allocate clients on the basis of worker caseload, case manager preference or skill in working with particular issues, however the client would not usually have this choice.

The relationship formed between the case manager and the client is a significant aspect of the case management process, particularly so with clinical approaches to case management. Case managers may be expected to do "whatever it takes" to support their client, and may often form intense and long-term relationships (Williams & Swartz, 1998). An understanding of counselling and therapy is integral to case management work (Williams & Swartz), however these skills are not necessarily part of a case manager's repertoire. Onyett (1998) observes that case management is not meant to be a life sentence. However for some people, case management is a long-term relationship and for many, this relationship is a key to their progress. Navarro (1998) has suggested that there is great potential for dependency to occur in such relationships. She suggests that the reliance on a "a two-person relationship as the fundamental basis of therapeutic practice" is inherently problematic as other workers often behave as if it is only the case manager who understands the client. Hence, in the absence of the client's case manager, the client loses access to an effective service. At a practical level, this two person relationship has two obvious problems — the case manager cannot always be available when the client needs support and clients requiring long-term case management support will have a series of case managers with the potential for numerous losses (Navarro). Each time the case manager changes, for the client the experience can be like "I am losing a friend" (UW, personal communication, 17 September 2003).

Figure 9.1: I am not making a lot of progress

"I sometimes feel like I am training case managers for this system. You get a good relationship established and finally get through that getting to know you phase, and then they are off to further their career or whatever. So here am I going over my story again, explaining why their new idea has been tried before, and telling them about the tricks of working around the impediments in the system. Sometimes I enjoy feeling like I am contributing to their development, but then I remember that I am the person supposedly getting the help here, and each time one of them moves on, it reminds me that I am not making a lot of progress."

(VX, personal communication, 8 January 2004)

Case management positions are usually "generic", that is, those who work as case managers may come from any professional or non-professional background. Case management is currently being provided by professionals including general practitioners, nurses, occupational therapists, physiotherapists, psychologists and social workers. Many of these professions have claimed they have special attributes that make them good case managers or that their profession has a philosophical alignment with case management to justify taking on case management roles (see, for example, Hafez & Brockman, 1998; Fisher, 1996). In many ways, it is not surprising that many professions have sought case management roles. These roles have been liberating for many professionals previously working in traditional health-care teams, as case management roles can provide greater breadth of responsibility and autonomy than more traditional clinical roles. However, different professions will bring differing models of health and illness, different value systems and different approaches and beliefs about what constitutes effective intervention to case management. Hence, case management will change according

151

to the focus of the person providing the case management service. The difference in case manager orientation can be disguised by the generic title of case manager.

Whether or not case management requires a professional background has been a topic of concern in the past, and the cost effectiveness of using professionals as case managers has been queried. For example, Rapp and Chamberlain (1985) suggested the system cannot afford "to use expensive, highly trained, experienced professionals as case managers" (p 422) and recommended that paraprofessionals who have no specific clinical skills but could have management skills would provide good case management services. However Schwartz, Goldman and Churgin (1982) suggested that good case managers require substantial clinical knowledge, skills and judgement even if they are not providing a direct clinical service. The need to have the expertise to manage the relationship in case management skilfully is also vital (Williams & Swartz, 1998). Furthermore, it has been suggested that paraprofessional case managers may not have the adequate assessment skills required to identify accurately clients' needs (Holloway, 1991) or the professional standing to have their opinions heard (Bachrach, 1993). Case managers also need to have an ability to understand and work with the differing philosophies in organisations, a role rather eloquently described by Rothman and Sager (1998) as spanning the "sometimes inhospitable borders between clinically oriented direct practice professionals and those with community organisation or administrative commitments" (p 13). Given this, some case managers report that it is to their advantage to promote their professional background as it enables them to be more effective as case managers.

Figure 9.2: I am a professional too

"Some people just think I am a 'pen-pusher', that is, simply someone who approves the budget. I find it helps if I make sure that health professionals know that I have a professional background too and I often make a point of including that in my introduction. This means they are more likely to communicate with me as an equal, and become more open about their recommendations. Ultimately this leads to a better outcome all round."

(JR, personal communication, 18 November 2003)

Along with the enthusiasm among professional groups to take on case management roles, there has been debate in some professions, for example in occupational therapy, as to whether the profession will lose their profession-specific skills if they do (Krupa & Clark, 1995).

Figure 9.3: Don't forget your role

"I don't think new graduates should work in this area. They need to consolidate their professional role first, and get some sense of the possibilities and options available for clients. I have seen some case managers become entirely focussed on the management aspects of the job — and that is very easy to do because the amount of regulation of our work. You cannot forget though that we have a therapeutic role. The relationships with multiple stakeholders mean you need to be very sensitive to a range of needs."

(JR, personal communication, 18 November 2003)

As increasing numbers of health professionals are moving into case management positions, this issue of the potential loss of profession-specific expertise would benefit from some further debate and discussion. Furlong (1997) suggested that "recasting" professionals as case managers is a strategy that aims to limit the discretion of professionals and to increase practitioner adherence to management decisions. Whereas professionalism gives autonomy and independence beyond the boundary of the agency, a case manager loses this autonomy, and greater control of their work is possible (Furlong). This view is particularly pertinent in the current environment where there are increasing demands both for professional accountability and strategies to regulate practice in order to increase certainty in the delivery of health and human services. However, while case management began as a process to manage the delivery of care, it is now developing very rapidly to a point where it is being presented as a profession in its own right. Significant in this increasing professionalism has been the establishment of professional bodies including the American Case Management Association, the Case Management Society of America and the Case Management Society of Australia. The impact of professionalisation on the role and allegiances of case managers remains to be seen.

Case management as a balancing act

Another challenge of case management is that health practitioners moving into case management roles often face the dilemma of balancing two disparate needs: the needs of the client or consumer and the needs of their organisation. As case management is often practised in profit-making services, a case manager needs to consider how to deliver the best possible service, as well as to ensure that service delivery remains profitable. Many practitioners who previously only focused on patient needs now need to consider the financial survival of their service (Joe, 1995). In the current environment, there is little argument that all practitioners must consider the cost and the cost effectiveness of intervention. However, what might be considered best for the client may not provide the best returns for the organisation. Some case managers create their own strategies for managing this dilemma. For example, it is not unknown in some systems for case managers to describe the client's need in terms that will fit the service brief, while it may in fact not strictly do this, in order to ensure the delivery of a service they believe the client needs. Hence the case manager's professional decision-making may override the restrictions of the organisation's guidelines.

Figure 9.4: It seems pretty unethical

"Maybe the client has personal reasons why they can't focus on return to work. For example their husband or one of their children might be really ill and so their concern and time is entirely taken up with the family. In this kind of case I'll report that the client is making maximum effort. It's a judgement call. From my perspective it is reasonable that the life issue be attended to before the client gets on with their own return to work rehabilitation. This explanation might not be acceptable to the insurer who wants the client back to work in the shortest time possible, but I think this is about being realistic and likely to have a better outcome in the long term."

(DR, personal communication, 30 December 2003)

"Our service was meant to only provide assessment and refer onwards for all therapy intervention. There are lots of times though when it seemed ridiculous for me not to provide some basic service. Especially when I know that that the client would have to go on to a waiting list if I didn't take some action. So sometimes I would see a client a few times and record it as assessment activity. We all do it, although it is not really discussed openly. It seems pretty unethical not to take some action when you know a little thing can make a huge difference in a client's life. I rationalise it by telling myself that funding for our assessment service comes out of the same pot as funding for the therapy services."

(NM, personal communication, 7 July 2003)

As well as balancing the needs of the client and the case manager's organisation, another challenge for case management is that some are "serving more than one master" when considering the client and this requires careful balancing of needs and interests. As observed by a case manager who works for a vocational rehabilitation service: "One of the problems for newer people coming into this system is that they become very focussed on the client, as in the injured worker. They forget that they need to consider they have other 'clients' as well. There is the insurer who is paying for the services the client receives, and there is the employer who may have major concerns that need to be addressed. You need to be able to balance these different demands as they are all 'the client'. You need to make sure there is a good outcome all round" (RB, personal communication, 16 February 2003).

A case manager aims to provide a central point of accountability within an increasingly dispersed service system. However, it has been suggested that case management would not be necessary if services were better designed and less inaccessible. In this vein, case management has long been criticised as indicating an inability of service planners and policy makers to create an integrated and co-ordinated service system (Rose & Black, 1985). Continuing from this criticism, defining case management as a service for clients with complex needs could be seen to place the "blame" on the client's "complexity" rather than on the real problem, which is the complexity of the service system. By creating case management as the core to service delivery, services shifted responsibility to the workers with the least power in the organisational structure, that is the "line worker" who is not in a position to influence service design or funding decisions (Rose & Black). Further, Rose and Black suggested that given their position within the system hierarchy, it is questionable as to whether case managers have the political and organisational power to manage a co-ordinated service plan which involves crossing the boundaries of various social service and mental health agencies. Concerns about the lack of power of case managers continue to be raised. For example, Furlong (1997) noted that in the mental health system in Australia, where a case management system has been introduced into clinical mental health services, doctors continued to maintain authority, and little changed except someone of lesser authority was given the title "case manager". Case managers in this situation cannot independently decide to provide hospitalisation for their clients and have been described as the least empowered workers in the service (Purtell & Dowling, as cited in Meadows & Singh, 2001). As some case managers have observed, they have substantial responsibility and little formal authority, but are someone to "blame" when there are problems.

Case management has been embraced enthusiastically as a service delivery system, and was implemented widely even as it was being described as being of questionable value (Marshall, Gray, Lockwood & Green, 2004) and of being a dubious, under-evaluated and ineffective practice (Marshall, 1995). Evaluations of case management are contradictory. They have shown it to increase rates of hospital admission and the cost of care, bringing about no clinically significant change in quality of life (Marshall, et al). They have also shown it to bring about positive changes such as reducing hospital admission (Ziguras & Stuart, 2000), improving quality of life and reducing the cost of people being discharged from hospital (Lim, Lambert & Gray, 2003). As with other areas of service delivery, more evidence is needed to support case management as an intervention, particularly from the perspective of the client receiving case management services.

Conclusion

The health and human service system is becoming more complex and more costly. Case management was implemented as a strategy to reduce complexity and to manage the costs of service delivery. It is an approach to service delivery that has been embraced enthusiastically by service planners and is now the cornerstone of service delivery in many sectors. Case management, however, places very high expectations on the role of the case manager. At one level, case management can be seen to be an extremely sensible response to problems in the human service system. It is difficult to argue that well co-ordinated service delivery is desirable, or that cost effective and efficient interventions are best. Whether those being case managed are quite so enthusiastic about the approach remains unclear.

References

Austin, C. D. & McClelland, R. W. (1996). Introduction to case management. Everybody's doing it. In C. D. Austin & R. W. McClelland (Eds), *Perspectives on Case management Practice*, pp 1–16. Milwaukee: Families International.

Bachrach, L. (1993). Continuity of care and approaches to case managment for long term mentally ill patients. *Hospital and Community Psychiatry, 35,* 465–468.

Burns, T. (1997). Case management, care management and care programming. *British Journal of Psychiatry, 170,* 393–395.

Case Management Society of Australia. (n.d.). *What is case management?* Accessed from http://www.cmsa.org.au/definition.html.

Clark, R. & Fox, T. (1993). A framework for evaluating the economic impact of case management. *Hospital and Community Psychiatry, 44,* 469–473.

Cohen, E. & Costa, T. (2001). *Nursing case management* (3rd ed.). St Louis: Mosby.

Crane-Ross, D., Roth, D. & Lauber, B. (2000). Consumers' and case managers' perspectives of mental health and community support service needs. *Community Mental Health Journal, 36,* 161–178.

Dill, A. (2001). *Managing to Care. Case management and service system reform.* New York: Aldine de Gruyter.

Felton, C., Stastney, P., Shern, D., Blanch, A., Donahue, S., Knight, E. et al. (1995). Consumers as peer specialists on intensive case management teams: impact on client outcomes. *Psychiatric Services, 46,* 1037–1044.

Fisher, T. (1996). Roles and functions of a case manager. *American Journal of Occupational Therapy, 50,* 452–454.

Furlong. M. (1997). How much care and how much control? Looking critically at case management. *Australian Journal of Primary Health-Interchange, 3*(4), 72–89.

Guransky, D., Harvey, J. & Kennedy, R. (2003). *Case management policy, practice and professional business.* Sydney: Allen & Unwin.

Hafez, A. & Brockman, S. (1998). Occupational therapists: Essential team members as service providers and case managers. *Journal of Care Management, 4*(2), 10–20.

Hagedorn, R. (1995). *Occupational perspectives and processes.* Edinburgh: Churchill Livingstone.

Holloway, F. (1991). Case management for the mentally ill: Looking at the evidence. *International Journal of Psychiatry, 37,* 2–13.

Human Services Victoria. (1998). *Victoria's mental health service resources for case managers. Individual service planning.* Melbourne: Aged, Community and Mental Health Division, Victorian Government Department of Human Services. Joe, B. (1995, October 12). Case managers confront managed care. *OT Week,* 14–15.

Krupa, T. & Clark, C. C. (1995). Occupational therapists as case managers: Responding to current approaches to community mental health service delivery. *Canadian Journal of Occupational Therapy 62,* 16–22.

Latini, E. (1998). Trauma critical pathways: A care delivery system that works. In C. Mullahy (Ed.), *Essential readings in case management,* pp 233–236, Maryland: Aspen Publishers.

Lim, W. K., Lambert, S. F. & Gray, L. C. (2003). Effectiveness of case management and post acute services in older people after hospital discharge. *MJA, 178*(6) 262–266.

Marshall, M. (1995). Case management: a dubious practice. Under-evaluated and ineffective, but now government policy. *British Medical Journal, 312,* 523–524.

Marshall M, Gray A, Lockwood A & Green R. (2004). Case management for people with severe mental disorders (Cochrane Review). In: *The Cochrane Library,* Issue 1. Chichester, UK: John Wiley & Sons, Ltd.

Mayer, G. (1996). Case management as a mindset. In C. Mullahy *Essential readings in case management, Quality management in healthcare, 5*(1), 7–16.

McDonald, R. (1989). The search for one-stop shopping. In M. Hubbard Linz, P. McAnally & C. Weick (Eds), *Case management: Historical, Current and future perspectives,* pp 39–46. Cambridge, MA: Brookline Books.

Meadows, G. & Singh, B. (Eds). (2001). *Mental health in Australia*. Melbourne: Oxford University Press.

Mullahy, C. (1998a). *The case manager's handbook* (2nd ed.). Maryland: Aspen.

Mullahy, C. (1998b). *Essential readings in case management*. Maryland: Aspen Publishers.

Navarro, T. (1998). Beyond keyworking. In A. Foster, V. Z. Roberts (Eds), *Managing mental health care in the community: Chaos and containment*, pp 141–153. London: Routledge.

Office of the Public Advocate. (1992). *Case management. A better approach to service delivery for people with disabilities*. Melbourne: Office of the Public Advocate.

Onyett, S. (1998). *Case management in mental health*. Case management in mental health. Cheltenham: Stanley Thornes Publishers Ltd.

Powell, S. (2000). *Case management. A practical guide to success in managed care* (2nd ed.). Philadelphia: Lippincott.

Raiff, N. & Shore, B. (1993). *Advanced case management*. Newbury Park: Sage Publications.

Rapp, C. & Chamberlain, R. (1985). Case management services for the mentally ill. *Social Work, 30*, 417–422.

Rapp, C. (1994). Theory, principle and methods of the strengths model of case management. In M. Harris & H. Bergman (Eds), *Case management for mentally ill patients: Theory and practice*, pp 143–164. Langhorne: Harwood Academic Publishers.

Rose, S. M. & Black, B. L. (1985). *Advocacy and empowerment*. Boston: Routledge & Kegan.

Rossi, P. (1999). *Case management in healthcare. A practical guide*. Philadelphia: WB Saunders.

Rothman, J. & Sager, J. S. (1998). *Case management. Integrating individual and community practice* (2nd ed.). Boston: Allyn & Bacon.

Schwartz, S., Goldman, H. & Churgin, S. (1982). Case management for the chronically mentally ill: Models and dimension. *Hospital and Community Psychiatry, 33*, 1006–1009.

Williams, J., & Swartz, M. (1998). Treatment boundaries in the case management relationship: A clinical case and discussion. *Community Mental Health Journal, 34*, 299–311.

Ziguras, S. & Stuart, G. (2000). A meta-analysis of the effectiveness of mental health case management over 20 years. *Psychiatric Services, 51*, 1410–1421.

CHAPTER TEN

Constructs of Allied Health: Making Considered Choices

Anne Cusick

Natasha Lannin

KEY WORDS

Identity

Interprofessional relations

Representation

Strategic planning

Workforce issues

Chapter Profile

Whereas other chapters in this book have tacitly included health professions as a collective grouping in the exploration of professional and practice issues, this chapter presents a critical discussion of allied health as a specific construct. Allied health is defined, described and deconstructed so that clear choices can be made by professions about allied health as a context for practice. To do this, the chapter explores six themes: allied health as a collection; the concept of allied health in chaos; customary uses; contradictions inherent in allied health; the challenge of allied health and individual professions with occupational therapy used as an example; and, finally, choices that can be made about the profession-allied health context relationship.

Introduction

Many professions are routinely described as "allied health". This description has been in common use since the 1960s (Committee to Study the role of Allied Health Personnel, 1989). It replaced the term "paramedical" which was previously applied most often during and following World War II, for example in occupational therapy (Anderson & Bell, 1988). Allied health has been a convenient way for the public, policy-makers, medical, nursing and non-health professions to categorise a range of diverse and distinct health professions. In spite of the common use, there is surprisingly little discussion or critical exploration of allied health in occupational therapy. Few textbooks index the term, research literature on occupational therapy and allied health is scant and most expert opinion derives from multidisciplinary panels often convened to inform policy rather than an occupational therapy knowledge base. This chapter explores the allied health context of occupational therapy first by critically analysing what it is, then exploring its attributes before finally considering what it means for occupational therapy in terms of choices that need to be made about the occupational therapy-allied health relationship.

Collection

There is an assumption that allied health professions "share a good deal of common ground" (Cole, 2002, p 2) which may encompass scope of practice, health care co-ordination and delivery, implications of government policy, funding, service accessibility issues, health-care priorities and common professional problems including identity and availability. There is also an assumption that the multidisciplinary nature of allied health is beneficial as it brings together "diverse skills and expertise to provide more effective, better co-ordinated, better quality services for clients" (Ducanis & Golin, 1979, p 1).

Allied health is a term that describes a collection of health professions and personnel grouped together in a systematic fashion. It is a convenient shorthand for professions that provide services in health which are distinct from nursing and medicine but beyond that may have little in common. The "allied health list" is a variable one and the diversity reflects the collective nature of the term. Like any collection, there is a need to identify and group particular items — in this case, professions. Like any collection, it changes, with new items being added and others discarded. As a collection, there needs to be some system for the grouping of items, and a purpose or audience that will make the collection meaningful.

Identifying, gathering and organising a collection of professions is a creative task. In any collection, there are collectors. In the case of allied health, they could comprise authors from any one of the professions, professional or government policy committees, hospital management teams or journalists. Someone needs to decide who, in any one instance, is "in or out" of the collection, its purpose and whether its benefits outweigh the demands of maintaining it. Within professions, opinion leaders make choices about whether or not to associate their group with the collective term allied health. Alternatively, outsiders can identify particular professions as belonging to allied health based on their views and preferences. Collectors themselves choose what allied health is and decide what attributes are needed to include a profession in the list. When that choice is made with a clear and unifying purpose in mind, the collection is meaningful. When there is no clear purpose, the collection risks fragmentation. Both clarity and fragmentation are apparent in allied health.

Concept in chaos

Allied health is a chaotic concept because of the continuous and situation-specific choice about whether or not to use it and who is "in or out". Little has changed since 1989 when it was identified that "there is not even consensus on what the term 'allied health means'" (Institute of Medicine/ National Academy of Sciences, 1989, p 336) and that "allied health was too complex and confusing an entity" (McTernan & Farber, 1989). Indeed, in a recent consumer guide to allied health, a commentator noted the mystery surrounding the utilisation of allied health as a term (Johnson, 2003).

Allied health has been proposed to be a "cluster" of professions and personnel (AMA Committee on allied health education and accreditation, 1987; Everson, 1999). A cluster, however, assumes "a close group or bunch of similar things growing together" (*Australian Concise Oxford Dictionary*, 1997, p 244). While allied health professions are no doubt continually growing and changing, the diversity of professions and personnel is so immense that even the most conservative of views suggests little similarity. If allied health is instead considered a "collection", as is proposed here, it helps to justify the term's lack of a consistent, precise definition. It also explains and legitimates the wild variation that occurs in professional listings of allied health, as collections do not require similarity. They can be fairly chaotic but still useful and meaningful.

Six types of allied health definition are apparent: lists that are related to policy; lists with categories; ad-hoc situation-specific lists; and definition by consensus, inclusion or exclusion. These are now described and examples provided.

Definition type 1

Allied health may be defined merely by lists collated in a pragmatic fashion for the general purpose of policy implementation. One North American example of this was cited by the Committee to Study the Role of Allied Health Personnel (1989). This involved the pragmatic formation of allied health coalitions as a result of federal programs designed to support allied health education: certain professions self-selected the allied health identity to obtain funding. Other examples from Australia demonstrate self-selection or top-down (usually government) inclusion in the allied health collection (Figure 10.1).

Figure 10.1: Pragmatic collections for policy implementation

Australian state or national government task forces and policy reports prov-ide examples of various allied health groups for the purpose of policy implementation. These include the National Allied Health Casemix Comm-ittee, the Allied Health Alliance and Allied Health Consultative Forum, Health Professions Council of Australia, the Australian Rural and Remote Allied Health Taskforce and National Allied Health Benchmarking Consortium. All these bodies include occupational therapy which is one of the largest professions represented. Other professions, such as audiology or nutrition, have variable membership.

Other lists are generated on an ad-hoc basis in reports designed to inform or influence policy, particularly policy relating to service provision and work-force planning. Membership and size of these pragmatic lists varies wildly (see Figure 10.2). These examples demonstrate that the size, scope and substance of allied health varies dramatically, and appears directly linked to the pragmatic purposes of the "list-makers".

Figure 10.2: Pragmatic collections for policy development

- The Council for Allied health in North Carolina, identified 100 occup-ational titles in allied health, and in Texas alone, 42 professions were cited as allied health (2003);

- The American Medical Association identifies 52 "verifiable" disciplines in allied health (http://www.ama-assn.org);

- The American Commission on Accreditation of Allied Health Education Programs accredits programs for 21 allied health professions although traditionally self-accrediting professions such as occupational therapy are excluded;

- the Institute of Medicine/National Academy of Sciences 1989 identified 10 representative allied health professions including clinical laboratory technologists, dental hygienists, dieticians, emergency medical personnel, medical record administrators, occupational therapists, physiotherapists, radiologic technologists, respiratory therapists, audiologists and speech pathologists;

- the Australian Institute of Health and Welfare collects allied health data on the basis of only three professions: podiatry, occupational therapy and physiotherapy (2003);

Pragmatic collections for policy development — *continued*

- Australian government population census data (Australian Bureau of Statistics, 2001);

- Individual authors vary in their allied health lists, for example, McTernan and Farber (1989) identified that allied health consisted of 85 small disciplines;

- The United Kingdom Department of Health (2000) identified 11 professions including arts therapists, chiropodists and podiatrists, dieticians, occupational therapists, orthoptists, paramedics, physiotherapists, prosthetists and orthotists, diagnostic radiographers, therapeutic radiographers, speech and language therapists;

- The Scottish National Health Service cites 13 professions making up the allied health workforce: arts therapists, drama therapists, music therapists, podiatrists, dieticians, occupational therapists, orthoptists, physiotherapists, prosthetists, orthotists, diagnostic radiographers, therapeutic radiographers, speech and language therapists.

Definition type 2

Some definitions of allied health list relatively arbitrarily and then categorise within the lists on the basis of particular features. Such features include: departmental affiliation; the relationship of the work to patient, laboratory, administration and community (Bureau of Health Manpower, 1967); job function such as primary care, health promotion or test work (National Commission on Allied Health Education); and whether or not, in the author's view, the professions are considered to be "traditional". For example, Smith and Crowley (1995) pronounced optometrists, physiotherapists, radiographers, podiatrists, occupational therapists, speech pathologists and dieticians as traditional allied health professions.

Definition type 3

Allied health definitions can also be entirely ad-hoc, based on the immediate and practical needs of the situation: for example those determined by management pronouncement as noted in organisational charts of hospitals or government health departments. Grouping individual professions together in something like an "allied health department" introduces another layer in organisational hierarchy. The creation of allied health departments was a common strategy in the 1980s (Duckett, 2000) and interestingly, most of the literature relating to allied health comes from the 1980s. This extra layer is often made to increase opportunities for consensual management through increased presence in decision-making and representation. These ad-hoc lists vary greatly. Figure 10.3 is one example which illustrates the ad-hoc nature of hospital allied health departments. While local variations in allied health may be expected, the lack of consistency is also apparent at a government level. For example, of eight 2003 state governments in Australia, six state health departments had identified allied health and relevant professions in their websites but none of them were the same. It ranged from 15 professions in the smallest state health department of Tasmania to only seven professions in Victoria, one of the largest states. At the national level, only six professions were identified in 2003 as allied health in the Commonwealth Department of Health. Although the range of professions included in these government lists varied considerably, occupational therapy, social work, physiotherapy, speech pathology and podiatry were consistently included.

Figure 10.3: Ad-hoc collections for health service management

One hospital described by Dawson (2001) exemplifies the ad-hoc and continuously changing nature of allied health: initially eight health professions (physiotherapy, occupational therapy, speech pathology, dieticians, social workers, podiatrists, pharmacists, hospital information management personnel) and untrained hospital volunteers were included in a new allied health grouping. This was then expanded with clinical psychologists, recreation therapists and catering staff. The group again grew with the addition of administrative functions of occupational health and safety, information technology, care planning and management of the hydrotherapy pool (Dawson). This allied health department is fairly typical of "on-the-ground" ad-hoc allied health arrangements. These are probably best characterised as allied health definition "by decree": as determinations are made using local processes to identify what is in and out of allied health, which are then confirmed through senior management authorisation of some kind.

Definition type 4

Some definitions of allied health bravely attempt consensus, and end up with a great deal of discussion but little precision in outcomes. For example, the AMACAHEA focused on the functions of professions and personnel, identifying that key functions included assisting or complementing the work of physicians or others. Another example is the North American National Commission on Allied Health Education which defined allied health as health practitioners who work towards common goals in care and health promotion (1980). Consensus attempts at definition can end up focusing more on the alliance aspect of allied health, seeing it as pragmatic collaboration which binds "together a disparate group of practitioners" (Committee to Study the Role of Allied Health Personnel, 1989, p 16).

Definition type 5

Consistent features or motivators can be used to identify groups which can be included as allied health professions. Here, particular features are seen as prerequisites to inclusion on allied health "lists" and Figure 10.4 provides examples. It could be argued that these features are not unique to allied health professions, and therefore do not really help define what is and what is not allied health. Regardless of this, whether or not a profession is allied health may relate simply to whether or not professions choose to include themselves in the group by using the term in relation to themselves (AMACAHEA, 1987; Committee to Study the Role of Allied Health Personnel ,1989). Self-inclusion is apparent when professions select membership of allied health associations (such as the Australian National Allied Health Benchmarking Consortium or the North American Association of Schools of Allied Health Professionals, or American Society of Allied Health Professions).

Figure 10.4: Including common allied health features

Some allied health definitions assume that there are particular aspects of professions that will be common and it is these that distinguish allied health from other professions. Examples of features include:

(a) Common properties (Everson, 1999) such as education, use of new technology;

(b) Common organisational interests such as communication, accreditation, professional development, budget and business planning (Dawson, 2001);

(c) Common education and workforce problems such as recruitment of students, financing of programs, supply of qualified faculty, retention of staff, compressed lifetime career salaries, effective and efficient services, realistic and satisfying career expectations, employment and education congruence, licensure, "jurisdictional struggles over scope of practice" (Institute of Medicine/National Academy of Sciences 1989);

(d) Common policy related characteristics, such as level of autonomy, dependence on technology, substitutability of personnel, flexibility in location of employment, degree of regulation, accreditation and standards (Committee to Study the Role of Health Personnel, 1989; Institute of Medicine/National Academy of Sciences, 1989);

(e) Common overarching treatment goals from a consumer perspective, for example "if you're feeling below par, they can play a vital role in optimising your day-to-day quality of life, degree of independence, and risk of further problems" (Johnson, 2003);

(f) Common usage by professions themselves.

Including common allied health features — *continued*

One example of an allied health definition which seeks to identify common features is the Australian National Rural and Remote Allied Health Advisory Service (2002) which states that allied health professionals "are involved in health care/health related care such as direct treatment, assessment, primary health care, community care, health promotion in either the private sector or the public sector; are tertiary trained at a recognized university course and required to obtain specific qualifications to be registered to join a professional association; [and] come together to form a collaborative position towards specific goals".

Definition type 6

Other approaches formulate a definition of allied health through a process of exclusion. The broadest of these definitions excludes medicine and nursing but usually includes everyone else in the health sector (Everson, 1999). This sweeping definition does not incorporate other attributes such as level or type of training, or accreditation. This definition assumes that allied health professions have taken over tasks that physicians no longer want to do (Committee to Study the Role of Allied Health Personnel, 1989) and assumes the continued dominance of doctors as they hold legal responsibility for patients (Mackay et al, 1995). Sometimes particular groups, in addition to medicine and nursing, are excluded. For example Everson, without explanation, identified that administrators, psychologists and social workers were excluded from the definition of allied health, although this is not the case in other definitions previously presented in this chapter. A more precise exclusionary approach is to exclude health-care workers who are covered by separate non-allied health legislation, who have general not health-specific expertise which could be applicable to other industries and who have roles which require little or no formal training in health care (US Department of Health Education and Welfare, 1979). Any further precision in exclusion is difficult and is not considered worthwhile: "pragmatism continues to prevail ... [it is more important] for old and new groups to draw what benefits they can from belonging to allied health than it is to have an accurate description of common characteristics that define the group" (Committee to Study the Role of Health Personnel, 1989, p 17). The pragmatic approach that emphasises benefits rather than commonality may be further driven by the limited understanding that allied health professions have of each other (Thomas, 1999).

Custom

The wide variation apparent in the concept of allied health has not prevented its continuing and customary use, although this use is relatively limited in comparison with other health professional category labels and varies from country to country. Newspapers provide an indicator of public usage (see Figure 10.5).

Figure 10.5: Public usage of the term allied health

An electronic newspaper search identified that the term was first used in newspapers in the United States of America in 1970 in the *New York Times*. This was followed by the United Kingdom in 1984, Australia and Canada (1986), Asian English language papers (1993) and New Zealand (1996) (LexisNexis Academic, search conducted November 2003, allied health in full text of article). Extent of usage varies widely in newspapers. In the 1960s, there was no identified use of the term in newspapers in the electronic search, there were 59 citations in the 1970s; 168 in the 1980s with the USA (N=133) and Australia (N=19) leading in use; and in the 1990s, 1627 citations, again with USA (N=1312) and Australia (N=211) leading. Interestingly, the use of the term by Asian English language newspapers appeared then for the first time and ranked third (N=63 citations) in usage. Overall patterns of usage reflect the increasing popularity of the term, however this needs to be considered in the context of other profession-specific terms which tend to have much greater exposure. For example, an electronic search of Australian newspapers for the month of August 2003 found the term allied health in 16 stories nationally. During the same time, however, there were 25 references to occupational therapy — so the professional term fared better. Both patterns of usage, however, were minimal when compared to those for nursing (598 references) and physicians (more than 3328 references) in one month.

Although allied health has minimal public usage, in professional discourse, it has widespread use, beginning in the 1960s (Committee to Study the Role of Allied Health Personnel, 1989). It is used to identify "peak" bodies convened to represent allied health professionals, for example, the North American Association of Schools of Allied Health Professionals. In addition, the term is useful in professional scholarship, with journals using allied health in the title of the *Journal of Allied Health* and the *Internet Journal of Allied Health Sciences and Practice* for example. A number also use allied health in their guidelines or information to suggest suitable readership, for instance the *Australian Journal of Rural Health*.

In service settings, allied health is also used to name and organise clinical departments. For example, an electronic search conducted while preparing this chapter found most university-affiliated teaching hospitals in Australia used the term within their organisation, even though there was little consistency about which professions were included. Internationally, the use of the term allied health within the structure of similar university-affiliated teaching hospitals was found less consistently than in Australia, with the term being more common in the USA and Canada than the UK. Allied health is also used to group together health professions for the purpose of legislation. The *Allied Health Professions Personnel Training Act* (1966) in North America is one example.

These examples demonstrate that while allied health is rarely used in public discourse, it is used commonly in professional, scholarship, service and legislative areas. In these areas, it is used to characterise a dynamic, expanding, service-orientated but vocationally diverse collection of health related personnel where the breadth and nature of that group can vary according to the situation. This is immensely useful in a volatile, high stake sector such as health where the strategic environment, services, organisational structures, technical capability and human capacity change so rapidly. It is no wonder then, that allied health is a customary term used in a wide variety of situations.

Contradiction

Although allied health is a convenient term, this convenience brings contradictions. These contradictions include the extent to which allied health is: small or large; specialised or similar; understood or little known; powerful or powerless; and co-operative or competitive.

Allied health has been identified to be both the smallest group within the health sector, and the largest. Size estimates depend upon which of the six definition types is being used in what particular circumstances. For example, in Australia, allied health is estimated to be about a fifth of the health professional workforce (Duckett, 2000) including medical practitioners (14 per cent), nurses (69 per cent) and allied health (17 per cent) (Smith & Crowley, 1995). Elsewhere, perhaps with a more inclusive definition of membership, it has been identified as the sleeping giant of the American health care system (McTernan & Farber, 1989), and majority (Institute of Medicine/National Academy of Sciences 1989) of the health care workforce at 60 per cent (Council for Allied Health in North Carolina, 2003). Allied health is also estimated to be growing dramatically in number (Western Australian Allied Health Taskforce on Workforces Issues, 2002).

Allied health has the internal contradictions of a group with highly diverse membership (National Rural and Remote Allied Health Advisory Service, 2002). Every professional group only belongs because it is unlike any of the others; indeed they have no specific links to each other (Everson, 1999). This is a potential weakness as it is unclear whether the allied health collective is representing a common ground or a patchwork of protected fields also known as "turf". Turf is created through separate consciousness, language, values and identity of health professionals which build up a sense of "tribalism" (Beattie, 1995). While tribalism may assist in developing professional identity, it does not serve the development of a collective identity for allied health. It can also backfire on individual professions when service goals and client needs are not met: for example, when highly specialised positions in disadvantaged areas are not filled; when services need to be provided by two or more highly paid staff instead of one; and so on. The narrow skill band of specialised allied health staff demonstrates uniqueness, but it can also make them vulnerable in resource-constrained settings (Beattie). This is particularly the case in settings where cost-cutting, multi-skilling, simplified job classification and flexibility is preferred (Everson; Smith & Crowley, 1995; Thomas, 1999). So, while allied health is a useful concept because it suggests commonality and perhaps versatility, the contradiction quickly becomes apparent; there is actually little commonality. Membership of allied health actually assumes specialisation and an inability to substitute skill. In spite of this, there are, in Australia for example, increasing examples of generic program or caseload-specific, rather than discipline-specific, allied health positions being advertised, with a patient, not provider, orientation. These positions assume substitutability, multi-skilling and a focus on service outcomes rather than on individual professions as providers. These positions challenge the marketability of narrow allied health skill bands and the future viability of discipline-specific service.

The customary use of the term within and outside the health professions is not backed by "appropriate, accurate and comprehensive allied health professional workforce data; instead, there is a remarkable lack of verifiable information" (National Rural and Remote Allied Health Advisory Service, 2002, p 2). This scarcity of data has been observed over a prolonged period (Bezold, 1989; Committee to Study the Role of Health Personnel, 1989; Institute of Medicine/National Academy of Science, 1989; Smith & Crowley, 1995). More recent studies also identify that data sources are limited, and are often restricted to official population census data (National Rural and Remote Allied Health Advisory Service, 2002). These sources provide insufficient information for meaningful allied health labour force analysis, planning or personnel management. Thus, allied health is a contradiction because it is both known and unknown; known as an entity but lacking comprehensive data. The need for better data to understand allied health is urgent. Factors such as gender, location and extent of employment, qualifications, career duration and trajectory are little understood, but potentially important for allied health professions. Figure 10.6 provides one example.

Figure 10.6: "Why aren't they working?"

One example which highlights the need for robust and sensitive information is found in Australian population census data. Here it is apparent that there is an astoundingly large percentage of people (62 per cent in 2001) who self-report that they have allied health qualifications and yet are not working as allied health practitioners (Australian Bureau of Statistics, 2001). This finding is consistent with 1991 Australian census findings (Smith & Crowley, 1995) and is thus indicative of a long-standing trend. Why is this occurring? Why do a significant proportion of trained allied health professionals not work as allied health practitioners? Where do they go and what do they do? Is the finding a result of data collection methods which mask career moves to other specialties within the health sector, or is it other factors that influence personal choices to leave health care? Currently, there are no answers to these questions as not enough appropriate information is collected, recorded and analysed about allied health as a workforce. For allied health to be a known part of health services, data regarding profile and participation is required, particularly as allied health has recognised workforce shortages with little evidence to explain this (Jones, Johnson, Beasley & Johnson, 1996).

Allied health is also characterised by the contradiction of being both powerful and potentially powerless. As an alliance, there are opportunities for greater input into decision-making and thus meaningful interprofessional work (Paul & Peterson, 2001). However, for health professionals who are "not doctors or nurses", the supremacy of the medical profession and the sheer size of nursing must be reckoned with, as it is their power that allied health is seeking to share (Figure 10.7). Little has changed since 1995 when Mackay et al noted:

> Without doctor's goodwill to listen, the contributions of other professionals can be marginalized. Interprofessional working ... is a question of the redistribution of power in health care. Other than in the interests of patients there seems little reason why doctors should accede to demands to power-share. Why should one professional group embark on a process of decision-making which reduces its power and makes decision-making a slower and more laborious process? The sometimes strident and resentful demands for equality from members of other occupational groups must strike a harsh note for doctors who are only too aware of the burden of responsibility they have to bear (p 8).

Figure 10.7: Power, politics, peak bodies and representation

Allied health erodes the power of doctors and nurses when it becomes a political force that needs to be accommodated in decision-making. This force can be exercised through: (a) influence, where the opinions and policy preferences of allied health are noted and acted upon; or (b) physical presence, where allied health has a "seat at the table" and exercises control in decision-making processes. Both methods of exercising power require representation (Phillips, 1995) and this one of the reasons that "peak bodies" such as allied health coalitions have emerged. They provide not only force of opinion through their sheer size, but they also provide a greater opportunity for gaining physical presence in decision-making arenas, which has been proposed to be critical in complex and volatile policy and resource landscapes (Phillips; Zappala, 1999).

The way in which allied health coalitions are constituted affects the amount of time and energy that needs to be invested: will professional representatives on allied health bodies act as "trustees" (Zappala, 1999) free to act as they think best for their profession and the allied health group? Or are they "delegates" (ibid) required to act according to their professions' interests and agendas? Each approach will require different internal professional processes and will assume different allied health collaborative structures — each making different demands in time and energy. If representatives are trustees, then who they are might be just as important as the professions they are representing; if they are delegates, then positions they represent need to have been worked through beforehand using processes that truly represent professional views (Zappala).

While achieving power is important in advancing allied health agendas, it erodes the time and energy allied health professions have to expend upon their individual professions and clients. This is because the politics of representation mean that time and energy must be spent on co-ordinating, monitoring and facilitating internal dialogue so that a professional position can be formulated. Having done this, time and energy must then be spent on co-ordinating, monitoring and facilitating the allied health group communication and determination of agreed political positions. This is even before the liaison with external stakeholders occurs!

The demands of representation are heavy but this is the price of maintaining power share and increased autonomy. As power increases for allied health, more people are involved in planning and decisions that affect the profession, and this increases internal and external politics. Political approaches necessarily involve control over resources; consequently, organisational structures, leadership and management strategies become increasingly important and intensive. More power also brings other duties: a need to market directly to clients and key stakeholders to maintain public trust; a need to participate more fully in the policy and administrative life of the health sector; and an obligation to provide a publicly recognisable efficient and effective high-quality service. These are responsibilities which doctors traditionally have had to bear as part of their dominant role. With greater power, allied health also has to undertake these responsibilities. For allied health, gaining power can therefore be a two-edged sword. On one side they can be involved in cutting edge decisions through ideological or physical representation, participative decision-making and consensual management, but on the other side the time, resources and energy required to do this can cut deeply into the goodwill and capacity of already overstretched staff and associations. Gaining power in the 21st century also brings particular ironies as there are fewer resources to exercise control over: health-service work is intensifying through increased numbers, severity and complexity of clients, and reduced staffing (Duckett, 2000).

While there are political benefits from increased power such as enhanced status, privilege, self-determination and autonomy (McTernan & Farber, 1989), the price for these benefits is high. This price needs to be practically as well as ideologically worthwhile. In some organisations, administration has determined it is not "worth it", abandoning the consensual approach and moving towards executive, centralised management. One example is the National Health Service which has implemented strategies for reducing professional autonomy and freedom, increasing financial accountability and monitoring indicators (Soothill et al, 1995). At this stage, there is little critical debate within occupational therapy or allied health literature to determine whether or not individual professions think the cost of power is "worth it".

The final contradiction in allied health is the simultaneous competition and co-operation that occurs among the professions. Adams and Jones (1989) characterise interprofessional practitioner competition well when discussing allied health practice. They remark on protected turf, the importance of trying to avoid stepping on the toes of other professions and the need to see how local professional roles are played out before making too many claims. If such rivalry and turf protection occurs in teams, there is no reason to believe that this ceases just because those professions are renamed allied health. So while the service needs of clients should be the primary focus and participatory practice desirable (Øvretveit, 1997), there are perceived risks when a competitive view is taken.

Figure 10.8: The thin edge of the wedge

Participatory interprofessional practice requires communication. Effective communication may require sharing knowledge and skills that can threaten perceived professional uniqueness (Øvretveit, 1997). Shared knowledge and skill could be the "thin edge of the wedge" of the generic allied health worker sword. Consequently, it has been vigorously opposed by many professions, and by educators who prepare entrants to them. Many educators prefer a hierarchical model of curriculum, where distinct fields of knowledge are collected together and separate disciplinary traditions are thus maintained (Bernstein, 1971). The traditional hierarchical approach differs to newer models, integrative in nature (Bernstein), which are more compatible with a co-operative interprofessional approach. Interprofessional approaches involve breaking down distinct disciplinary boundaries, seeking relevant knowledge and skills, and then applying them to the real world. The contradictions between hierarchical and integrative models of curricula may well underpin the simultaneous competition and co-operation within allied health, caught between traditional and more flexible emerging modes of learning for practice.

Allied health as a collection may thus merely be the child of traditional collective curricula (Bernstein, 1971). If this is the case, moving towards real co-operation, intrinsic commonality and genuine collaboration may be a revolutionary rather than evolutionary process. Real co-operation in allied health may require a substantial change in professional preparation curricula from models which are discipline-specific, compartmental and hierarchical to models which stress integration, interdisciplinary knowledge and application (Wolf, 1999). Commonality may require a sustained, scholarly and practical assault on deeply-held professional values and knowledge. Genuine collaboration may require the development of decisive, interprofessional goals which serve an integrated purpose. Given the highly competitive, discipline-specific, resource-constrained nature of many allied health educational institutions, service settings and market segments, this is a substantial challenge and an unlikely occurrence in the short term. Apart from rhetoric of enhanced patient care, interprofessional contribution and team effectiveness, there is little or no incentive for individual professions in allied health to confront these issues, as rhetoric does not translate to resources. If change occurs at all, it is likely to be externally driven by agendas of inter-disciplinary efficiency in education and health-care sectors, not by professions themselves which have a mandate to sustain and enhance their own distinct contributions.

Challenge

If we consider a specific profession such as occupational therapy, the challenges of its relationship to allied health become apparent as it differs considerably in collective nature, customary use, inherent conceptual chaos and contradictions. Indeed, occupational therapy is more of a cluster than a collection, as members share common characteristics. Occupational therapy is a relatively consistent group, unique because of attributes such as specified training programs, restrictive accreditation and so on. Even on a global scale, there is a remarkable lack of chaos in the profession of occupational therapy, illustrated by achievements such as benchmark accreditation processes, a world association and occupational therapy scholarship. Occupational therapy as a term is more commonly used than allied health in public discourse, although it is less common in policy. Occupational therapy is also less wracked by internal contradiction than allied health. Occupational therapy appears to be everything allied health is not. These differences challenge occupational therapy to adopt a position on allied health: either to elect to be within it or outside it. If the election is to be within allied health, then the issue is raised of how to manage the relationship.

A literature search of professional journals and standard occupational therapy texts has revealed that scholarly literature to date has been relatively silent on the matter of occupational therapy as allied health. Rather than arguing a position one way or the other, it appears that professional literature tends towards customary usage. Occupational therapy is therefore presumed to be part of allied health, a presumption by occupational therapy itself and others (Committee to Study the Role of Allied Health Personnel, 1989; Duckett, 2000). Foundational texts on occupational therapy (Hagedorn, 1995; Kielhofner, 1997; Turner, Foster & Johnson, 2002), for example, do not index allied health, which suggests that it is a concept of little direct interest to readers.

Occupational therapy in the real world appears to have overcome this silence by establishing a position of identifying with allied health. Numerous practical examples exist from health service and university departments, health policy consultative groups, multidisciplinary and interprofessional outcome measures and evidence-based practice resources (Figure 10.9). These practical examples suggest that occupational therapy has made a choice to be identified as, or with, allied health. Having made that choice in practical terms, more complex issues then arise in relation to the way in which the relationship between allied health and occupational therapy is to be managed.

Figure 10.9: Occupational therapy as allied health

Occupational therapy is found within allied health service departments in hospitals. An electronic search of the large university-affiliated hospitals in Australia, USA and Canada while preparing this chapter found many examples of occupational therapy within allied health departments. In universities, there are numerous examples of occupational therapy within allied health academic departments in English speaking countries. Occupational therapy as a member of formal allied health consultative groups for health policy and procedure is common, such as the Australian National Allied Health Casemix Committee or the Allied Health Consultative Forum of the NSW Health Department in New South Wales, Australia. Occupational therapy as part of multidisciplinary allied health outcome instruments occurs, such as the Australian Therapy Outcome Measure, which not only has subscales for individual professional use (occupational therapy, physiotherapy and speech pathology), but also subscales (participation and wellbeing) which can be scored consensually or by any one of the three identified allied health professions (Morris et al, 2004; Perry et al, 2004; Unsworth et al, 2004). There are also policies in which occupational therapy is identified as allied health. Consultation has occurred with the profession to generate the policy, such as the National Allied Health Benchmarking Consortium. Occupational therapy is also included under allied health in statutes, for example the North American *Allied Health Professions Training Act 1976*. Further, occupational therapy is an identified target profession of the Centre for Allied Health evidence, a collaborating centre of the Joanna Briggs Institute, part of the electronic database facility for evidence-based practice. The Centre provides a knowledge resource of evidence-based research for allied health workers, researchers, educators, clinicians, policy makers, administrators and patients which aims to produce evidence-based solutions to allied health problems (Walker, 2003).

Considered choices

There are three choices open to occupational therapy if it continues to identify with allied health. These are to:

1. continue with the relationship of convenience;

2. develop a more formal relationship in the nature of a "covenant" based on agreed understandings and undertakings; or

3. revise and reinvent the relationship to move away from a collection and toward a cluster of professions growing together with an integrated purpose.

Each of these choices will now be explored.

Occupational therapy can choose to continue what has been essentially a relationship of convenience where the profession is one of many in a collection of health professions. This relationship emerged as there was "no other viable alternative to this collaborative path" (Jones et al, 1996, p 230). There is nothing wrong with this choice; indeed it has been strategic and continues to bring benefits in policy, administration, statute, status and prestige. But if this choice is made, then a purpose, consistent with occupational therapy goals, needs to be clear. This purpose needs to go beyond vague references to "political advocacy" (Council for Allied Health in North Carolina, 2003) or platitudes such as "communication amongst disciplines, government lobbying, consideration of standards, formal representation particularly in relation to policy and legislation formation and review" (Health Professions Council of Australia/The Australian Council on Allied Health Professions, 2003). Such statements mask the very real costs of representation, liaison, co-ordination and risk management. Occupational therapy goals in a relationship of convenience with allied health need to be explicit and operational, derived from professional concerns. The goals need to be "worth it" and to reflect the functions of peak occupational therapy bodies including representation, legal compliance, strategy and policy, accountability, public relations and risk management (Oke, 2003). Currently, the risks and costs of the allied health–occupational therapy relationship have not been debated in the literature, even though there are clearly great benefits from the relationship of convenience. Otherwise the use of the term allied health would not have proliferated, membership of associations would not have continued, allied health departments would have acrimoniously split and there would be a great deal less collaboration than is currently observable.

The choice to stay in a relationship of convenience with continued benefits is not unreasonable, but it is risky. Too many things are assumed, unsaid and unwritten. Thus, the second choice is to restructure the relationship to one where there are clear mutual understandings, formal agreements, integrated goals and a sense of growing together. This can be characterised as a covenant. If the profession chooses this option, the relationship between allied health and occupational therapy needs to be reformed so that it works better. To do this occupational therapy needs to:

- Know more about allied health as a collection and debate the desired role in it.

- Identify a clear purpose for the relationship with allied health. This purpose must align with professional strategic priorities and be supported by key internal stakeholders. This is critical as it is the purpose which will guide whether or not representation should be ideological or physical and whether representatives should be trustees or delegates.

- Determine the extent to which occupational therapy will welcome or reject diversity in allied health membership, where the limits of diversity lie and what criteria will be used to identify membership — whether it is ad-hoc, by exclusion, inclusion or consensus. It is no longer reasonable to continue in a haphazard fashion accommodating anyone and everyone who self-selects or has allied health thrust upon them. Determining criteria for membership is necessary to protect and enhance the status and identity of occupational therapy as the profession will inevitably have overarching allied health characteristics associated with it.

- Decide on the appropriate level of time, energy and resources that can be diverted from profession-centred tasks and priorities towards interdisciplinary pursuits where the benefits will be collective rather than profession specific.

- Determine whether or not size matters. First, an assessment is required of whether or not there are advantages in growing allied health as a collection by taking a wide sweep of professions into the fold, or whether there are advantages from remaining smaller through restricted entry. If the latter approach is taken, mechanisms for restricting use of the term and entry will be needed. Secondly, as one of the two largest professions in allied health (the other being physiotherapy), determine whether occupational therapy can or should use its strength in numbers to influence the strategic directions and priorities of the collective.

- Determine the extent to which competition or collaboration will predominate in the pursuit of disciplinary and interdisciplinary goals through allied health. Collaboration can be frustrating and time-wasting or rewarding and productive, and in any one instance it is difficult to anticipate which will occur. Determining whether or not competition or collaboration predominates will, in a worst case scenario, provide a default position from which occupational therapy can try and obtain benefit from participation.

- Engage with other allied health professions to obtain agreement on identity, strategic directions, priorities, norms of participation, desired benefits, understood acceptable risks, processes and goals.

These recommendations require the discussion of uncomfortable, and possibly taboo subjects, within occupational therapy with other professions. These subjects include power, politics, resource scarcity, priorities, tactics and organisational change to name a few. These recommendations are, however, merely stating the obvious, as these issues are already at work and will inevitably destabilize the relationship of convenience if not addressed in an informed manner. Implementing these recommendations will improve the current relationship between allied health and occupational therapy, moving it from one of convenience to covenant.

The third choice is the most difficult. This is to transform rather than reform the relationship. Occupational therapy could elect for an entirely new view of allied health. It can choose to reinvent the relationship from a diverse collection towards an integrated cluster. This means not only understanding allied health better — its characteristics and contradictions — but also setting specific interdisciplinary goals in addition to those of occupational therapy. To reinvent the relationship, occupational therapy will need to:

- adopt a visionary position, looking at what allied health could be rather than what it is now;

- set and/or support an agenda for change;

- identify factors at work in maintaining a collectivist status quo and engage in organisational development strategies to manage these;

- develop compelling reasons to change towards a more integrated view of allied health;

- propose, support and even lead strategies to move integrative change forward; and

- identify consequences for power, identity, knowledge and skill capacity, and current structures.

This third choice, being a change of such magnitude, seems unlikely in the short term as the investment would be enormous, current structures could not carry the level of direction and leadership required and professional tribalism is alive and well, making the politics of integration risky. This choice also implies organisational change and development on a grand scale and currently there is little structural incentive for integration. Symbolically, any professional leader advocating integration would be viewed as either naïve or foolhardy in "selling off" hard won turf for uncertain returns. Therefore, reinvention of the relationship on this scale may therefore either not come at all or only as a response to changes in the terrain upon which professional turf lies. And these changes may well be underway. Health care is moving inexorably away from a provider focus towards a patient focus, from diversity to integration, from rigidity to flexibility, and from input and process to outcome focus. In this new landscape, allied health as an integrated cluster may be the only way individual professions have a sustainable future. The knowledge and skills of occupational therapy as a large, established, strategic profession within allied health may be critical to the new map that charts a way through this unfamiliar land.

Conclusion

This chapter has explored the nature of allied health both as a concept and a practical reality so that this context of occupational therapy can be better understood. It has presented varying definitions and assumptions that underpin them. It described the conceptually chaotic nature of the term and continuing usage in spite of this problem. Contradictions inherent in allied health, and the pragmatic way in which most professions including occupational therapy use it whenever and wherever it appears beneficial, were explored. This chapter concluded with three choices that provide occupational therapy with ways forward in an allied health context. The first is to continue as a significant part of the allied health collection, maintaining the relationship of convenience. The second is to formalise the relationship through an explicit understanding of the purpose, process and promise of allied health from an occupational therapy perspective but with the engagement and agreement of other parties. This second option is characterised as a covenant. The third choice is to reinvent the relationship, abandoning the collective nature of allied health and forming a cluster, genuinely integrated, with interdisciplinary goals. Any one of these three choices can work: it just depends upon the goals occupational therapy wishes to pursue, the investment it wishes to make in collaboration and the situation at the time. Allied health is an enduring context for occupational therapy. It provides an opportunity for the profession only if control is exercised through strategic considered choice.

References

Australian Bureau of Statistics. (2001). 2001 Census of Population and Housing Australia: Selected Social and Housing Characteristics. ABS Cat. No. 2015.0.

Adams, C. H. & Jones, P. D. (1989). *Interpersonal skills and health professional issues*. Mission Hills: Glencoe Publishing.

AMA Committee on Allied Health Education and Accreditation (AMACAHEA). (1987). *Allied Health Education Directory* (15th ed.). Chicago: Committee on Allied Health Education and Accreditation.

American Commission on Accreditation of Allied Health Education Programs. (2003). Retrieved 25 November 2003, from http://www.caahep.org/caahep/default.asp

Anderson, B. & Bell, J. (1988). *Occupational Therapy: Its Place in Australia's History*. Sydney: NSW Association of Occupational Therapists.

Australian Institute of Health and Welfare. (2003). Retrieved 25 November 2003, from http://www.aihw.gov.au

Beattie, A. (1995). War and peace among the health tribes. In K. Soothill, L. Mackay & C. Webb (Eds), *Interprofessional relations in healthcare*, pp 11–26. London: Edward Arnold.

Bernstein, B. (1971). *Class, codes and control*. Vol 1. London: Routledge.

Bezold, C. (1989). The future of health care: Implications for the allied health professions. *Journal of Allied Health*, Fall, 437–457.

Bureau of Health Manpower. (1967). Report of the National Advisory Commission on Health Manpower, Vol. II. Washington D.C.: U.S. Government Printing Office, November 1967.

Cole, J. H. (2002). Australian perspectives and challenges. *Journal of Allied Health, 31*, 2–3.

Council for Allied Health in North Carolina. (2003). What is Allied Health? Retrieved 16 November 2003, from http://www.alliedhealthcouncilnc.org

Dawson, D. (2001). Carving an identity for allied health. *Australian Health Review, 24*, 119–127.

Ducanis, A. J. & Golin A. K. (1979). *The interdisciplinary health care team: A handbook*. London: Aspen Systems Corporation.

Duckett, S. (2000). *The Australian health care system*. Melbourne: Oxford.

Everson, C. (1999). Kathleen Mears Lecture: Allied health issues and actions, *American Journal of Endocrine Technology, 39*, 131–137.

Hagedorn, R. (1995). *Occupational Therapy Perspectives and Processes*. Edinburgh: Churchill Livingstone.

Health Professions Council of Australia (formerly The Australian Council on Allied Health Professions). Retrieved 24 November 2003, from http://www.agd.com.au/browse/Organisation s%20&%20Associations/Medical?state=VIC&page=4

Institute of Medicine, Committee to Study the Role of Allied Health Personnel. (1989). *Allied Health Services: Avoiding Crises*. Washington: National Academy Press.

Johnson, C. (2003) Health matters — allied health services — consumer guide. Retrieved 12 December 2003, from http://www.abc.net.au/health/regions/cguides/alliedhealthservices.html

Jones, W. J., Johnson, J. A., Beasley, L. W. & Johnson, J. P. (1996). Allied health workforce shortages: The systemic barriers to response. *Journal of Allied Health, 25*(3), 219–232.

Kielhofner, G. (1997). *Conceptual foundations of occupational therapy* (2nd ed.). Philadelphia: F. A. Davis Company.

Mackay, L. (1995). The patient as a pawn in interprofessional relationships. In K. Soothill, L. Mackay & C. Webb (Eds), *Interprofessional relations in health-care*, pp 349–360. London: Edward Arnold.

McTernan, E. J. & Farber, N. E. (1989). Allied health education: An overview. In N. E. Farber, E. J. McTernan & R. O. Hawkins (Eds), *Allied health education: Concepts, organisation, and administration*, pp 5–12. Springfield: Charles C. Thomas Publisher.

Moore, B. (Ed.). (1997), *The Australian concise Oxford dictionary* (3rd ed.). Melbourne: Oxford University Press.

Morris, M., Perry, A., Unsworth, C., Duckett, S., Dodd, K., Skeat, J. & Riley, K. (2003). (under review). *Reliability of the Australian Therapy Outcome Measures* (AusTOMs).

National Commission on Allied Health Education. (1980). *The future of allied health education: New alliances for the 1980's*. San Francisco: Jossey-Bass.

National Rural and Remote Allied Health Advisory Service. (2002). Unveiling the secrets of the allied health workforce in Australia. Retrieved 16 November 2003, from http://www.sarrah.org.au/NRRAHAS/reports.asp

Oke, L. (2003). Review of the composition of national council. *AusOTnews: A publication of OT Australia, Vol 10*(11), 1–2.

Øvretveit, J. (1997). How patient power and client participation affects relations between professions. In J. Øvretveit, P. Mathias & T. Thompson (Eds), *Interprofessional working for health and social care*, pp 79–101. Hampshire: Macmillan.

Paul, S. & Peterson, C. Q. (2001). Interprofessional collaboration: Issues for practice and research. *Occupational therapy in health care, 15*, 1–12.

Perry, A., Morris, M., Unsworth, C., Duckett, S., Dodd, K., Skeat, J. & Riley, K. (2003) (in press). Therapy outcome measures for allied health practitioners in Australia: The AusTOMs. *International Journal of Quality in Health Care.*

Phillips, A. (1995). *The politics of presence*. Oxford: Clarendon.

Smith, C. S. & Crowley, S. (1995). Labour force planning issues for allied health in Australia. *Journal of Allied Health*, Fall, 249–265.

Soothill, K., Mackay, L. & Webb, C. (1995). Troubled times: The context for interprofessional collaboration? In K. Soothill, L. Mackay, & C. Webb (Eds), *Interprofessional relations in healthcare*, pp 5–10. London: Edward Arnold.

The American Medical Association. Retrieved 16 November 2003, from http://www.ama-assn.org

The Scottish National Health Service. Retrieved 16 November 2003, from http://www.show.scot.nhs.uk

Thomas, L. (1999) Images within the allied health professions. *Journal of Allied Health, 28*, 91–96.

Turner, A., Foster, M. & Johnson, S. E. (2002) *Occupational Therapy and Physical Dysfunction — Principles, Skills and Practice* (5th ed.). Edinburgh: Churchill Livingstone.

United Kingdom Department of Health. (2000). Meeting the challenge: A strategy for the allied health professions. Retrieved 25 November 2003, from http://www.doh.gov.uk/pdfs/meetingthechallenge.pdf

Unsworth, C., Duncombe, D., Duckett, S., Perry, A., Morris, M., Taylor, N. & Skeat, J. (2003) (under review). *Validity of the AusTOM Scales: A comparison of the AusTOMs and EQ–5D.* Disability and Rehabilitation.

U.S. Department of Health Education and Welfare. (1979). *A report on allied health personnel.* Washington DC: Government Printing Office.

Walker, H. R. (2003). UniSA Centre for allied health evidence, *Occupational Therapist: Newsletter of the OT Australia NSW*, December 2003, p 13.

Western Australian Allied Health Taskforce on Workforces Issues. (2002) Allied Health Taskforce on Workforces Issues Report. Retrieved 4 November 2003, from www.alliedhealth.health.wa.gov.au/documents

Wolf, K. N. (1999). Allied health professionals and attitudes to teamwork. *Journal of Allied Health, 28*, 15–20.

Zappala, G. (1999). *Challenges to the concept and practice of political representation in Australia.* Research Paper 28, Politics and Administration Group Commonwealth of Australia, Retrieved 11 November 2003, from http://www.aph.gov.au/library/pubs/rp/1998-99/99rp28.htm

CHAPTER ELEVEN

Cultural Power in Organisations: The Dynamics of Interprofessional Teams

Marion Jones

KEY WORDS

Interprofessional practice   Teamwork
Cultural capital   Health-care systems
Cultural power   Ethnographic research

Chapter Profile

This chapter explores the notion of cultural power within organisations and the influence it has on interprofessional team practice. Its meaning is discussed as a guiding philosophy for the day-to-day functioning of health professional teams in today's practice settings. Initially, the changing context for health services in Australasia lays the foundation for critiquing practice against the backdrop of the move to client-centred care. Through examining the findings of an ethnographic study, the distinction between the different types of power and their place in understanding how health professional disciplines shape interprofessional team practice is explored. In particular, the relationship between each discipline and interprofessional practice is analysed in relation to cultural power and the resultant professional and organisational tensions. Interprofessional practice therefore is a balancing of discipline, team and context-driven practice that uses the opportunities and challenges to counter the tensions and struggles that occur. The vision for the future of interprofessional team practice is considered in relation to the capabilities that need to be developed including effective communication, adaptation to change, valuing each other's diversity and therefore overall team development (Jones, 2000).

Introduction

Health-care systems are made up of complex structures and are responsible for providing the services and personnel to meet the health needs of society through both the private and public sectors. While exploring the political, legal and management implications of interprofessional practice is important, the notion of interprofessionalism must also be considered from the perspective of the work interface. Interprofessional team practice needs to be considered within the context in which it occurs along with the make up of the team, the degree of integration that occurs and how the team is led. The place of interprofessional team practice is important to consider as it represents the different professional discipline responses to consumer expectations and the emergent public policies aimed at delivering integrated, quality services for targeted consumer groups. Confusion and multiple expectations can arise from the way teams work and how they are perceived. Interprofessional practice provides the means by which the client's needs can be met more effectively through the collaborative pooling of knowledge, skill and expertise from all disciplines required in each specific client care situation (Jones, 2000). It is at this point where team members' practice, professional cultures and interprofessional assumptions shape team practice. Therefore, "interprofessional" refers to the nature of the relationship between different professional groups. Clearly, the tension between professional identity, discipline, team and the system is complex (Jones; Biggs, 1997).

In common with much of the Western world, the major restructuring of the New Zealand and Australian health-care systems during the 1980s and 1990s was driven by an increased consumer demand for health care, the introduction of new technologies and the financial constraints these issues presented (Bloom, 2000). In Australasia, the successive health sector reforms and the newly competitive, consumer-oriented environment have challenged the practice of professionals within the system. The restructuring and re-engineering of the system included the rationing of health care, rationalisation of the workforce and the introduction of new ways of working. Integrated teamwork was seen to be at the centre of effective health-care delivery and interprofessional practice became the focus for team development.

For teams in today's health care environment, respecting and understanding each other's philosophical views is central to interprofessional practice. Team members must understand and complement other's contribution to the team function and service provision. For many practitioners living through the sector changes and the practice challenges, uncertainty, confusion and perhaps chaos in the social construction of their day-to-day activities in delivering health care is experienced (Youngson, 1999). Under such circumstances, health professionals may be more likely to seek and gain power through asserting their professional voice and "turf guarding" rather than collaborate in interprofessional ways. Working to maintain one's own professional identity builds a territorial focus on the set of boundaries that differentiate each discipline. This in turn sets up the power and authority interplay that in itself legitimates the separate entity of the each discipline. As a consequence, health professionals caught up in these changes have often been torn between wanting to cling to familiar habits and customs while also being excited by the possibilities offered.

However, despite the significant and well-publicised success of work teams in other industries, the health industry has only recently moved to incorporate formal team structures in health-care functions and operations (Manion, Lorimer & Leander, 1996). This raises the question of whether the same teamwork constructs can be applied across all industries, or whether the health industry is, or ought to be considered as, fundamentally different. When team members are more accepting of each other, they are inclined to help each other, suspend judgement of others and listen to the other's professional voice (Wilson & Porter-O'Grady, 1999). This suggests that when health professionals value the diversity of each discipline capability, they may more readily respect and understand others' professional and philosophical views which in turn leads to delivering complementary, inter-professional health care.

Power in organisations

The distribution of power influences how effective teams are in their work function within the organisation. Organisational structures therefore can act to constrain or facilitate team functioning, depending on the tensions present. For example, while wanting to deliver quality care, a lack of resources can create tension and conflict between health professionals. Bourdieu (1977; 1985; 1990) sees power as capital and as being the very basis of domination as it can both be accepted as legitimate while producing conflict. Power can be embedded in government policy and law as well as organisational policy, hierarchical positions, traditional ways of practising and the language of different professionals (Figure 11.1: see next page). Power as capital is a multifaceted concept and a resource and is best seen in relation to particular organisational activities (Calhoun 1995; Harker, Mahar & Wilkes, 1990).

An imbalance of power within organisations can inhibit team achievement of the intended outcomes. Moreover, where any type or source of power is in imbalance, personal and professional conflict, work dissatisfactions and perceived powerlessness can occur (Bourdieu, 1977; Kanter, 1979; Pfeffer, 1992; Swartz, 1997). Gaining understanding about the complexity of culture in relation to individuals and groups presents as one way forward for developing effective teamwork in contemporary health-care organisations.

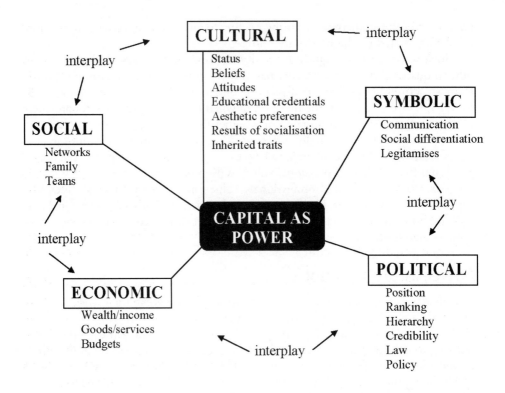

Figure 11.1 Capital as power and the unequal distribution of capital

Cultural power and teams

Teams and the interprofessional discourse are the medium within which cultural capital and its power are negotiated. Each discipline or health professional group has a specific culture.

> It is significant that "culture" is sometimes described as a map; it is the analogy which occurs to an outsider who has to find his way around in a foreign landscape and who compensates for his lack of practical mastery, the prerogative of the native, by the use of a model of all possible routes.
>
> (Bourdieu, 1997, p 2)

Therefore, culture informs the definitions of reality held in common by a group of individuals who share a distinctive way of life (Strasen, 1992). Culture is to the group what personality is to the individual. It is a product of history and a continual process that exists as a consequence of personal and interpersonal actions and interactions. Bourdieu (1977) introduces the notion of cultural power to describe the nature of a group's interactions and its relationship to social structures. Cultural power, which can exist within individuals, groups or organisations, is therefore not a separate domain of health professions but is considered to be at the heart of all social life (Bourdieu; Swartz, 1997).

For health-care teams, cultural power relates not only to each discipline and the accumulation of power within a specific team, but also to the team culture itself. Cultural power, as with other cultural constructs, incorporates a group's beliefs, traditions, values and language. Thus, professional education, socialisation and experiences in belonging to a health discipline all underpin the struggle for domination and recognition through the use of cultural status, beliefs and attitudes. For health professionals, their own professional culture is thus embedded in the everyday world of practice (Bourdieu, 1997). Culture as power is therefore interpreted as influencing interprofessional practice and the competitiveness and social distinctiveness that may exist. It is the concern of Bourdieu (1985, 1990) that capital, or power, from a cultural, symbolic or social perspective, can create "tunnel vision" which acts to maintain the status quo rather than promote change. His understandings may inform the development of interprofessional practice in teams made up of many disciplines.

A health discipline, or professional group, may be identified by its beliefs, knowledge and language as well as by its unique skills and scopes of practice. Such forms of cultural capital influence how each discipline is likely to relate to and influence other discipline members (Lovell, 1981; Street, 1992; Sohier, 1992; Jones, 1993). When members of diverse disciplines come together within work groups, interprofessional discourse becomes one medium through which cultural power is expressed and negotiated. As a consequence, health professionals are frequently socialised into seeking a place within the perceived hierarchies, which further develops tensions and competition over access to limited resources.

Bourdieu's work focuses on how cultural socialisation places individuals and groups within competitive status hierarchies, with different fields interlocking and conflicting over resources, while pursuing their own interests and social order (Swartz, 1997). Within every organisation one can gain a sense of "how things are done here and what is really important" (Garner & Orelove, 1994, p 28). Therefore the cultural capital, or the aggregate of individual, group and team power within health-care organisations, has a major impact on practice. Accordingly, interprofessional conflict and tension provides a rich environment for the self-interested or individual discipline pursuit of social status within the health arena (Swartz).

Cultural power is thus lived and internalised as the norm, providing the social signposts for professional and interprofessional behaviour (Jones, 1993). However, the practice reality of working within complex health-care organisations, with multiple structural and functional components, means that cultural power is often not explicit, discussed or even recognised. If this is so, it has major implications for effective health-care delivery particularly with the promotion of integrated teamwork within today's organisational context. Cultural power can be seen as enabling or disabling for practice depending on the practice context and tensions that exist between the team, discipline, organisation or system. Culture in this way mediates practice by connecting individuals and groups to institutionalised hierarchies (Swartz, 1997).

Interprofessional practice and team interplay

Working interprofessionally means crossing the boundaries of occupations, actively listening to what each other says and ensuring the focus of concern is quality client care (Soothill, Mackay & Webb, 1995). Interprofessional practice implies that health professionals from diverse disciplines collaborate within their team practice that is underpinned by effective communication, resolution processes for conflict and is shaped by a commitment to a common objective (Leathard, 1994; Øvretveit 1995). It has the potential to meet client needs more effectively through the collaborative pooling of knowledge, skill and expertise, thus avoiding duplication of care (Øvretveit, 1995; Calman, 1994). Organisational efficiency along with cultural and clinical safety is jeopardised if interprofessional communication is not effective (Henry & LeClair, 1987; Farley, 1989; Shortell & Kaluzny, 1994; Clinton & Scheiwe, 1995). Not only does interprofessional practice demand collaboration and effective communication systems but also the organisational structures to support it (Soothill, Mackay & Webb, 1995; Walby & Greenwell, 1994). It is difficult for health professionals to co-operate and collaborate when the accepted working practices, organisational structures, decision-making processes and occupational positions are being restructured and seem to threaten the very integrity of the health professional. In such circumstances, survival tactics may be the priority and interprofessional practice an ideal unable to be reached.

The evident tensions between the coexistence of the old and new forms of health care delivery in New Zealand are well documented (Malcolm, 1994; Blank, 1994; Ashton, 1995; Ashton, 1998; Youngson, 1999). Working within teams, the disciplines need to represent their own needs continually while simultaneously considering the needs and scopes of practice of each health professional as well as maintaining a client focus. While team members may be centralised or dispersed geographically, each person is likely to have a different interpretation of what it means to work interprofessionally in a team. For interprofessional practice to flourish in the new health environment, practice must be infused with a spirit of openness (Salmond, 1998). Achieving this while maintaining each discipline's identity, and recognising the inherent potential for professional territorialism, poses real challenges for balancing the different types of power within team and organisational management (Figure 11.1). Therefore, understanding how professional diversity and cultural power may impact on interprofessional practice presents as a critical question.

A study in which data were gathered from health professionals of diverse disciplines working in a team structure is presented in the next section. The findings illustrate the interplay of cultural power in practice within the organisational context.

Interprofessional practice and the research journey

As a researcher, I was aware as I began a journey of working with health professional teams that I wanted to try and capture the very essence of team practice and the dynamics of teamwork when many disciplines work together. Data were gathered in relation to health professional teams and interprofessional practice. Given the worldwide trends of health reforms that have encouraged inter-disciplinary or interprofessional teams to be developed, it was important to examine the concept of team and how it may influence the interprofessional practice process. Therefore, the study was developed to explore how different health professional disciplines working within a team influenced or shaped interprofessional practice.

The makeup of the three teams included social workers, doctors (including the specialties of anaesthesia, dentistry, gerontology and psychology), nurses, occupational therapists, physiotherapists and speech therapists. Each of these discipline representatives held different positions in the team in relation to being full-time or part-time in their specific team role. Some were managers of the team; others were professional co-ordinators of a discipline, or practitioners within the team. Each team had a different combination of health professionals in relation to numbers of each discipline. In total, there were 21 participants in the study. How each health discipline was perceived as contributing to interprofessional team practice was the essence of exploration within the study.

Gathering the data

Data collection occurred over eighteen months and involved individual interviews, observations and team focus groups. The multi-dimensional data collection process was chosen in order to improve the credibility of findings through gathering different types of data and allowing for concurrent data collection and analysis (Swartz, 1997). Each interview, either individual or focus group, was approximately 60 minutes long. At the end of each initial interview, a time was set to observe the team meetings that were called multidisciplinary, any specific discipline meetings, case conferences and the individual disciplines in their practice setting.

Uncovering the team, discipline and organisational cultures was a central aim of the research. In line with Bourdieu's theory of practice, the culture of the teams was examined and the power relations were explored in relation to "whose interests were being served by such a value or position" (Edwards, 1995, p 34). The unacknowledged dimensions of power distribution, resource allocation and discipline beliefs were explored in relation to the shaping of each team's interprofessional practice. The participants had the opportunity to think about their practice world, to reflect critically on their thinking about the influence of organisational structures and contexts and to imagine how interprofessional practice might develop over time. This reflective process is seen as moving from "what is" to "what could be" (Thomas, 1993). Therefore, through the data, the participants provided glimpses of their professional cultures as they interacted within a contextual setting of a complex organisation. Any team interplay was interpreted from the perspective of the different forms of cultural, social, symbolic, economic and political power. The power struggles within health professional teamwork from an individual and team perspective showed how these dimensions influenced and shaped interprofessional practice.

Summarising the findings

Discipline culture as power was emphasised by all three teams as being critical in relation to influencing a role within the team and in maintaining an individual professional identity. Inter- and intra-organisational conflicts were emphasised. A change in structure and name of the team, as often occurred, did not always indicate that a change in processes or practices would follow. That is, inter-professional practice does not naturally evolve from the naming of a group of health professionals as a team. Hence, it was particularly important to understand the difference between the types of power and how they influenced inter-professional relations within the teams and the organisation itself.

> The title, I guess, indicates to the patient what they might expect from that particular person. It is the way we have been educated, doctors do this and the idea people have that nurses are kind, understanding people and physios are going to do hands on and massage and move your limbs. I don't think people have a clear idea about what occupational therapists are going to do. It is almost like if people have a good experience with nurses then I often feel like I have a head start because of the way people perceive a nurse should be. I think they do have a stereotype image and I don't fit it here and so even though I say I am the nurse practitioner, quite often group members will say "Oh I didn't realise you were a nurse". (Nurse)

The participants recognised that interprofessional practice required an investment of effort by all team members as well as having the organisational structures to support it. Without the right supports, things would stay the same or change more slowly.

> In preserving professional identity I think it comes from the individual. I don't really support protection of professionalism when there is no point and I think we can be precious and sensitive about things that have nothing to do with the client. I hear groups talking "people don't understand us, they don't know what we do" and stuff like that. I think if it was clear you had a purpose and people know what you do, you meet the need and you are being useful. (Occupational Therapist)

The health system's structural changes, both intra- and inter-organisationally, and each discipline's understanding of team practice, were a major influence on how each team developed, practised and achieved a harmony of direction. The participants expressed difficulties in changing the circumstances within which they worked due to the decreased resources (economic capital) and perceived limited power (cultural capital). They felt helpless as though effecting changes, such as the length of waiting lists, wheelchair availability and the wait for ongoing assessments, were beyond their control. In addition to the varying levels of perceived powerlessness experienced, each team evidences power struggles between the disciplines and the organisation. Working within a context undergoing continual, systemic change compounded the sense of being engaged in a power struggle. Teams perceived the ongoing shift in the goal posts influenced the parameters of their practice. For Bourdieu (1977), power is fundamental as it is always present in some form, is used and involves domination or marginalisation in some sense and/or differential distribution of it (Calhoun, 1995). The data demonstrated that power dynamics may both facilitate new opportunities and therefore positive change, as well as inhibit them when the status quo would probably remain.

> The good thing is each subgroup listens to each other and it is extraordinary that they talk to each other; a lot of the time it seems to me that the different disciplines will work in their patch, do their job and there isn't enough cross-communication. Mostly communication happens in the corridors or informal conversations. (Physiotherapist)

The teams used inservice education as a means of promoting effective teamwork. However, this often maintained a discipline-specific focus. For example, in two teams the physiotherapists conducted seminars for physiotherapists focusing on the physiology of physiotherapy applications. It seemed difficult for participants to let professional traditions go and some "turf" battles were seen between the disciplines and between medical specialties. Such illustrations reflect the power of cultural capital for the different professions as underpinned by the discipline-specific knowledge, beliefs systems and domains of concern. Nevertheless, the cultural and symbolic power held by each discipline was justified by the participants as being paramount to their existence within an inter-professional setting.

> There are some people who have maybe territorial behaviour where they say this is my patient. I handle that my way and other people say this is our patient and we try to find the best way for the patient. It can create a lot of tension in the team. (Doctor)

In the teams, it was evident that any decisions were perceived as being led by the doctors rather than being a shared function of the team as a whole. In itself, this served to preserve professional identity but perhaps caused tunnel vision and resulted in a discipline not a team decision. In most instances, the initial plan of care was a discipline decision and the involvement of any other disciplines depended on who received the initial referral and how the client need was perceived that influenced when referrals were made to another health professional.

> Sometimes I find I don't see them [the patients] as soon as I would have liked. As for getting referrals early enough, the district nurses are the ones we have the most problems with. (Speech Therapist)

How integrated a team is depends on whether a team is accountable in its own right for all services it provides, or just for specific services delivered by particular health professionals. The decisions made depend on whether there is a central allocation process or individual discipline referral. Individual discipline referral is very dependent on the discipline-specific health professional recognising early enough that ongoing referral and case conferencing is necessary or believing that they can give all care required without turf guarding. Not only is the type of team important to contextualise but also the team membership. Teamwork does not just happen in a universal pattern. It is dependent on the framework used, context and collaboration that exist along with the nature of team development. It would appear a balance of discipline-specific and team input could be appropriate depending on the contextual issue and problem that exists. Interprofessional practice as a way of working challenges professionals to rethink their occupational practice model and to discover a more effective one for practice.

Reflections of the participants

The feedback from each team, on presenting the research findings and interpretation of the data at the final analysis stage, was affirming. The processes identified and needs for setting directions for team development were recognised as being representative of their team practice in a time of ongoing change. One team was surprised with the analysis in that, the previous day they had discussed their directions for the future and had covered the same areas of need, including team building, clinical supervision and ongoing education. They had raised similar issues to be addressed such as overcoming the traditional ways of thinking, providing the support in understanding team practice, improving communication processes and understanding whose interests were actually being served through their actions and interactions. Another team, having shifted location just prior to engaging in the focus groups, was still in the process of adjustment. In the new premises, the nurses were separated from the rest of the team by locating them on a different floor. This was already seen as an obstacle to interprofessional practice and created a tension in relation to team member's interpretations of symbolic capital. Intra-team communication, including written and verbal interactions and case conferencing, was seen as a major area for improvement. The discipline culture was seen as predominant but, apart from nursing, major strides had been achieved in working more effectively together.

In two teams, even though they were labelled multidisciplinary, exclusionary boundaries continued to exist, in that nursing stayed outside most activities and functioned as a separate entity. In spite of team members holding a vision of developing the characteristics of interprofessional practice, the separateness of one discipline, constrained both the interprofessional exchange and continuity of care for clients.

Team interplay: Opportunities, challenges, and constraints

The overall categories conceptualised as patterns of power struggles were:

1. Discipline culture as power.

2. Inter-organisational and intra-organisational conflict.

3. Team representations of practice and power struggles.

4. Shaping interprofessional practice through team development.

How discipline, team and organisational power are understood depends on the philosophical view taken by the person perceiving it. In this study, the perceived position of the different disciplines within the team structure, as identified by each discipline, was interpreted as an effective means of building and distributing cultural capital. Where communication between team members was mostly informal, the shaping of interprofessional practice was inhibited as the social capital, or strength of networking and collaboration, occurred outside the formal decision-making in relation to client care. Not surprisingly, informal patterns of communication strengthened the perceived prestige and social differentiation of each of the disciplines.

In this study, practice structures reinforced parallel working within team functioning more than integrated, interprofessional ones. In one team, client referral was to a specific discipline, not to a team for assessment and planning and triage was by a doctor. Øvretveit, Mathias and Thompson (1997) would refer to these as a mixture of network meeting teams and co-ordinated professional teams with some attempt at being collective teams who took responsibility together as a team.

How then can interprofessional practice be promoted and does it need to be? The potency of symbolic and social capital as power in relation to the separate disciplines precludes boundaries being broken down, joint goals being developed and health professionals working together on client care. The strong professional orientation in their roles has the team wanting to practise to meet the needs of the clients without the complexity of the budget demands and intra- and inter-organisational conflict.

Anderson (1997) re-emphasises this important point when she talks of being less fixed on structure and more concerned with having the ability to adapt. She stated "the new successful organisation will encourage empowered teams to move the business of the organisation to newer heights and produce better improved outcomes for customers" (p 334). One of the most important functions is to cultivate the human capital in organisations that is otherwise stifled by the existence of an organisational hierarchy. In considering this, team members need to think about what sort of interprofessional practice is really wanted, given the context within which each team works, and the change and adaptation demanded by health-care reform (Wilmot, 1995).

The complexities of health team practice and the necessity of considering the sociopolitical context and different types of clients who present is a constant challenge for teams. Interprofessional practice is a balancing of discipline, team and context-driven practice that uses the opportunities and challenges to counter the tensions and struggles that occur between the different types of capital evident in health-care organisations.

The dominant controller of all resources has the greatest influence on the structure and processes of team practice. In this way, the prestige of doctors over the other disciplines was legitimated through position and ranking within teams. Where this is seen to occur, the disciplines function in parallel, which in turn constrains the potential for integration and a shift to an interprofessional world-view. As a consequence, the continued power struggles between disciplines exist in spite of management changes to team structures and titles. While cultural power of the disciplines remains a dominant force for team members, the professional boundaries are reinforced and collaborative, integrated practice is inhibited.

While most participants in the study saw themselves as relatively autonomous in some decisions related to day-to-day practice, there was evidence of a struggle between autonomy and accountability both as a health professional and as a team member. Engagement in the struggle challenges the identity and cultural power of the health professional and constrains the development of team culture. Case conferences are one context in which cultural capital and team relationships are played out. The doctors were typically perceived by the other disciplines as being the dominant group, acting to maintain the status quo by controlling the timing of case conferences or their attendance at them. In two teams, the nurses felt the case conferences were scheduled when they were busy, and one occupational therapist believed the doctors chose not to attend when it was her turn to present. Making the time to attend case conferences and participate in team learning and discussions was seen as a further challenge when workloads are high. Some participants stated that there is no time to do anything else as their caseload was excessive and they would never get their work completed if they had any more meetings to attend.

The complexities of health team practice and the necessity of considering the sociopolitical context for a range of clients is a constant challenge for teams. Inter-professional practice is a balancing of discipline, team and context-driven practice that uses the opportunities and challenges to counter the tensions and struggles that occur between the different types of capital evident in health-care organisations. Interestingly, an interprofessional focus was more evident in the context of a more complex situation. Therefore when client's needs and clinical circumstances present as complex, three or more disciplines are often involved in the care and team interplay increases.

The active shapers of team practice, the policy makers and corporate managers, are seen by the health professional participants to be distant from the day-to-day practice they consider as the workface. From this position, health professionals believe they have difficulty in influencing macro decision-making and the competing discourses that exist in relation to what they can do and what they need to practise. While economic control is seen to lie with senior management, the context is set for perpetuating the belief that the institution's interests are being served, rather than the clients. Furthermore, the evidence from this study indicates there is a lack of cohesion in relation to team practice. The existence of competing discipline cultures inhibits team development, thereby maintaining the status quo. Paradoxically, the push towards interprofessional teams has seemingly promoted discipline territoriality.

Overall, discipline culture is especially strongly evidenced by the reality that each profession continues to define and build its territorial boundaries that make it a unique group. While practitioners may consult their team colleagues with problems of practice, the actual decision-making for client care remains discipline specific. Such practice is "multidisciplinary" in its nature, implying that more than one profession may be involved in a particular scenario without effective collaboration. In reality, discipline-specific solutions evolve and practice is delivered by disciplines operating in parallel. Can members of different professional disciplines working in teams realise the importance of sharing knowledge and expertise so complex problems do not fall between the cracks? The implications for professional and economic accountability evolve from these issues. "Collaboration requires a commitment to the relationship between partners who agree in essence to work through any barriers and sustain the relationship despite impediments" (Wilson & Porter-O'Grady, 1999, p 150).

Capabilities for team development and interprofessional practice

The teams and individual health professionals cannot change the health-care system itself but they can work together in an integrated care continuum to develop a common purpose to channel their energies. This way, they will utilise their expertise effectively and efficiently to provide the quality care the participants aimed to achieve. This in itself may filter down to influence the organisation. The challenge for teams is to create new ways of working in the world of health care that in turn will influence the context of team practice and the distribution and balance of the different forms of capital or power.

The capabilities for developing effective interprofessional practice include effective communication, adaptation to change, team development and valuing difference. In this way, the different forms of capital can be used to balance the tensions evident in the dispersion of capital power. Achievement of quality client care that is efficient as well as effective needs to incorporate professional and team satisfaction.

For interprofessional team practice to occur, each discipline should be clear about its practice scope and foundations. The volume of cultural, symbolic and social capital present influences the shaping of this scope. In addition, a framework, mission and goal statements for the team to work towards is required. These would include role expectations and relationships together with expectations of team performance and evaluation policy (Porter-O'Grady & Krueger-Wilson, 1998). It is, therefore, important that teams learn how to develop processes to build a team. Professional boundaries and traditional ways of delivering health care remain the reality for many teams. This suggests a strategic, long-term approach is needed to effect real change.

Practice within a team structure does not mean dominance by any one discipline. Rather it is important to value differences, to use differences constructively, to maximise on common areas of interest and to plan for interprofessional practice. Team development is dynamic and influenced by context including changing public policy, health-care needs and the challenges and constraints of health-care delivery.

Effective communication, professional identity, complexities of health-care systems, expectations of management and external agencies in the form of different forms of capital all influence the shaping of interprofessional practice in the day-to-day work of teams. Moreover, the everyday way of being in the practice world for an individual practitioner and a discipline group is challenged in the process of striving to develop an integrated, interprofessional team. When there is a change in structure but not a change in process, the practice sequences and traditional ways of working stay the same. The ongoing contextual changes posed by the health reforms and the perceived absence of support systems to cope with them have strengthened the perceived need for strong discipline cohesiveness and the perpetuation of symbolic and cultural power.

Team practice is always going to have tensions and power struggles, but what makes the difference is how the tensions and power are processed and with whom. There are opportunities and constraints, barriers and challenges, and benefits and losses in all practice settings in differing proportions. Support for ongoing professional development in interprofessional practice competencies is necessary to effect real change. Strategies need to be compelling and motivational while promoting change and new directions. The development of integrated interprofessional teams will evolve over time as the power struggles that exist in practice come more into balance. Power balancing provides the foundation for building interprofessional opportunities rather than constraints.

Conclusion

A change of thinking is required in order to mobilise health professionals' divergent forms of cultural power and resources of practice in the pursuit of ongoing team development. Strategies are required to motivate health professionals to use change and economic tensions as an opportunity and challenge to work differently. The development of a collaborative, decision-making framework that expedites successful outcomes within a complex practice continuum will facilitate this. It must be remembered, however, that past experiences influence how people respond to new ideas. If the recent push towards interprofessional team practice has acted to strengthen discipline, symbolic and social culture, a new and different response is needed to move health practitioners towards an interprofessional team culture.

Interprofessional team practice implies a commitment to a common purpose and goals and a mutual respect together in the context of effective communication systems and complementary and overlapping skills. Capability for interprofessional practice, therefore, needs to include the ability to adapt and participate in change, along with demonstrating effective communication and an intact self and discipline integrity. The challenge in today's health-care environment is to respect and understand each other's philosophical view and to concentrate on how each other's contribution to a health-care team is complemented. The challenges, opportunities and benefits for interprofessional practice are there to be taken up by the health care professionals along with provision being made for professional development requirements. Talking the same language creates an exciting new impetus for interprofessional practice. There needs to be recognition that in a dynamic context, tensions will always exist. However, health professionals need to experience tensions and take the opportunity to change, investing the time to create new directions and ways of working. Holding a belief in what is possible can make interprofessional practice happen.

References

Anderson, R. (1997). Future organisational leadership. *Journal of Professional Nursing, 13*(6), 334.

Ashton, T. (1995). From evolution to revolution: Restructuring the NZ health system (Chapter 5). In D. Seedhouse (Ed.), *Reforming healthcare; the philosophy and practice of international health reform*. West Sussex, UK: John Wiley & Son Ltd.

Ashton, T. (1998). Implementing the Coalition health policy: The baby and the bath water. *Health Manager, 5*(1), 5–7.

Biggs, S. (1997). Interprofessional collaboration: Problems and prospects. In J. Øvretveit, P. Mathias & T. Thompson (Eds), *Interprofessional working for health and social care*. London, UK: Macmillan Press Ltd.

Blank, R. (1994). *New Zealand health policy: A comparative study*. Auckland: Oxford University Press.

Bloom, A. C. (2000). *Health reform in Australia and New Zealand*. Melbourne: Oxford University Press.

Bourdieu, P. (1977 – reprinted 1997). *Outline of a theory of practice*. Cambridge: Cambridge University Press.

Bourdieu, P. (1985). The social space and the genesis of groups. *Theory and society, 14*(6), 723–764.

Bourdieu, P. (1989). Social space and symbolic power. *Sociological Theory, 7*(1), 14–25.

Bourdieu, P. (1990). *The logic of practice (English translation)*. Cambridge, UK: Polity Press.

Bourdieu, P. (1997). The forms of capital. In A. H. Halsey, H. Louder, P. Brown & A. S. Wells (Eds), *Education: Culture, economy and society*. Oxford: Oxford University Press.

Calhoun, C. (1995). *Critical social theory*. Oxford, United Kingdom: Blackwell Publications.

Calman, K. (1994). Working together, teamwork. *Journal of Interprofessional Care, 8*(1), 95–99.

Clinton, M. & Scheiwe, D. (1995). *Management in the Australian healthcare industry*. Sydney: Harper Educational (Aust) Pty Ltd.

Edwards, M. (1995). *Ethnography: A View of Qualitative Research*. Adelaide: Document Services, University of South Australia.

Farley, M. (1989). Assessing communication in organizations. *Journal of Nursing Administration, 19*(12), 27–31.

Garner, H. G. & Orelove, F. P. (1994). *Teamwork in Human Services*. Boston: Butterworth-Heinemann.

Harker, R., Mahar, C. & Wilkes, C. (1990). *An Introduction to the Work of Pierre Bourdieu: The Practice of Theory*. London: The Macmillan Press Ltd.

Henry, B. & LeClair, H. (1987). Language, leadership and power. *Journal of Nursing Administration, 17*(1), 19–25.

Jones, E. M. (1993). *Shaping nursing praxis. Unpublished MEd Admin thesis*, Massey University, Palmerston North, NZ.

Jones, E. M. (2000). *Shaping team practice in the context of health reform: Opportunities, tensions, benefits. Doctoral thesis*, Flinders University of South Australia.

Kanter, R. (1979). Power failure in management circuits. *Harvard Business Review, 57*(4), 65–75.

Leathard, A. (1994). *Going interprofessional: Working together for health and welfare.* New York: Routledge.

Lovell, M. C. (1981). Silent but perfect partners: Medicine's use and abuse of women. *Advances in Nursing Science*, 25–40.

Malcolm, L. A. (1994). Managed care in NZ — making it happen. *Health Manager, 1*(4), 9–12.

Manion, J., Lorimer, W., & Leander, W. (1996). *Team Based Health Care Organisations: Blueprint for Success.* Gaithersburg: Aspen Publishers.

Øvretveit, J. (1995). Team decision-making. *Journal of Interprofessional Care, 9*(1), 41–51.

Øvretveit, J., Mathias, P. & Thompson. (1997). *Interprofessional working for health and social care.* London, England: MacMillan Press Ltd.

Pfeffer, J. (1992). *Managing with power: Politics and influence in organisations.* Boston: Harvard Business School Press.

Porter-O'Grady, T. & Kruger-Wilson, C. (1998). *The healthcare team book.* St Louis: Mosby Inc.

Salmond, G. (1998). Integrated care — the ethical debate: The role of professionalism in pursuit of health system improvement. *Healthcare Review — Online TM, 2* (7 May), from http://www.enigma.co.nz/hcro_articles/9806/vol 2 no 7_003.htm.

Shortell, S. & Kaluzny, A. (1994). *Health Care Management: Organizational Design and Behavior* (3rd ed.). New York: Delmar Publishers Inc.

Sohier, R. (1992). Feminism and nursing knowlege: Power of the weak. *Nursing Outlook, 40*(2), 62–66.

Soothill, K., Mackay, L. & Webb, C. (1995). *Interprofessional relations in health care.* London: Edward Arnold.

Strasen, L. (1992). *The Image of Professional Nursing.* Philadelphia: Lippincott Company.

Street, A. F. (1992). *Inside nursing: A critical ethnography of clinical nursing practice.* New York: State University of New York Press.

Swartz, D. (1997). *Culture and power: The sociology of Pierre Bourdieu.* Chicago: The University of Chicago Press.

Thomas, J. (1993). *Doing Critical Ethnography.* Newbury Park, London: Sage Publications.

Walby, S., Greenwall, J., Mackay, J. & Soothill, K. (1994). *Medicine and nursing: Professions in a changing health service.* Thousand Oaks: Sage Publications Inc.

Wilmot, S. (1995). Professional values and interprofessional dialogue. *Journal of Interprofessional Care, 9*(3), 257–266.

Wilson, C. & Porter-O'Grady, T., (1999). *Leading the Revolution in Healthcare* (2nd ed.). Gaithersburg: Aspen Publishers Inc.

Youngson, R. (1999). Leadership in health: The role of clinical leadership in New Zealand — patient centred health reform and the challenge for health professionals. *Healthcare Review — Online TM, 3*(3), from http://www.enigma.co.nz/hcro_articles/9903/Vol 3 No 3_002.htm.

The Sociocultural Context of Practice

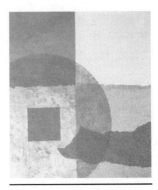

CHAPTER TWELVE

Gender, Occupation and Participation

Alison Wicks

Gail Whiteford

KEY WORDS

Gender

Occupation

Social structures

Occupational participation

Occupational strategies

Occupational tensions

Chapter Profile

This chapter explores the impact of gender on occupation and occupational participation and, from a feminist perspective, considers how being a woman creates occupational tensions throughout the life course. The chapter begins with a discussion of occupation as a human phenomenon and gender as a socio-cultural construction. Next, drawing upon data from a recent life history study of older women undertaken by the authors, the chapter examines the influence of gender on the women's occupational opportunities and how this impacted upon choices for personally meaningful occupation across their life course. In addition, extracts from the study are presented to illuminate strategies developed by the women to negotiate barriers created by gender, so they could satisfy their occupational needs. The chapter concludes with a discussion of what consideration of occupation as a gendered construct means for occupation-focused practice.

Introduction

> Women make their own lives, but do so in conditions not of their own making.
>
> (Personal Narratives Group, 1989, p 5)

Gender influences the way life is experienced (Hess, 1990; Wearing, 1996) as it is a key dimension of culture, social relations and personal life (Connell, 2002). Indeed, this understanding lies at the core of the feminist movement, which has sought to address inequities experienced by women in social, economic and political life (Lake, 1999). Yet, although central to our everyday existence, the influence of gender has been relatively unexplored from an occupational perspective. Such lack of exploration is despite the fact that most contemporary theoretical models currently guiding occupation-focused theory and practice emphasise the dynamic interaction between the person, the environment and occupation (Chapparo & Ranka, 1997; Christiansen & Baum, 1997; Kielhofner, 2002; Townsend, 1997). One of the possible reasons for its relative invisibility in the occupational science literature and other literature focused on occupation, is that gender, like occupation, tends to be taken for granted in everyday life (Connell) unless it is perceived to be problematic.

A recent doctoral study, which analysed life stories of older women from an occupational and a feminist perspective, has highlighted the influence of gender on occupation across the life course (Wicks, 2003). The findings of the study inform this chapter, which focuses on two issues relevant to occupation-focused practice:

- how gender facilitates and constrains women's occupational choices and participation; and
- how women respond to the gendered nature of occupation.

Extracts from the life stories of the women who participated in the study are presented in this chapter as they illustrate how gender constrained their occupational opportunities, and choices that impacted on their everyday life in a profound way. The stories also reveal some of the strategies the women developed to satisfy their occupational needs and desires. Collectively, these women's narratives, which express their frustrations and disappointments over the course of their lives, provide a cogent vehicle for understanding human occupation as a socially and politically situated phenomenon. Accordingly, recognition of the complexity of occupation as socially and culturally mediated, reinforces the need to view occupation from a socio-critical rather than just an individualistic perspective, which has been the tendency to date. Practitioners have traditionally adopted an individualistic perspective as a way of maintaining a historical alignment with biomedicine.

In order to appreciate the dynamic relationship between occupation and gender, the chapter begins with a review of related literature on human occupation and gender as a socio-cultural construction. This is followed by a description of the study upon which this chapter is based and a presentation of two of the study findings that are relevant to the discourse on occupation as a gendered construct. These finding are: gender as a source of occupational tensions; and women's ways of doing. Discussion on the implications of the gendered nature of occupation in respect of occupation-focused practice concludes the chapter.

Understanding human occupation

In this chapter, the term "occupation" does not refer just to the commonly held notion of paid employment. Rather, this chapter refers to occupation as it is described in the occupational science literature, that is, as a complex, multi-dimensional phenomenon embodying time, purpose, meaning, form and context. Occupational science assumes that humans need occupation, and that they are shaped by their daily patterns of occupational participation (Wilcock, 1993; Zemke & Clark, 1996).

Since the renaissance of interest in occupation in the postmodern era (Whiteford, Townsend & Hocking, 2000) and the establishment of occupational science in 1989 to study occupation and humans as occupational beings spec-ifically (Zemke & Clark, 1996), numerous definitions of occupation can be found in the occupational science literature (AOTA, 1997; Christiansen, 1991; Kielhofner, 1995; Sabonis-Chafee, 1989; Townsend, 1997; Yerxa et al, 1990). Recently, a range of definitions of the term occupation was compiled for the Occupational Terminology Interactive Dialogue in the *Journal of Occupational Science* (Dunn, 2001). A selection of these definitions by Yerxa et al, Christiansen and Kielhofner are presented and critiqued, highlighting important conceptual points of alignment and differentiation:

> Occupation is a general term that refers to engagement in activities, tasks and roles for the purpose of productive pursuit (such as work and educ-ation), maintaining oneself in the environment, and for the purpose of relaxation, entertainment, creativity, and celebration.
>
> (Christiansen, 1991, p 26)

> Occupation refers to specific "chunks" of activity within the ongoing stream of human behavior which are named in the lexicon of the culture. These daily pursuits are self initiated, goal directed (purposeful), and socially sanctioned.
>
> (Yerxa et al, 1990, p 5)

> We can define human occupation as doing culturally meaningful work, play, or daily living in the stream of time and in the contexts of one's physical and social world.
>
> (Kielhofner, 1995, p 3)

Each definition refers to all the things that people do in their daily lives as occupations. Both Yerxa et al (1990) and Christiansen (1991) refer to the purposeful and meaningful nature of occupations. The definition by Kielhofner (1995) incorporates an important temporal dimension of occupations. Yerxa et al make reference to the cultural and social aspect of occupation, whereas Kielhofner considers the physical and social environments in which occupations occur. For the purpose of this chapter, occupation refers simply to the things people do in their daily lives, within and in response to their environments (Townsend, 1997). In this definition, the environment, when considered broadly, includes the socio-cultural environment, in which gender constructions are situated and experienced.

Understanding gender as a socio-cultural construction

Gender, considered a social structure, refers to the social division and cultural distinction between men and women, rather than their natural or biological differences (Jackson & Scott, 2002). Social structures determine the patterns of social interaction (Germov, 1998), defining possibilities and consequences, and conditioning practice. As such, gender influences the social arrangements, patterns and relationships between men and women (Connell, 2002) and exerts a significant influence over the way we live our lives, in particular influencing what we do. Connell (1987) contends there are two levels of gender politics: the gender order, which encompasses institutional policies and practices, thereby influencing the power relations between men and women at the macro level; and the gender regime, which influences relationships between men and women and patterns of everyday activities at the micro level, that is, within homes, workplaces and communities. The gender regime, however, is largely influenced by the gender order.

To a greater or lesser extent, gender reflects the values and power relationships of the society in which it is constructed (Germov, 1998). Accordingly, gendered arrangements and patterns of participation may differ strikingly from one cultural context to another. The narratives recounted by Makler (2003) in her book titled *Our woman in Kabul*, and Macdonald's (2002) colourful description of Hindu marriages, highlight contemporary gendered patterns in Afghani and Indian cultures respectively. Interestingly, the comments made by Makler and Macdonald reveal their personal difficulties in understanding and accepting gendered patterns and arrangements that vary greatly from those of their own Australian culture. Langford's (1988) autobiography provides an understanding of gendered patterns of occupational participation in Australian Aboriginal families during the period 1940–1980. In these particular societies and in other societies, where patriarchal ideology exists, women are associated with nature and men with culture, and men have more power and economic privilege than women, for no reason other than their maleness. An outcome related to patriarchy is the sexual division of labour in which men are allocated the role of breadwinner, while women undertake childcare and domestic roles (Alston, 1995).

Not only do the meanings associated with gender vary between societies and cultures, they may also vary within societies. For example, in Australian society gender patterns vary between urban and rural communities (Alston 1995; 2000).

Additionally, meanings and expectations change as gender intersects with other social structures. Such is the case in relation to age, according to Rosenthal (1990) who maintains that "for women as they age, the intersection of ageism with sexism can be devastating, in circumscribing their activities and controlling their self image" (p 1).

Adding to the complex nature of gender is the fact that gender patterns are not only imposed from the outside by social norms or by pressure from authorities. People construct themselves as masculine or feminine, personally responding to their place in the gender order by the way they conduct themselves in everyday life (Connell, 2002). The interaction between the personal and social dimensions of gender is revealed in the life stories of the women who participated in the study. The women shared a common socio-cultural milieu, in that they all lived in Australia during the last two-thirds of the twentieth century. As a result, each woman's occupational life course was shaped by the Australian gender order and regime that prevailed during this period. In essence, it was Australian gender politics that largely determined what they could do, what was expected of them and to what they were entitled. Yet each woman's occupational life course was unique, due to her personal response to the gender order, as influenced by her own occupational persona (Whiteford & Wicks, 2000).

In order to understand the relationship between the narrative extracts presented in this chapter and the discussion on gender as a socio-cultural influence on occupational participation, the study informing this chapter is now described in brief.

Researching occupational potential

The purpose of the qualitative doctoral study was to explore the concept of occupational potential and its development across the life course. Occupational potential refers to a person's capacity to do what is personally meaningful. In particular, the study focused on understanding the influences that facilitated or constrained the development of occupational potential over time from the perspective of a small group of older women. The six women who comprised the group were all aged over sixty-five years and living in the Shoalhaven community in New South Wales, Australia.

The study had ethical approval, inclusive of informed consent processes, through Charles Sturt University. Using a life history approach, the three-year project generated thick, rich data illuminating the occupational lives of the six older women. Methodological triangulation was achieved through use of preliminary focus groups and thorough documentary analysis. Participant checking, continual dialogue throughout, the use of detailed field notes and a researcher journal, in addition to peer and expert supervision ensured trustworthiness. Anonymity and confidentiality of the women have been maintained through use of pseudonyms and textual changes to any identifying details.

The six women in the study, born between 1924 and 1935, recounted widely diverse occupational experiences. For example: Sylvia's earliest memories include listening to the opera and playing her grandmother's pianola; Maureen, the eldest daughter of four children, was obliged to leave school and go to work instead of training to be a teacher; Fran grew up in the inner city, in very heart of the working class; Doris' parents were Jehovah's Witnesses (her father left when she was eight and her mother died young, leaving Doris to manage alone); as a young woman, Mary travelled around the United Kingdom and Europe, working as a nurse; and Alice was a country girl who married a dairy farmer.

When the study data, which were the life stories of these six women, were interpreted from an occupational perspective, generic features of the concept of occupational potential were illuminated. Gender-specific understandings about occupational potential also became apparent when a feminist perspective was applied to the data. Such gender-specific understandings are informing this chapter, which focuses on how gender constrains women's occupational participation and how women respond to the gendered nature of occupation.

Selected from the study data for inclusion in this chapter are extracts that reveal gender as a source of occupational tensions for women and highlight unique ways in which women deal with such tensions throughout their life.

Gender as a source of occupational tensions

In this chapter, the term "occupational tensions" refers to people's experiences when they are denied the opportunity of doing what they want to, or when they have to choose between what they want to do and what is expected of them. When the study data were analysed, it was apparent that each woman experienced occupational tensions at different stages of her life course. The following extracts and accompanying interpretive commentaries highlight some of the themes associated with the women's occupational tensions, effectively revealing the influence of gender on the direction of the women's occupational life course, as well as the feelings engendered by such an influence.

Being denied an occupation of choice

Two of the women in the study were denied their careers of choice because of the established views regarding education for women, which infiltrated Australian family values, beliefs and practices in 1940s and 1950s. When the study participants went to school, most students left school at the age of fourteen years and nine months, or upon completion of the Intermediate Certificate. The small percentage of students completing their Leaving Certificate, which involved another two years of schooling and enabled admission to university, were predominantly male. It was the commonly held belief that most women did not need additional formal education for the work they were expected to do.

The following extract from Maureen's life story highlights not only the power of the gender regime and how it infiltrates family values and practices, but also people's need to do what is personally meaningful. It is also apparent that such occupational deprivation (Whiteford, 2000) when Maureen was young subsequently impacted upon her occupational participation over time and her overall level of satisfaction with her life course.

Maureen:

I liked school. I was good at school. I applied myself to it, too. I wouldn't say I was brilliant, but I studied hard and I did well, until I got up to the Intermediate. I was almost fifteen when I sat for the Intermediate. I think we sat for the exams in early November, and I was fifteen on the eighteenth. Then my father informed me that I was going to Business College, which I didn't want to do. I said I wanted to be a schoolteacher. No, he said, you can't do that. That is too hard. You have to put up with unruly children and all sorts of things. I said, well, I want to be a dressmaker. He said, no, you have to put up with people changing their minds and all this sort of thing. It was going to be office work. So, I went to Business College for about a year, just over I think. … it was St Luke's in Sydney. And then the nuns found me a job as a shorthand typist. … I had been there about six months and Mother's brother said that if I wanted to go back to school, he would help. And I realised then, that it was partly financial that my parents didn't want me to go on, because I was the eldest of the family of four. But my parents were still against that. And then I got a bright idea. To become a teacher, I could become a nun. My parents were against that too. But I went and saw the nuns that had been teaching me at Stanmore and they talked to my mother, and they said, give it a go. They talked her into it. So then I ended up at Granville Convent, at school, and we lived in the Convent at Rosehill. But I got so homesick after about six months there, that I couldn't stand it. Because I had never been away from home before, so I decided that I would give that up. So I went home again.

As this extract reveals, Maureen was so keen to participate in her chosen occupation of teaching that she was prepared to lead an occupationally restrictive life in a convent for a period. It was the gender regime within the family, influenced by the gender order (Connell, 1987) that was responsible for constraining her occupational participation by limiting her choice of career. Maureen is still unforgiving for being denied the opportunity of doing what she wanted, to the extent that she said, in another part of her life story interview, "I feel as though something has been wasted".

Being constrained by explicit policies

In addition to the constraints on women in relation to education, certain Australian governmental regulations and policies clearly limited the occupational options available to women in the 1940s–1980s. But it was not just government policies that disadvantaged women during this period. Some large public institutions also created occupational barriers for women, the explicit social prescriptions associated with the profession of nursing being an excellent example.

A career in nursing was only available to single women, primarily because trainee nurses were required to live in nurses' residences. Now, at that time, it was quite common for women to marry when they were in their early to mid-twenties because, post-World War II, marriage was considered a source of critical support as it provided financial security (Elder, 1999). Therefore, for many young women at that time, nursing as a career was not an option. The following extract from a focus group discussion highlights the determination of one woman at that time to pursue her career of choice, in spite of the deception and personal sacrifices entailed.

Ellen:

I always lived on the farm, but I wanted to go off the farm, so I decided to go nursing. In those days, you had to pay to be a nurse. You had to pay for your uniforms. We worked for six months without pay and then we got four and tuppence for the next six months ... I was not going to get married or have children until I had "done my thing" or, those times, it was "live my life". But I did get married, at twenty, but I had to keep that secret for my nursing. And of course we were not going to have children for years and years to come. But I did start to have a child. And it was so evident, of course, I had to give up my nursing.

Being constrained by implicit social expectations

In addition to governmental regulations and explicit social exclusions, it is apparent that implicit social expectations also limited options for some of the women in the study. For example, it seems that Mary felt she had no choice other than to have an abortion when she became pregnant during her nurse training. As the next extract reveals, it appears that her decision to abort was primarily based on the tacit social and familial expectations that prevailed at that time.

Mary:

[Nursing] Sisters were all unmarried. You could not be married, or be known to be married. As we were talking earlier, you did find that people did put on weight and left or had to leave. Lots of us had abortions when we fell pregnant because not only could you not continue your work, but you couldn't tell your parents. Well, you could tell your parents, I suppose, but I could never have told my mother. My mother was a Victorian, through and through. I could never have told my mother I was pregnant, I really couldn't. And I have thought over the years, I wonder if it was a boy or a girl, or how old it might be now ... but it was a necessity ... Actually, I didn't even think of my career. It was the thought of telling my mother ... and telling the family. I could imagine, oh, my God, what my brothers would have said ... So, for me, it was personal and, I suppose, mores of the day. And I would say, for nearly all of us, it was more the mores. I mean, Nell, her parents were Methodist ministers. You didn't tell them you were pregnant. *Laugh.* Actually, I think they knew, but Mother never did, I don't think.

Indeed, this is a moving account of the pressures and the tensions experienced by young, unmarried women who fell pregnant during the mid-1900s. So powerful were these expectations that it seems Mary was prepared to risk her health and wellbeing, and to quell possible biological instincts to be a mother. Although Mary states that the primary reason she decided to have an abortion was the fear of her family's reaction to her being pregnant out of wedlock, other pressures may well have influenced her decision. Considering the frequent references in her story to her need for a regular income, perhaps she had also considered the financial implications for a single woman of having to leave work due to being pregnant.

Not only did Mary suffer personal loss as a result of such social pressures, but also it seems there were ongoing consequences that impacted on her social occupations, as shown by her following comments.

Mary:

It was a relief, but I was very wary. I didn't want to go out with men for quite a while. I was very wary. I did go out, but I didn't want to be kissed. I didn't want to be touched. That was a no, no. I didn't want to go through it for a while. Not forever, but for a while.

Certainly, young, unmarried women at this time seemed to pay dearly in order to abide by the established conventions, albeit silent ones.

Having obligations

The obligations associated with being an adult woman during this period in Australian life also determined the direction of the women's occupational life course, consequently influencing their occupational participation. Shaped by personal values, an obligation is a strong emotional disposition to do what is perceived as right. To what extent values and obligations are personally or socially determined depends on philosophical perspective. For example, in existentialism, emphasis is placed on the inner experiences of individuals in their dealings with social issues, while an interpersonal perspective maintains that there are social roles which prescribe what people do and not do (Coleman, Butcher & Carson, 1980). This chapter adopts the viewpoint that personally determined obligations are inextricable from social prescriptions, which include gendered roles.

As revealed in the women's stories, obligations, regardless of their origin, can provoke strong occupational tensions. In the extract that follows, it is possible to sense Sylvia's agony as she was pulled in two directions. Should she go and work, fulfilling her personal occupational needs? Or should she stay with the family, to which she apparently felt strongly obligated? In this instance, it seems Sylvia's sense of obligation overrode her personal needs and, as a result, her career in the film industry did not eventuate.

Sylvia:

If you come up to the mid-1980s, through to the 1990s, you have already by then got a different breed of women, generally speaking, the ones who say, yes, I am going to do it. But we weren't like that really, in the 1970s. Not too many of us. Although, I did have a friend who worked as a scriptwriter at the Film and Television School at Lindfield. She was pretty single-minded. And she went into film production and she was extremely successful. And she made films in New South Wales, and then she got funding for a film crew in South Australia to make [a new film], and she had to go on location in South Australia for, she estimated at that time, six months. And nothing held her back. Joyce was going to go. And how I knew her in the first place, was because her daughter and my daughter in primary school were best friends. And she asked me if I would go to South Australia with her and be her production assistant. Oh, what a temptation. Oh, and I didn't do it, of course. Naturally. Joyce went, and she was the talk of the North Shore. How could she leave those children! And that was nothing, that wouldn't influence me in the slightest, because I knew that was a load of rot. But I personally couldn't have made that choice, because it was everybody: the children, the mother, the grandmother, the husband. I just couldn't do it. But, mind you, when I get bitter and twisted, *laugh*, sometimes, I think, God, I was a fool. But I would have been a fool if I had gone, because if I had come back and things were unhappy, if the olds were lonely, or something like that, I wouldn't have felt guilty, I don't like that very much, but I certainly would have felt sad. So, all I am saying is that I think that is pretty much the difference between many, many women today, to what they were thirty years ago. They are not quite so torn, are they, between responsibilities? But it is like all sweeping statements, it is not totally true.

This powerful extract highlights some important issues that are relevant to this discussion on the influence of gender on occupational participation. First, it underscores the tensions involved with doing what one could and what one should: "Oh, what a temptation". Secondly, it is another example of the taken-for-granted limited choices available to women at this time: "I didn't do it. Of course. Naturally". Thirdly, it illustrates what was socially expected of women at that time: "How could she leave those children?" Finally, it raises a significant question regarding women today: "They are not quite so torn, are they?" Perhaps women today are equally as torn, but those who choose to work are more readily accepted than those who did so thirty years ago.

Although all of the women in the study reported experiencing occupational tensions at various stages of their lives, they reported different levels of satisfaction when they reflected on their occupational life course. It became apparent that such satisfaction was related directly to the occupational strategies they developed.

Occupational strategies: Women's ways of doing

Just as women have ways of knowing (Belenky, Clinchy, Goldberger & Tarule, 1986) and ways of learning (Pamphilon, 1997), the study revealed that the women had unique ways of doing. It became apparent that the women developed various occupational strategies as responses to the explicit and implicit exclusions they experienced in relation to occupational participation within familial and social contexts. Such strategies enabled the women to cope with, and adapt to, interruptions to their patterns of occupational participation and overcome some of the occupational deprivations they experienced on account of being female.

Although the analysis of the stories revealed that each woman in the study developed unique strategies in response to her own occupational needs, there are some features of their occupational strategies that were common. Some of these common features are similar to those described by Frank (1996) in her discussion of adaptive strategies, which was grounded in the concept of adaptation (King, 1978). When the women's strategies were considered collectively, four significant features were revealed.

First, the primary purpose of the strategies was to create opportunities for meaningful occupational participation. Such a purpose is understandable given the many constraints that reduced their occupational options at different stages of the life course. Secondly, the occupational strategies were developed by the women in the early stage of their life course and gradually refined over time. Thirdly, there was a relationship between the quantity and quality of effective strategies and the level of participation in meaningful occupations. The final feature of the women's occupational strategies was the relationship between satisfaction with their occupational life course and the effectiveness and refinement of their strategies.

Essentially, the women developed and implemented occupational strategies as a way of coping with and adapting to, the interruptions to their patterns of occupational participation and overcoming some of the occupational deprivations they experienced. Their occupational strategies were tools of improvisation that may be interpreted as assertions of self-determination in the face of covert oppression. The following extracts, selected from the life stories of the study participants, illustrate some particular occupational strategies developed by the women.

Pursuing personal leisure interests

Alice:
I don't mind going in and joining organisations on my own. Vince was a quietish person. He never wanted to go out. Farmers are often like that anyway ... But I just had to have more in my life than that, so I used to go and do my own thing, anyway.

This extract reveals that for Alice, pursuing her own leisure interests was a means of enhancing her occupational opportunities and acknowledging her personal occupational interests, independent of her husband's. To ensure she was not constrained by doing only what her husband wanted, Alice needed to find avenues for meeting her personal occupational needs.

Getting out of the house

"Getting out of the house", away from their everyday occupations, is another strategy adopted by some of the women. A break in routine, or doing something completely different from mundane activities, if only for a short while, can be a way of reducing occupational tensions. Maureen presents as a woman who enjoys doing things and being involved with other people. She finds staying at home with her husband, who is content doing very little, unenjoyable — in fact depressing. As the next extract shows, Maureen has learnt over time to structure her weekly timetable so that she gets out of the house at least once a day.

Maureen:

But I have to get out of the house. I can't sit at home all day. My husband just sits in a chair reading a book or watching TV, or he goes and lies down or sits out on the front veranda. He was sitting out there smoking like a chimney, but he got on these [nicotine] patches and he gave it up. But then last week, he has taken it up again.

Well, this week I have only got tomorrow at home. I was home Monday. Next week I have only got one day home. Mostly only half days. Ron is not real happy about it. But I just *have* to go out. I can't stay there all the time. It is too depressing … He won't do anything for himself if I am home. I have got to the stage where I have to [look after myself]. If I crack up … And there is not as much friction at home when I am out a bit, either. If I am home all the time, I get irritable.

For Maureen, when she gets away for short periods, the occupational benefits outweigh the emotional costs, if only marginally. Yes, she gets to do what she wants, but has to endure her husband's displeasure. She is aware this is a crucial strategy for her general wellbeing and mental health because she fears "cracking up" if she stays at home all the time in an unsatisfying occupational and emotional environment.

Likewise, Fran, who chose to stay at home most of the time when the family was young, found there were some personal benefits in getting away at times. When she got her driver's licence at the age of fifty, she realised that it increased her occupational participation by broadening her occupational choices.

Fran:

What did I do? I played tennis. I had started to play tennis by that time. I wasn't any good. It was just a matter of getting out and meeting people and having a hit. And I learnt to drive the car at that time. Yes, it did [make a difference]. Yes. From then on if I was lonely, I would just hop in the car and go to Roselands or Bankstown. I would just walk around and then come home. Yes, it did make a big difference.

Enriching occupational experiences

"You know, wherever you are in life, I think you just make life interesting for yourself". This quote by Alice embodies what has emerged from the stories as a distinctive female way of participating in obligatory and self-chosen occupations. Some of the women realised that enriching what may be considered ordinary or mundane occupations was a successful means of increasing their occupational opportunities. In some respects, this strategy was akin to accepting what they had to do, yet managing to get the most out of it. This pragmatic strategy that accomplishes what needs to be done, but enhances the women's occupational participation in the process, is illustrated by the following extract.

Alice:

While the children were involved with their interests, I also took an active part in their organisations. I was on the committee of the Nowra Athletic Club and held various offices including Secretary and organiser of the Festival ... I was also a member of the Nowra Dance School ... on the committee, eventually Treasurer, Secretary and finally President ... and I was awarded Life Membership. I was also on the committee of the Tennis Club, became Treasurer and helped raise funds at fetes. Also, the ladies in the Tennis Club committee catered for the official luncheon of the local Show, in the club rooms, and at other times served luncheons to members of the public in the pavilion next to the "added area" at the showground. Also, one year we worked in a tent. In the Girl Guides, I have served as Secretary, Cultural Officer, International Officer, Delegate to State Conference for three years and then Publicity Officer.

Becoming immersed in the children's organisations had long-term benefits for others, as well as for Alice. Not only was she helping the community groups in which she participated, but also she was acquiring additional skills and knowledge.

Adopting enlightened self-interest

Sylvia's strategy of adopting what she called "enlightened self-interest" appears to be an attempt at satisfying personal occupational needs as well as meeting the needs of significant others. The following extract explains her particular strategy for enabling participation in occupations of her choice.

Sylvia:

I suppose I started thinking about it twenty-odd years ago, really, at least. I had a reputation within the family of being fairly forthright. The kids would sort of laugh and always say, you always know where you stand with Mum. And I thought, does that mean that I am domineering, formidable, or bossy, or is this a good thing, that they always know where they stand with Mum? And I decided that it was a good thing. ... If everyone knows where they stand with you, and if you say, no, I am not going to have you for the weekend of the Queen's birthday, I would rather go down the coast and walk along the beach or something like that, that is the enlightened bit. It's the bit where they know where they stand with you. And the self-interest is being met at the same time. There is no devious, hidden agenda in me saying that I don't want you to come to me for that weekend. It is not that I don't love you, or I am cranky with you for any reason. I am not sulking. It is just that I would rather do something else. I think it [enlightened self-interest] appeals to me, because I like to be upfront, but I also don't like to always do what somebody else thinks I should do. *Laugh.* So, it is a nice little two bob each way, I suppose you could say. And it works. It works for me.

Enlightened self-interest is about firstly recognising your own needs, accepting that at times your needs may conflict with the needs of others, and finding a way in which all parties are satisfied and no one is hurt. It is very much like a "win-win" situation.

Pursuing personal interests, getting out of the house, enriching experiences and adopting enlightened self-interest are just four examples of women's ways of doing. For the women in the study, their personal occupational strategies instilled within them a sense of control over the direction of their occupational life courses.

Having discussed how gender influences occupational participation across the life course, and given that occupation-focused practice endeavours to enable people to participate in shaping their own lives, it is now timely to consider what occupation as a gendered construct means for occupation-focused practice.

Consideration of the gendered construct of occupation in practice

Primarily, the gendered natured of occupation, as illuminated by the doctoral study informing this chapter, strengthens and supports the person–environment–occupation theoretical models that guide contemporary occupation-focused practice. The influence of the socio-cultural environment on a person's doing, being and becoming is particularly highlighted. Consequently, it is important that practitioners adopt a broad view of the individual, a view that recognises individuals are embedded and embodied (Fay, 1987) within their societies and that the social organisation is the locus through which individuals find expression (Mumford, 1967).

By revealing the social and political influences on occupational participation, this chapter has also highlighted the need for practitioners to become more socially responsive and politically aware. Some ways in which practitioners can do this include moving beyond traditional roles and becoming part of health promotion, public health and community development teams. Within such teams, practitioners will have opportunities to develop working relationships with politicians, social planners, research bodies and the media. The development of these relationships will broaden the dissemination of understanding and ideas about occupation, health (Wilcock & Whiteford, 2003) and gender. Once practitioners become entrenched within the public health domain, they can use available opportunities to focus debate on the underlying factors that limit people's occupational opportunities and prevent them from participating in occupations of choice. Such debate is essential in public health given the relationship between occupational participation and health and wellbeing (Wilcock, 2001).

Finally, given the apparent influence of the socio-cultural environment on occupational participation, it is essential that the socio-cultural context, in addition to the historical, economic and political contexts within which people live, work and recreate is considered in practice (Wilcock & Whiteford).

These recommendations for practice are presented for consideration and reflection. The dominant theme underpinning each recommendation is the dynamic interaction between the person, environment and occupation. Acknowledging and employing the dynamic interaction in everyday practices has the potential to emancipate marginalised groups and enhance occupational participation in society at large.

Conclusion

In summary, this chapter has illuminated the influence of gender on occupational participation. Gender has been explained as a complex, socio-cultural construction that reflects the values and power relationships of the society in which it is constructed. Specifically, the chapter has revealed how being a woman can limit occupational opportunities and prevent participation in occupations of choice across the life course. The implications of the influence of gender on occupational participation in respect of occupation-focused practice have been discussed and some recommendations for practice presented for consideration.

Understanding the socio-cultural influences that affect what people do in their everyday life is essential for effective occupation-focused practice. Such influences may be explicit, such as social policy, or they may be implicit, for example, social expectations. Regardless of their origin, appreciation of how socio-cultural influences shape people's occupational life course is essential if practitioners are to adopt an holistic approach to practice and thereby enable occupation. Traditionally, practitioners have adopted an individualistic perspective of what people do. If practitioners adopt a critical social perspective of what facilitates and constrains occupational participation and consider the contexts in which people engage in occupation, they will enhance the potential of occupation-focused practice.

References

AOTA (American Occupational Therapy Association). (1997). Statement: Fundamental concepts of occupational therapy: Occupation, purposeful activity and function. *American Journal of Occupational Therapy, 51*(10), 864–866.

Alston, M. (1995). *Women on the land: The hidden heart of rural Australia*. Kensington: University of NSW Press.

Alston, M. (2000). *Breaking through the grass ceiling*. Amsterdam: Harwood Academic.

Belenky, M., Clinchy, B., Goldberger, N. & Tarule, J. (1986). *Women's ways of knowing. The development of self, voice and mind*. New York: Basic Books.

Chapparo, C. & Ranka, J. (1997). *Occupational performance model (Australia): Monograph 1*. Sydney: Occupational Performance Network, School of Occupation & Leisure Science University of Sydney.

Christiansen, C. (1991). Occupational therapy. Intervention for life performance. In C. Christiansen, & C. Baum (Eds), *Occupational therapy: Overcoming human performance deficits*, pp 3–43. Thorofare: Slack.

Christiansen, C. & Baum, C. (1997). Person-environment occupational performance: A conceptual model for practice. In C. Christiansen, & C. Baum (Eds), *Occupational therapy. Enabling function and well being* (2nd ed.), pp 47–70. Thorofare: Slack.

Coleman, J., Butcher, J. & Carson, R. (1980). *Abnormal psychology and modern life* (6th ed.). Glenview: Scott, Foresman & Co.

Connell, R. (1987). *Gender and power. Society, the person and sexual politics*. Stanford: Standford University Press.

Connell, R. (2002). *Gender*. Malden: Polity/Blackwell.

Dunn, T. (Ed.). (2001). Occupational terminology dialogue. *Journal of Occupational Science, 8*(2), 38–41.

Elder, G. (1999). *Children of the great depression. 25th Anniversary edition*. Boulder: Westview Press.

Fay, B. (1987). *Critical social science: Liberation and its limits*. Cambridge: Polity Press.

Frank, G. (1996). The concept of adaptation as a foundation for occupational science research. In R. Zemke, & F. Clark (Eds), *Occupational science: The evolving discipline*, pp 47–55. Philadelphia: F. A. Davis Company.

Germov, J. (1998). *Second opinion: An introduction to health sociology*. Melbourne: Oxford University Press.

Hess, B. (1990). Preface. In E. Rosenthal (Ed.), *Women, aging and ageism*. New York: Haworth Press.

Jackson, S. & Scott, S. (Eds). (2002). *Gender. A sociological reader*. London: Routledge.

Kielhofner, G. (1995). Introduction. In G. Kielhofner (Ed.), *A model of human occupation: Theory and application* (2nd ed.). Philadelphia: Williams & Wilkins.

Kielhofner, G. (2002). *Model of human occupation*. Baltimore: Lippincott Williams & Wilkins.

King, L. (1978). Toward a science of adaptive response — 1978 Eleanor Clarke Slagle Lecture. *American Journal of Occupational Therapy, 32*, 429–437.

Lake, M. (1999). *Getting equal — the history of Australian feminism*. Sydney: Allen & Unwin.

Langford, R. (1988). *Don't take your love to town*. Melbourne: Penguin.

Macdonald, S. (2002). *Holy cow*. Sydney: Bantam.

Makler, I. (2003). *Our woman in Kabul*. Sydney: Bantam.

Mumford, L. (1967). *The myth of the machine*. London: Secker & Warburg.

Pamphilon, B. (1997). *Making the best of life: Aged women's (re)constructions of life and learning. Unpublished doctoral dissertation*, University of Wollongong, Australia.

Personal Narratives Group (Ed.). (1989). *Interpreting women's lives: Feminist theory and personal narratives*. Indianapolis: Indiana University Press.

Rosenthal, E. (1990). Women and varieties of ageism. In E. Rosenthal (Ed.), *Women, aging and ageism*, pp 1–6. New York: Haworth Press.

Sabonis-Chafee, B. (1989). *Occupational therapy: Introductory concepts*. St Louis: Mosby.

Townsend, E. (Ed.). (1997). *Enabling occupation: An occupational therapy perspective*. Ottawa: CAOT Publications ACE.

Wearing, B. (1996). *Gender. The pain and pleasure of difference*. Melbourne: Addison Wesley Longman Australia.

Whiteford, G. (2000). Occupational deprivation: Global challenge in the new millennium. *British Journal of Occupational Therapy, 63*(5), 200–204.

Whiteford, G., Townsend, E. & Hocking, C. (2000). Reflections on a renaissance of occupation. *Canadian Journal of Occupational Therapy, 67*(1), 61–69.

Whiteford, G. & Wicks, A. (2000). Occupation: Persona, environment, engagement and outcomes. An analytical review of the Journal of Occupational Science Profiles. Part 2. *Journal of Occupational Science, 7*(2), 48–57.

Wicks, A. (2003). *Understanding occupational potential across the life course: Life stories of older women. Unpublished doctoral dissertation*, Charles Sturt University, Australia.

Wilcock, A. (1993). A theory of the human need for occupation. *Journal of Occupational Science: Australia, 1*, 17–24.

Wilcock, A. (2001). *Occupation for health: Volume 1*. United Kingdom: College of Occupational Therapists.

Wilcock, A. & Whiteford, G. (2003). Occupation, health promotion and the social environment. In L. Letts, P. Rigby, & D. Stewart (Eds), *Using environments to enable occupational performance*, pp 55–70. Thorofare: Slack.

Yerxa, E. J., Clark, F., Frank, G., Jackson, J., Parham, D., Pierce, D., Stein, C. & Zemke, R. (1990). An introduction to occupational science. A foundation for occupational therapy in the 21st century. *Occupational Therapy in Health Care, 6*(4), 1–17.

Zemke, R. & Clark, F. (Eds). (1996). *Occupational science: The evolving discipline*. Philadelphia: F. A. Davis Company.

CHAPTER THIRTEEN

The Family as a Unit in Postmodern Society: Considerations for Practice

Karen Stagnitti

Family

Collaboration

Values

Intervention

Chapter Profile

Families provide a context in which we are simultaneously individuals and social beings. Families can meet emotional needs, provide patterns of socialisation, provide role models for decision-making and resolution of conflicts, provide intimacy and security, instil a sense of belonging and give us our moral starting point (Porter, 1995). The ordinary can take on special significance when associated with the family. For example, a child's teddy bear may bring special comfort to that child in hospital. The family is crucial to understanding people in the health-care context as clients are part of a family. The values, beliefs and culture of the client's family can directly impact on the services offered.

This chapter begins with defining the notion of family and exploring its forms before considering the importance of family as a contextual feature for practitioners within the health sector. The impact of postmodern society on families in Western culture is briefly considered, particularly in relation to advances in communication technologies and the resulting influences on families seeking health and disability information. Beliefs, values and culture of a family are examined in general and specifically with respect to families that have a member who is disabled. In considering what families mean in the applied practice context, two models of working with families are presented, followed by a self-reflective exercise and an overview of suggested principles for working with families. The chapter concludes with a case study to illustrate the principles put forward. While the discussion is founded within the Australian context, the types of family and notions considered are not unique to Australian families.

Introduction

The family lies within a cultural context that gives meaning to physical markers such as lactation, menstruation and semen; sexuality markers such as courting behaviour, prohibitions and permissible behaviour; religious markers such as procreation or divorce; and law markers such as division of property, custody and adoption (Porter, 1995). Within the family, social, religious, political and cultural values are instilled through celebrations, routines, rituals and traditions.

Defining family

The traditional concept of a family is the blood relationship between people (Porter, 1995). With the exception of the relationship between partners, blood family relations are uniquely different from all other relationships because they are involuntary and are not interchangeable (Porter). As a Western construct, family types are frequently compared to the nuclear family. The nuclear family, typically thought of as consisting of a man and a woman committed to each other for life and living in the same residence with their biological children, has been the root of kinship ties. In Australia, couple families with children increased by 3 per cent from 1986 to 2001 and comprised 47 per cent of all families in 2001 (Australian Bureau of Statistics, 2003). Social trends are toward later partnering and childbearing, with the woman likely to be working in paid employment, and partners negotiating the division of labour within the household. Each nuclear family has developed its own traditions, negotiated family roles, financial arrangements and boundaries between it and the extended family members. Nuclear families are diverse in ethnic and racial background, politics, occupations, cultural practices, religious and spiritual beliefs and community affiliations. Between 1986 and 2001, the number of families in Australia increased by 19 per cent (4.9 million families), which was slightly less than the population growth in the same period (Australian Bureau of Statistics).

Currently, the structural components of family vary to include families that are nuclear, single parent, foster, ageing, same sex, extended, stepfamily, based on a compound or tribe, or units of people that share a commitment to care, provide a sense of belonging, and degree of intimacy to the members within that group (Porter, 1995). To some, this seems as if the family is breaking down but Porter makes the point that it is not the family that is breaking down in modern society but rather the stereotypical versions of family based on strict sexual divisions of labour. Social trends in Australia are toward people marrying later, couples living together before marriage, couples having children later in life (if at all), children living at home for longer, smaller families, negotiated division of labour between the sexes or partners and women engaging in the labour market (Australian Bureau of Statistics, 2003; Porter). With these social changes comes freedom of choice and an increase in individualism as each family member asserts his or her rights. Individualism and increases in mobility can negatively impact on maintaining extended family ties, support from the extended family and being responsive to the needs of ageing, disabled or sick relatives (Porter). Social mobility and freedom of choice within families have impacted on health service provision. Health services have responded to these changes by increasing services to include respite care, home carers, parent support groups and interchange families.

Forms of family

In the early 21st century, the nuclear family is only one form of family among a diversity of family forms (Australian Bureau of Statistics, 2003; Hanna & Rodger, 2002; Laird, 1995; Porter, 1995). Differences in ethnic and racial backgrounds, politics, occupations, cultural practices, religious and spiritual beliefs and community affiliations are evident across the forms of family. Each disparate form of family has unique characteristics. The diverse forms of family include but are not limited to:

- childless couples;
- families with adopted children;
- stepfamilies in which at least one of the adults has a child from a previous relationship living together in the household (Kelley, 1996);
- de facto relationships;
- teenage parents;
- same sex lesbian or male gay couples who choose to make a permanent home together (Laird, 1996);
- single parent families in which one parent and child/ren of that parent live together in the household following divorce, separation, death of a spouse, or never married persons who chose or unexpectedly had a child (Jung, 1996);
- foster care families in which children are taken in from other families; either foster parent families in which non-related children are taken into the family

unit, or kinship care families in which children of relatives are cared for (McFadden, 1996); and

- separated couples where children spend time between the residences of the two parties, and so on.

A "family" can also comprise people who live together for a long time, lived together during significant life stages, and those who live together and share a kindred spirit (Porter, 1995). Llewellyn (1994) quoted the New South Wales Social Policy Directorate as stating that a family was "a matter of emotional closeness, mutual support, caring, and creating and passing on values and traditions to the next generation" (p 175).

Postmodern society

Postmodern or (post) modern society is a term that refers to the recent and current time, that is, the late 20th century and early 21st century. Literature about postmodern society grapples with features of the world in which we now live such as globalisation, diversity, integration and disintegration, social change, measurement, information revolution, individualism, consumerism, morals and mobility. There is no uniform opinion regarding these concepts; for example, Crang (1999) noted differences in the interpretation of the theme of globalisation. Laird (1995) regarded the modernist era as a period of time when emphasis was on scientific thought, rationality and objectivity of the researcher and clinician. "The modernist practitioner ... was to assume the stance of the value-free, objective expert" (Laird, 1995, p 152). Laird then argued that the postmodern clinician must be aware of social and political values in themselves, the client and the larger society.

Pressures on families in postmodern society

Globalisation, a contextual dimension explored in a later chapter in this book, has impacted on families in numerous respects but particularly in the form of consumerism. A poignant illustration of this impact over time is the possession of toys by children. More than 150 years ago, children made their own toys, including dolls, from what they could find (Mergen, 1982). With World War II came the invention of plastics and this invention, coupled with the invention of television, the introduction of toy catalogues and strategic marketing during prime time children's television, have resulted in a situation today where parents feel they are neglecting their children unless they buy them toys or the latest gadget (Mergen). The pressure to buy toys for children has overshadowed the fact that everyday objects are effective and valuable playthings (Stagnitti, 2000).

Globalisation has also influenced the division of labour as male and female roles are now open to negotiation within a family. Women are often in the paid workforce, house-husbands are becoming more common and increasingly fathers are taking a primary role in rearing their children. Despite these changes, equitable sharing of household work between the sexes has not occurred with women still carrying out more tasks than men (Esdaile, 1994).

The information revolution has impacted on families through computer technology, the internet and telecommunications. In 2000, 61 per cent of Australians had access to the internet with the trend towards access increasing (Aisbett, 2001). Families now have access to knowledge that was unavailable to them in the past. Internet access has meant that families with members who are disabled are able to access information relating to their condition and to communicate with other families with similar conditions on a global level. One parent reported that, upon her son's diagnosis, downloads from the internet flowed in from relatives (Baird, Cass & Slonims, 2003). Not all information downloaded is accurate or useful information.

The availability of knowledge has changed the dynamic between the therapist and family. Increasingly, families are well versed with their child's condition, know where resources are on a global level and communicate with people on the other side of the world who have a child with a similar disability. The internet, being available 24 hours a day and offering a wealth of information via websites, chat rooms, mailing lists and so on, has become a resource on disability information, equipment, leisure and public policy for families with members who are disabled (Hayes, 1998). Because not all information is accurate or useful, resources are now available for therapists and families that summarise disability-related information available on the internet (Hayes, 1998; Strudwick, Spilker & Arney, 1995) or that are dedicated to particular disabilities, for example, traumatic brain injury (Vaccaro, Hart & Whyte, 2002).

The internet is also being used as an education tool for people who have disabilities. For example, a pilot study found that a dedicated website was effective in increasing the knowledge of reproductive health of women with a mobility impairment (Pendergrass, Nosek & Holcomb, 2001). Increasingly, the role of the therapist is to give a balanced view to parents on the quality of information found on the internet. It is also an opportunity to learn from parents who find useful, valuable information.

Disability in the family context

Families who care for a disabled member are not a homogeneous group (Hanna & Rodger, 2002). Families' reactions to a disabled family member vary in emotional responses, interactions with the family member, ability to adapt in times of crisis, ability to express concerns and ability to adapt to role changes (Hanna & Rodger). The grief and loss model (that is, denial, bargaining, anger, depression, acceptance) has been well documented and has influenced how professionals have interacted with families (Shonkoff & Meisels, 2000). Parental behaviours have been matched to the first four stages of the model, for example, shopping around, labelling the family member "lazy" or "unco-operative", looking for cures, blaming others and themselves, low energy levels, depression and no follow-through. However, the grief and loss model is limited when applied to families as families continually experience a range of emotions as birthdays and special events can bring back memories of loss, grief and mourning.

When a family member has been diagnosed with a disability or delay, the family enters a new world. This world is one of appointments, professionals, programs to carry out, new ideas to consider, debating the diagnosis or value of the intervention with other family members, new regimes to follow, alternative residential arrangements or even new food to introduce to the family menu. Within this new world, a parent of a disabled child can find him or herself in a situation (such as a team meeting) where he or she is the only parent facing a "formidable force" of professionals to discuss the child they know so well (Lyons, 1994, p 28). At another extreme, a diagnosis of a family member can mean being added to a waiting list of overstretched services (Baird, Cass & Slonims, 2003).

The involvement of families with health professionals has not always been satisfactory as Hayes (1994) noted when she and her family were trying to care for an aged parent. She was left thinking that procedural manuals were really to warn professionals about families and how to keep them at bay. Families caring for people with mental illness have reported similar frustrations (Ohaeri, 2003). A diagnosis can result in health professionals viewing a person as a problem to be managed. Parents can find themselves being chastised by grandparents for being too negative about their children because lifelong conditions are accepted as lifelong (Baird et al, 2003). Parents may not always have specialist knowledge of their child's assessment, treatment or condition, but they do know their child in a way that a professional never will (Lyons, 1994).

> It would be unrealistic for us [that is, occupational therapists] to think that we who see a person for an hour or two a week have more potential impact than those who live with or care for that person on a daily basis.
>
> (Hayes, 1994, p 151)

Family caregivers

In Australia, family caregiving has largely fallen to women (Schultz, Smyrnios, Carrafa & Schultz, 1994). Schultz et al reported that caring for an elderly relative who is cognitively impaired brings a greater emotional burden than caring for a family member who is physically disabled. Family members who cared for elderly or disabled family members have been reported to have higher levels of depression and anxiety (Chambers & Connor, 2002; Cummins, 1997). Schultz et al carried out a study in Australia with 461 caregivers and 454 care-recipients examining factors that contributed to anxiety in caregivers. Results of their study showed that male caregivers who were unemployed and had fewer responsibilities were likely to be more anxious than women caregivers. The results of the study supported programs that addressed the emotional and psychological factors in caregiving. Esdaile (2004) also advocated programs for parents that addressed emotional and psychological factors.

Factors that help parents with children who have a disability cope and adapt to care-giving were examined in a study carried out in Hong Kong (Yau & Li, 1999; Li, Yau & Yuen, 2001). They found that families with a small, intense social network, the attitude of the community, a higher education level of parents, a stable personality, realistic expectation of the child with disabilities, active seeking of resources, creativity in parental role and problem-solving and time management skills contributed to parents' adaptation and coping "successfully" with a child with a disability. Parent support groups were found to be very beneficial to parents because the groups allowed shared experiences and knowledge, an increase in personal sense of achievement and a strengthened positive attitude and coping ability in daily life (Yau & Li, 1999; Li et al, 2001).

Mothers
Mothers of children with disabilities share traits with all other mothers such as limited leisure activities due to employment and/or household tasks, fatigue and need for time-out from care-giving (Esdaile, 1994). In addition, mothers of children with a disability have been reported to experience isolation, social discomfort, increased stress and role strain (Esdaile, 1994; Llewellyn, 1994; Warfield, Krauss, Hauser-Cram, Upshur & Shonkoff, 1999). Australian mothers have reported that they felt that therapists failed to consider other demands or roles placed on them within the family. Thus, considerable adjustments were made in personal and family routine to accommodate their child's early intervention program (Hanna & Rodger, 2002). Research from others (Esdaile, 1994; Llewellyn) and my own clinical experience have found that parents find it difficult to carry out a home program and if it is carried out at all, it is carried out in a way that suits the family environment where the "therapy" is part of the family routine.

Fathers
In Western society, there have been many challenges to the historical pattern of male dominance such as the feminist and gay rights movements and women's increasing financial independence (Curran, 2003). The impact on fatherhood has been paradoxical. Some men take on traditional female roles by becoming more involved in child care while other men disengage from family life altogether (Curran). Fathers are thought to be more distanced from the stresses of a child with a disability as they often have a greater participation in work and other activities outside the home; however, this has not been researched adequately (Esdaile, 1994). It is estimated that fathers spend approximately 25 per cent of the time that mothers spend with their children and that during this time they make important contributions to daily routines of their children such as playful interactions, teaching of skills and shaping conversations (Primeau, 2004). Yau (2003a) reported that fathers wished to be involved with their children but often did not know how to do this. A strategy suggested by Yau was to give fathers specific tasks to carry out, for example, instead of saying "Can you take care of 'Johnny' this afternoon?" saying "How about taking Johnny to the park and throw the ball around?".

Siblings
Strohm (2002) has written of her experiences as the sibling of a family member with a disability. She discussed the feelings of embarrassment as strangers stared at her family as they walked down the street and feelings of being restricted in what she could do at home. Some siblings of children with disabilities have found the

experience a positive one, while others have been constrained in leisure and social activities, experienced difficulty in bringing friends home to play, been at risk of having problems with their emotional adjustment and engaged in more household chores than peers (Esdaile, 1994). Siblings should be encouraged to express themselves about their unique situation otherwise they are at risk of developing psychological problems (Scelles, 1997).

Models of working with families

People who access health and disability services are part of a family. The process of "assessing" and "diagnosing" reflects a medical model, a hierarchical relationship where power resides with the professional. The sole use of this model is often disempowering for a family and brings feelings of inferiority. However, there are alternative ways of working with families that develop effective collaborative relationships. Two approaches are presented in Text Box 1. By working collaboratively with clients and their families, practitioners can assist family members to become actively engaged in life activities and build healthy communities (Baum & Law, 1997).

CASE STUDY

Text Box 1: Two Models of Family Practice

Family-centred practice: Model overview and key elements

Family-centred practice is a collaboration between family and professionals. The focus of intervention is influenced by the needs of all the family, not just the mother of a child who accesses health and disability services (Hinojosa, Sproat, Mankhetwit & Anderson, 2002). In family-centred practice, the family choose, that is, the family makes the final decision. Choices made can cover family membership, nature of professional-family relationship, sharing of information and limits of choice. In family-centred practice, every family is regarded as having strengths that come from values, hopes, talents, oppression, trauma and capacities (Turnbull, Turbiville & Turnbull, 2000). By focusing on strengths of the family rather than weaknesses, family-centred practice "depathologises" the family unit (McFadden, 1996).

Power

Family-centred practice is a "power-with partnership" between parents and professionals (Turnbull et al, 2000, p 639). The practitioner and the family each have some power to determine issues.

Two Models of Family Practice — *continued*

Assumptions

The family is a constant in a person's life. Family-professional collaboration is facilitated at all levels of care. The diversity of families is recognised and honoured. Family strengths are recognised. Unbiased information is shared with families on a continuing basis. Family to family networking is encouraged. The needs of all family members are considered. Health care provided is flexible, culturally competent and responsive to families' needs and strengths (Turnbull et al, 2000).

Health practitioner perspective

The health practitioner is the agent of the family in promotion of family decision-making and focuses on family strengths by facilitating environments where the strengths of the family can be recognised and used. Services provided by the health practitioner aim to enhance the family's knowledge, skills and abilities to make decisions about the family member, and mobilise resources.

Family perspectives

The family can choose the team members to work with it, family members can look for resources and include their own issues in treatment planning. The family shares power with the professional and maintains its role of ultimate decision-maker. Parents report a greater sense of control as sharing information and decision-making helps maintain a collaborative partnership.

Expected outcome

Families are more able competently to meet the needs of family members and there is involvement of family and kin in health-care decisions.

Limitations

Family-centred practice still primarily includes only the mother or primary care giver (Turnbull et al, 2000). Most services and support for families come from formal rather than informal networks.

Collective empowerment model: Model overview and key elements

Collective empowerment is when families and professionals "increase their capacity and mastery over the resources needed to achieve mutually desired outcomes" (Turnbull et al, 2000, p 641). Families, professionals and the context of their interaction and collaboration are the beneficiaries.

Power

Power is through the family-practitioner partnership. Power is synergistic. The collaboration itself creates its own power. Power becomes capacity building with participants gaining in competence, abilities, resources and

Two Models of Family Practice — *continued*

capabilities without taking power from others. Power is the ability to get things done.

Assumptions

Assumptions are the same as in family-centred practice with the addition of the assumption that participants are knowledgeable about resources and make decisions about resource allocation.

Participation

Informal networks are encouraged such as family members, friends, neighbours and community providers. The partnership between families and professionals develops at the pace of family involvement.

Changing community ecology

Needs reside within an ecological context of families relationships (microsystem), professional-family relationships (mesosystem), corporate relationships (exosystem) and relationships with society (macrosystem).

Health practitioner perspective

The health practitioner assumes the role of facilitator, collaborator and partner rather than expert or specialist and facilitates equality between him or herself and the family. The health practitioner feels appreciated by the family.

Family perspective

Parents feel appreciated and respected by professionals.

Expected outcomes

Synergy results in effectiveness of the group being greater than the participants. Increases in participant satisfaction as individuals feel they are able to meet their needs and creatively problem solve are more self-efficient.

Limitations

Power becomes related to the role of participant and not to the collaborative relationship.

Practical applications

In this section of the chapter, some of the practical applications of working with families are explored. The internet has changed the knowledge balance between health professionals and parents but even before the internet was available, parents had concerns about the practitioner-family relationship. Equality was one of these issues (Lyons, 1994). Parents have reported that they were not treated with respect and this sense of inequality can allow an adversarial relationship to develop (Lyons). Professional distance and objectivity have also been criticised by parents (Lyons). Stepping outside the mask of professionalism makes the practitioner vulnerable but it also allows a more collaborative relationship with families. To work effectively with families, it is important to take time to reflect on one's own family's values, beliefs and culture and how this impacts on work with families.

Principles when working in the context of families

The following are suggested principles when working collaboratively with families. They are based on clinical experience as well as understandings of cultural competence (Yau, 2003b; Rounds, Weil & Bishop, 1994).

1. Acknowledge and value diversity in families

No two families are the same so an attitude of openness, acceptance and respect toward families is a beginning to start to build up trust. Come to the family open to learn how it operates and what is valuable to it. However, there is a limitation to this principle which is that when the safety of the family member with the disability is at risk in the family, the health practitioner must act on behalf of the client, not the family. Usually though, collaboration can occur by finding common ground and common values between the practitioner and family that affirm human dignity. Finding this common ground sounds simple, but it can be very difficult if, for example, the family views the child's disability as punishment and the health practitioner views it from a biological and neurological viewpoint. Common ground in this situation could mean that an action is agreed upon but for different reasons. For example, the therapist works with the child to increase the child's independence and the family allows this because the child quietens down when this happens.

2. Be prepared to understand and appreciate other types of families

Be aware of your own family structure and values and how your family has shaped your beliefs and behaviour. The health professions are an avenue to meet a diverse range of people that we may not normally meet in our daily lives. In this process the practitioner may be called upon to suspend what he or she thinks is "right" because it may not be right for that particular family.

3. Recognise and understand the dynamics of difference

Health professionals come to a family with specialised knowledge and skills. Families come to the practitioner with knowledge of the client as a family member. Professional training influences our understanding of disability and best practice.

With some families, best practice may be working at the family's pace of acceptance of disability within their family. For example, in paediatric occupational therapy, simply the presence of an occupational therapist assessing and treating their child may convey to a family the meaning that there is something wrong with him or her. For some families, this is confronting while for others it is a relief. For families where this is confronting, the practitioner may "lose" the family if the pace of therapy and intervention is beyond what the family can cope with. As the family accepts their child's condition, they may want more services more quickly, or request another practitioner. The family's request for another practitioner should not necessarily be seen as an insult to the practitioner because the original practitioner may be a reminder to the family of the trauma of coming to terms with a child with a disability. Hinojosa et al (2002) found that parents' adjustment to their child's disability and interest in the progress of their child were common issues faced by the occupational therapists.

Consideration of the clinic environment is also important. For example, relevant issues may include whether the space is welcoming, the chairs comfortable or, if the family has travelled a long way, whether tea, coffee or a cool drink are offered. For indigenous families, relevant issues may include whether there is enough room for all the family, the colours are welcoming, the ability to see outside and the availability of information in the family's language. Consideration should also be given to appropriate dress. For example, if working with families who struggle to feed their children, health professionals wearing designer clothes and power suits may give the impression to the family that they are in a more powerful position and come from a different culture.

4. Gather relevant information about the family and validate this information

In clinical work, it is important to find out how families have made sense of their experience of having a disabled family member, how they have interpreted this and what effects those interpretations have had on their lives (Laird, 1995). Involve significant family members. These members usually have power within the family structure.

5. Communicate your understanding of the family's values, beliefs and culture by clarification

Families may either not view their situation as problematic or define problems differently from the health professional's views of the situation. In these situations, find the common ground to work on. For example, if a family's concern is a child who is noisy, the therapist could stimulate cognitive development (the therapist's goal) and in so doing the child quietens and begins to learn to play. Sometimes families communicate their values non-verbally. For example, a parent who continually cancels or misses appointments may not want therapy. Such actions need to be clarified.

6. Understand issues relevant to the profession of the health practitioner

In working with families, there will be times when the best course of action is to collaborate with the family and refer them to another health professional or service. It is not the role of the health professional to be all health professionals in one. Teamwork can offer best practice to families because the expertise of several members can be utilised.

7. Determine the goals of the interaction, assessment and intervention from the perspective of all family participants

The view of the family situation from another family member can change how a situation is perceived. For example, one mother at an early intervention service obstructed access of health professionals to the child's father with excuses such as "he's busy" or "he's not interested". A family meeting to discuss the goals of the child's program with both parents was insisted upon by the health professionals. The father came to the meeting, and contrary to the impression given by his wife, he was very interested in his children and had a very realistic view of his child's abilities and potential.

8. Establish goals and objectives that meet the needs of the family from their perspective

Use the language of the family to frame goals and objectives. This principle will allow maximum effectiveness of the intervention because the family and the practitioner will have an agreed goal and be supportive of each other. This principle should ensure that home programs (if applicable) are part of the family's needs and routine. If a home program or exercise regime will not be used in a family, then alternatives should be worked through with the family, such as integration of an exercise into bathing or dressing, or bringing the family member to a clinic more often.

9. Engage in continual assessment of the level and appropriateness of intervention for the family

Therapy that is appropriate and timely is effective therapy. Families change and have crises. Life can become overwhelming for some families. In collaboration with the family, alternative arrangements may need to be made such as seeing the client in a centre-based setting, having extended family members accompany the client or professionals monitoring each other's goals and so maximising therapy input. If a family is being seen by more than one health professional, then monitoring of overload of appointments should be undertaken. In collaboration with the family, the length of involvement in therapy for a family member is dictated by the identified need in addition to consideration of the stress to the family, the therapist's experience and evidence that has been documented about the technique used. It may be that the "non-compliant" family is really a family that cannot cope with any extra pressures. In that case, therapy should focus on easing stress for the family or having a break from therapy. For families where common goals were, for example, keeping the child quiet (as discussed above in point 5), the practitioner and family may negotiate another goal as trust builds between them, for example, the child attending playgroup.

The above principles of working with families are put forward as a guide only. There will be some families where collaborative working arrangements between them and the health practitioner are not possible and other families where the health practitioner becomes an important aspect of their life. The case study below is given as one illustration of working with a family.

CASE STUDY

Jill and Mark are in their early 20's. They have four children, all boys, and the eldest, Bill, who is four years' old has spastic quadriplegia cerebral palsy. He gets around by walking on his knees. Jill and Mark live on a property several kilometres from the nearest shop and Mark is a farm hand on the surrounding property. Jill and Mark's parents live in mobile homes four hours' drive away. Bill was referred to the local early intervention team when he came to the notice of his preschool teacher when he was four years old. There had been no prior health-care intervention. A home visit was made by the occupational therapist. Jill and Mark wanted Bill to walk and to use his hands more than he currently was doing. Apart from these aims, they did not express any other goals. A program was established in collaboration with the family that involved regular visits by the occupational and physiotherapist to work with Bill at kinder and to see him at home on alternate weeks. On home visits, enough toys were taken to include Bill's siblings in the sessions. As trust built up, Jill expressed her concerns about her next eldest son who was very active. On assessment, this boy's results showed that his skills were within typical range for his age and Jill was reassured that he was developing in a typical way. She concluded that she was so used to Bill, it was difficult having an active boy. In conjunction with Jill, arrangements were made to have her second son involved in a playgroup and a local neighbour transported him each week. During the intervention period, Jill and Mark had the phone and electricity cut off at regular intervals due to non-payment of their bills. On a trip to an agricultural show, they took out a subscription on an encyclopaedia because they thought it would be good for the education of their boys. Suggestions of financial counselling were not seen as important by the couple. Before their eldest boy turned 6 years, Jill was diagnosed with breast cancer and had to undergo chemotherapy and their parents' mobile homes were flooded in a storm. Jill and Mark were inconsistent with home programs and often appointments times were difficult to make as either the phone was cut off or they were out when a therapist called in to the home. Before Bill began school, a program-planning meeting was held at the home of Jill and Mark with the occupational therapist, physiotherapist, the playgroup co-ordinator, and the preschool teacher. Jill and Mark were commended on the strength of their courage and relationship as they had managed to maintain

Case Study — *continued*

a home through a very difficult time. Mark smiled and changed his posture, as this family was everything he had ever wanted. During the meeting, targets were made for Bill's school commencement and in collaboration with Jill and Mark, visits were made to the school to organise programs for the following year.

When working with families such as Bill's family, it could be easy to be critical. However, when working with this family over time, it became apparent that Jill and Mark made every effort to maintain a family life that they both wanted and never had themselves. Among the lack of support by their own parents, Jill's breast cancer, a flood, numerous financial crises and a child who was disabled, Jill and Mark made adjustments to family routines to fit in aspects of home programs and they were grateful for support through preschool, playgroup, community and school. They were young themselves and learning along with their children.

All families are diverse and as health practitioners we come to them with our own experiences of what a family is and "should" be. Supporting Bill's family was equally as important as therapy intervention for Bill. Recognising my own values of family, and then seeing what Jill and Mark were coping with, seeing the family they were nurturing, feeding and sheltering, and recognising that they themselves needed support, taught me what it was to truly work with a family.

Conclusion

When considering contexts of practice, the family context of the person seeking health or disability services is presented as central to providing relevant services. While health and disability services may typically take an individualistic focus on the client, clients are part of a family. The values, beliefs and culture of the client's family can directly impact on the relationships entered into by health practitioners and the nature of services offered. In understanding family as a practice context, the chapter has presented a discussion on what makes a family and the different forms of family in postmodern society. While some forms of family are not new, some of the influences on family and their position and relationships within the health sector are new. The technological revolution and ready access to information and resources through the internet and telecommunications necessarily brings a different dimension to understanding families, particularly where disability is present. The dynamic interaction between a family and a health practitioner is changed. Increasingly families are well versed with their child's condition, know where resources are on a global level and communicate with people on the other side of the world who have a child with a similar disability.

While the notion of the nuclear family may still underpin social structures and systems throughout the Western world, practitioners must be open to understanding the disparate forms families can take as well as the difference that family structure, role definitions, division of labour, intergenerational connections and communication patterns mean to working effectively with them to meet a health or disability need within that family. Working collaboratively with families is rewarding. Together, health practitioners and families collaborate for better health and well being of the client and the family. Attitudes of the family or the practitioner can hinder or advance intervention but with a good working relationship, health professionals can find common ground with diverse family types to bring about the best outcomes in health care.

References

Aisbett, K. (2001). *The Internet at home. A report on Internet use in the home*. Sydney: Australian Broadcasting Authority.

Australian Bureau of Statistics (2003). *Australian social trends: Family and community — living arrangements: Changing families*. Australian Social Trends 2003. From http://www.abs.gov.au/Ausstats/abs%40.nsf/94713a

Baird, G., Cass, H. & Slonims, V. (2003). Diagnosis of autism. *British Medical Journal, 327*, 488–493.

Baum, C. M. & Law, M. (1997). Occupational therapy practice: Focusing on occupational performance. *American Journal of Occupational Therapy, 51*, 277–288.

Chambers, M. & Connor, S. (2002). User-friendly technology to help family carers cope. *Journal of Advanced Nursing, 40*, 568–577.

Crang, M. (1999). Globalization as conceived, perceived and lived spaces. *Theory, Culture & Society, 16*, 167–177.

Cummins, R. A. (1997). The subjective well-being of people caring for a family member with a severe disability at home: A review. *Journal of Intellectual and Developmental Disability, 26*, 83–100.

Curran, L. (2003). Social work and fathers: Child support and fathering programs. *Social Work, 48*, 219–227.

Esdaile, S. (1994). A focus on mothers, their children with special needs and other caregivers. *Australian Occupational Therapy Journal, 41*, 3–8.

Esdaile, S. (2004). Toys for shade, and the mother–child co-occupation of play. In S. A. Esdaile and J. A. Olson (Eds), *Mothering occupations: Challenge and agency and participation*, pp 95–114. Philadelphia: F. A. Davis Company.

Hanna, K. & Rodger, S. (2002). Towards family-centred practice in paediatric occupational therapy: A review of the literature on parent–therapist collaboration. *Australian Occupational Therapy Journal, 49*, 14–24.

Hayes, M. (1998). Individuals with disabilities using the Internet: A tool for information and communication. *Technology and Disability, 8*, 153–158.

Hayes, R. (1994). Editorial. *Australian Occupational Therapy Journal, 41*, 151.

Hinojosa, J., Sproat, C. T., Mankhetwit, S. & Anderson, J. (2002). Shifts in parent–therapist partnerships: Twelve years of change. *American Journal of Occupational Therapy, 56*, 556–563.

Jung, M. (1996). Family-centered practice with single-parent families. *Families in Society: The Journal of Contemporary Human Services, 77*, 583–592.

Kelley, P. (1996). Family-centered practice with stepfamilies. *Families in Society: The Journal of Contemporary Human Services, 77*, 535–544.

Laird, J. (1995). Family-centered practice in the postmodern era. *Families in Society: The Journal of Contemporary Human Services, 76*, 150–162.

Laird, J. (1996). Family-centered practice with lesbian and gay families. *Families in Society: The Journal of Contemporary Human Services, 77*, 559–572.

Li, C. W. P., Yau, M. K. & Yuen, H. K. (2001). Success in parenting children with developmental disabilities: Some characteristics, attitudes and adaptive coping skills. *British Journal of Developmental Disabilities, 47*, 61–71.

Llewellyn, G. (1994). Parenting: A neglected human occupation. Parents' voices not yet heard. *Australian Occupational Therapy Journal, 41*, 173–176.

Lyons, M. (1994). Reflections on client–therapist relationships. *Australian Occupational Therapy Journal, 41*, 27–29.

McFadden, E. J. (1996). Family-centered practice with foster-parent families. *Families in Society: The Journal of Contemporary Human Services, 77*, 545–558.

Mergen, B. (1982). From "play pritties" to toys: Artifacts of play. In B. Mergen, *Play and playthings: A reference guide*, pp 103–123. Westport: Greenwood Press.

Ohaeri, J. U. (2003). The burden of caregiving in families with a mental illness: A review of the 2002. *Current Opinion in Psychiatry, 16*, 457–465.

Pendergrass, S., Nosek, M. & Holcomb, D. (2001). Design and evaluation of an Internet site to educate women with disabilities on reproductive health care. *Sexuality and Disability, 19*, 71–83.

Porter, E. J. (1995). *Building good families in a changing world*. Melbourne: Melbourne University Press.

Primeau, L. (2004). Mothering in the context of unpaid work and play in families. In S. A. Esdaile and J. A. Olson (Eds), *Mothering Occupations. Challenge, agency, and participation*. Philadelphia: F. A. Davis Company.

Rounds, K. A., Weil, M. & Bishop, K. K. (1994). Practice with culturally diverse families of young children with disabilities. *Families in Society: The Journal of Contemporary Human Services, 75*, 3–15.

Scelles, R. (1997). The impact of a person's disability on his or her sibling. International *Journal of Rehabilitation Research, 20*, 129–137.

Schultz, C. L., Smyrnios, K. X., Carrafa, G. P. & Schultz, N. C. (1994). Predictors of anxiety in family caregivers. *Australian Occupational Therapy Journal, 41*, 153–161.

Shonkoff, J. P. & Meisels, S. J. (Eds). (2000). *Handbook of early childhood intervention* (2nd ed.). Cambridge: Cambridge University Press.

Stagnitti, K. (2000). *Playthings. 101 creative ideas for everyday objects*. Ballarat: Wizard Books.

Strohm, K. (2002). *Siblings: Brothers and sisters of children with special needs*. Adelaide: Wakefield Press.

Strudwick, K., Spilker, J. & Arney, J. (1995). *Internet for parents*. Bellevue: Resolution Business Press.

Turnbull, A. P., Turbiville, V. & Turnbull, H. R. (2000). Evolution of family–professional partnerships: Collective empowerment as the model for the early twenty-first century. In J. P. Shonkoff and S. J. Meisels (Eds), *Handbook of early childhood intervention* (2nd ed.), pp 630–650. Cambridge: Cambridge University Press.

Vaccaro, M., Hart, T. & Whyte, J. (2002). Internet resources for traumatic brain injury: A selective review of websites for consumers. *Neurorehabilitation, 17*, 169–174.

Warfield, M. E., Krauss, M. W., Hauser-Cram, P., Upshur, C. C. & Shonkoff, J. P. (1999). Adaptation during early childhood among mothers of children with disabilities. *Journal of Developmental and Behavioral Pediatrics, 20*, 9–16.

Yau, M. K. & Li, C. W. P. (1999). Adjustment and adaptation in parents of children with developmental disabilities in two-parent families: A review of the characteristics and attributes. *British Journal of Developmental Disabilities, 45*, 38–51.

Yau, M. K. (2003a). *Adjustment, adaptation and participation: Parents of children with developmental disabilities*. Public seminar paper. Seminar series Greater Green Triangle University Department of Rural Health. Warrnambool and Mount Gambier.

Yau, M. K. (2003b). *Cultural Competence in Health Care Practice*. Workshop paper. Seminar series Greater Green Triangle University Department of Rural Health. Warrnambool and Mount Gambier.

CHAPTER FOURTEEN

Practice in an Indigenous Context

Mihi Ratima

Matiu Ratima

KUPU MATUA: KEY WORDS

Indigenous peoples
Determinants of health
Disparities
Indigenous paradigm
Māori health and development
Self-determination

Whakarāpopototanga: Chapter Profile

Homogenous approaches to health development have failed to meet the health needs and aspirations of indigenous peoples, and to address disparities between their health status and the health status of other population groups. This provides a powerful equity and needs-based argument in support of indigenous approaches to addressing health status disparities. Alternative approaches located within a distinctly indigenous paradigm and consistent with an indigenous philosophy should be used to complement culturally safe mainstream approaches. New Zealand Māori experience is drawn on in discussing a distinctly indigenous approach to health service provision. A Māori paradigm and philosophy for practice is identified and the way in which it has been operationalised within Tipu Ora, a Māori health promotion initiative, is highlighted. The way in which the paradigm and philosophy might be applied to guide practice in other indigenous contexts is discussed as a basis for practice that is responsive to the needs and aspirations of indigenous peoples.

Kupu whakataki: Introduction

The vitality and resilience of indigenous peoples has been demonstrated by their very survival in the face of the relentless pressures of colonisation that even today continue to undermine the expression of their unique identities. The impacts of introduced infectious disease, systematic land alienation and political oppression have been costly, and indigenous peoples remain marginalised relative to the general population. The extent of that marginalisation is often most clearly reflected in the disparities between the health status of indigenous peoples compared to other population groups. While the disparity is largely attributable to differences in the social, economic, cultural and political determinants of health, there is much that can be done to enhance the responsiveness of health structures, systems and practice to indigenous peoples' aspirations and needs and thereby to improve health outcomes. It is usual for practitioners to tailor their ways of working to meet the needs and preferences of particular populations. The way a practitioner works with elderly middle class women will differ from the style adopted when working with male, lower socioeconomic group adolescents. These differences are likely to be reflected in the service orientation, stakeholder relationships, staff profiles, promotional material and the language used in consultations. In the same way, practice in indigenous contexts should be tailored to the needs and preferences of indigenous peoples.

This chapter is based on the premise that while homogenous approaches to health development can lead to health gains for indigenous peoples, those approaches in isolation are insufficient to address disparities. Instead, alternative approaches located within a distinctly indigenous paradigm should be applied to complement generic ways of working. The experience of New Zealand Māori is drawn on in discussing an indigenous approach to practice.

Te ariā o te "tangata whenua": The concept of "indigenous peoples"

There is some controversy surrounding the term "indigenous peoples" which relates to the rights that the term might engender. Under international law, use of the term "peoples" recognises organised societies with a distinct identity and implies the right to secede from countries in which they live. The concept of indigenous peoples is therefore a sensitive area for non-indigenous governments who themselves claim sovereignty and governance rights over the customary territories of indigenous people (Centre for Human Rights, 1997). Many governments, particularly in the Pacific, American and Arctic regions, recognise indigenous peoples within their countries' borders though the status of these groups is often unclear. Indigenous peoples are diverse in terms of culture, heritage, language and a wide range of other characteristics. Despite this diversity, there are common threads that run through the experiences of indigenous peoples around the world.

Work has been carried out under the auspices of the United Nations Sub-Commission on the Prevention of Discrimination and Protection of Minorities on the concept of indigenous peoples. Five factors were identified as essential to considering the concept of indigenous peoples:

1. self-identification and recognition by other groups as a distinct collective;

2. historical continuity with their territory that predates settlement by other groups, including colonising powers;

3. attachment to a particular territory, expressed in the special nature of their relationship to their lands;

4. an experience (past or present) of marginalisation, dispossession, exclusion or discrimination; and,

5. the choice to perpetuate cultural distinctiveness (Daes, 1996).

The need for flexibility and respect for the right of each indigenous people to self-definition was stressed.

These factors are useful to consider in understanding the concept of indigenous peoples. It is safe to say that while there is still no absolute consensus on a definition of indigenous peoples, they have shared characteristics that distinguish them from other population groups, they choose to identify as indigenous peoples and they oppose any moves to subsume their issues within those of wider categories (for example minority groups or vulnerable populations).

Te tangata whenua o Aotearoa: Māori — the indigenous peoples of New Zealand

Māori are the indigenous peoples of New Zealand and participate regularly in global indigenous peoples' forums, including the United Nations Working Group on Indigenous Populations.

At the time of first contact with Europeans in 1769, the Māori population was estimated at approximately 100,000 (Poole, 1991). The post-colonisation experience of Māori has been characterised by dispossession, discrimination and marginalisation. Māori continue to have poor access to many of the benefits of New Zealand society and this is reflected in, among other things, high unemployment, low income levels and poor educational attainment relative to other New Zealanders (Te Puni Kokiri, 1998). In health terms, there are gross ethnic inequalities in health outcomes in both quantitative (for example mortality and hospitalisation rates) and qualitative terms (for example independent life expectancy and self-reported health status) (Ministry of Health, 1999). Moreover, there is evidence that these disparities are due to avoidable causes. Socioeconomic inequalities are major determinants of health, but they do not account for the full extent of the disparities. Further, there is sound international and local evidence of ethnic disparities in health care (Kressin & Petersen, 2001), and this is associated with disparities in health outcomes.

As an example of disparities, comparing Māori to non-Māori non-Pacific ethnic groups, there has been a progressive widening of the gap in life expectancy at birth for the 20-year period 1980–1999 (Ajwani et al, 2003). This has largely been the result of increasing differences in chronic disease mortality. There is an urgent need within the health sector for improvements in the prevention and management of chronic diseases for Māori.

Despite the challenges facing Māori, they make up close to 15 per cent of the total population, and are a growing section of the population. By 2051, it is projected that Māori will comprise 22 per cent of the New Zealand population (Health Workforce Advisory Committee, 2002). Therefore, it is in New Zealand's best interests to ensure that this group of New Zealanders is well equipped to make a full and positive contribution to New Zealand society.

The determination of Māori to perpetuate their cultural distinctiveness and to improve their position in New Zealand society is reflected in a range of Māori-driven initiatives across sectors. There is evidence to support Māori-specific approaches to health development. Ethnic concordance between the health consumer and the health service provider are linked to increased consumer participation in care, greater satisfaction and adherence to treatment (Cooper-Patrick et al, 1999). At a wide range of fora, and at all levels, Māori have repeatedly called for recognition of their own unique worldviews, concepts of health and approaches to health practice.

There are currently over two hundred Māori-specific health interventions that are largely controlled by Māori. Currently, Māori are under-represented in the health workforce. While Māori make up around 15 per cent of the New Zealand population and have a disproportionately high health need, they comprise only 5.4 per cent of the regulated health workforce. Further, Māori are under-represented across the range of health disciplines. For example, Māori make up 3.4 per cent of midwives, 6.3 per cent of nurses, 2.3 per cent of medical practitioners, 0.6 per cent of occupational therapists, 0.7 per cent of physiotherapists, 1.6 per cent of podiatrists and 1.3 per cent of registered psychologists (Health Workforce Advisory Committee, 2002). Therefore, while Māori health interventions are mainly delivered by Māori, non-Māori practitioners make a critical contribution both in mainstream services and in Māori-specific interventions. The key element, from a Māori perspective, is that the services are located within a Māori worldview. Therefore, Māori concepts of health are central and Māori preferences for service delivery take precedence.

He tirohanga, he whakaaro Māori: A Māori paradigm and philosophy

It is since the beginnings of the indigenous peoples' movement in the 1970s that the notion of a distinctly indigenous approach to development across sectors has gained a profile, based on the commonalities of indigenous peoples and the shared goal of self-determination. Work in this area is grounded in indigenous peoples' aspirations for self-determination, is a critique of Western approaches and, most importantly, arises from "within".

"Development" is an academic area in which some discussion and debate around a distinctly indigenous paradigm has begun. From an indigenous perspective, the major criticism of the dominant development paradigms is that historically they have exacerbated the marginalisation of indigenous peoples, have been dismissive of the aspirations of indigenous peoples and have not given due consideration to cultural factors (Loomis, 2000; Puketapu, 2000; Young, 1995). Indigenous peoples contend that they have their own approaches to development that are distinct from Western development (Loomis).

Within New Zealand, unique Māori paradigms have not yet been articulated in the literature in a comprehensive way. However, a number of themes have been identified in the Māori health literature as providing an indication of the essential features of a Māori paradigm (Ratima, 2003). In the sense used here, the themes are fundamental tenets that are based on values or moral attributes and help to make a belief system explicit. The themes recognise that: Māori understand the world in holistic terms (interconnectedness); that practice should lead to positive health outcomes and increased opportunities for Māori to achieve their potential (Māori potential); Māori-specific interventions should be controlled by Māori (Māori control); Māori collectives such as iwi/tribes are key stakeholders in Māori health (collectivity); and that there is an important link between culture and health (Māori identity).

The themes and linked implications that guide practice approaches are listed in Table 14.1 opposite. Understanding in each of these areas will be important in informing practice that is relevant and able to contribute effectively to improved Māori health outcomes.

Health practice located within a Māori paradigm will be founded on a Māori concept of health and will be consistent with the themes of a Māori paradigm.

He kaupapa whakaaro Māori mō te take ka māuiui, mō ngā ariā hauora, me te rapunga whakaaro mō te mahi hauora Māori: A Māori theory of disease causation, concepts of health and a philosophy for Māori health practice

From a Māori perspective, health and disease are attributed to spiritual factors, alongside individual, social and environmental factors (Buck, 1950; Gluckman, 1976; Henare, 1988; Macdonald, 1973). Durie (1998c) has conceptualised Māori theories of disease causation in terms of mana. Mana has been variously described, but is essentially a form of power or authority (Barlow, 1994). The mana theory of disease causation attributes health, or a lack thereof, to one of four areas: mana atua (supernatural forces); mana tangata (human activities or genetics); mana whenua (access to tribal lands); and mana Māori (opportunities for Māori control).

Those diseases that could not be explained by natural or obvious causes, such as epidemics that were rare prior to colonisation, were attributed to supernatural forces (mana atua). Injury or diseases that could be attributed to human activities or genetics (mana tangata) include those resulting from lifestyle factors, war and some inherited disorders. Ill-health was also attributed to loss of access to tribal land (mana whenua), perhaps through land alienation or urbanisation. Finally, a lack of opportunities for Māori control over their own destiny (mana Māori) was considered to be a source of ill-health (Durie, 1998c).

The mana theory of disease causation has much in common with Western theories and the links are made explicit in Table 14.2. The mana theory of disease causation is holistic, bringing together many of the categories that are treated separately in most Western theories.

Themes	Implications for practice approaches
Interconnectedness (Cunningham, 1998; Durie, 1996; Royal, 1992)	– recognition of links to Māori development – cognisance of determinants of health – holistic Māori concepts of health applied
Māori potential (Bishop, 1994; Cram, 1995; A. Durie, 1998; Durie, 1996; Te Awekotuku, 1991)	– lead to positive health outcomes for Māori – contributes to Māori health workforce development – contributes to development of Māori providers
Māori control (Bishop, 1994; Durie, 1998b; Glover, 1997; Pōmare et al., 1995; Tuhiwai Smith, 1996)	– interventions led and controlled by Māori – priorities defined by Māori – contributes to expanded and enhanced Māori health workforce
Collectivity (Durie, 1998a; Irwin, 1994; Pōmare et al., 1995)	– incorporate mechanisms for accountability to Māori collectives – opportunities for meaningful input by Māori collectives – produce positive outcomes for Māori collectives
Māori identity (Durie, 1998a; Irwin, 1994; Pōmare et al, 1995)	– consistency with Māori cultural processes – personnel have Māori cultural competencies and/or access to quality Māori cultural advice – Māori concepts of health underpin practice

Table 14.1 Themes of a Māori inquiry paradigm and implications for practice approaches

The mana theory of disease causation underlies Māori models of health. The most widely quoted Māori model of health is Te Whare Tapa Whā (the four walls of a house) (Durie, 1998c). The model, which outlines the ideal of good health, proposes that health is the balance between four interacting dimensions:

1. te taha wairua — spirituality;

2. te taha hinengaro — thoughts and feelings;

3. te taha tinana — the physical side; and

4. te taha whānau — the extended family.

Realm of influence	Māori categories	Western categories	Common themes
Extraordinary	Mana atua	Hippocrates' environmental theory, Germ theory	Unseen forces can cause ill-health
Human	Mana tangata	Lifestyles theory, Gene theory	Behaviours and hereditary factors influence health
Environmental	Mana whenua	Determinants theory	Access to land is linked to good health
Political	Mana Māori	Determinants theory	Opportunities for control over one's future promotes good health

Table 14.2 Māori and Western theories of disease causation

Te taha wairua acknowledges spiritual awareness as an essential component of wellbeing, and emphasises the connection between the human situation and the environment. Te taha hinengaro is the mental dimension and refers to the capacity to communicate, think and feel. The capacity to feel is the ability both to recognise emotions and to express those emotions appropriately. Te taha tinana, the physical dimension, is similar to Western understandings of physical wellbeing. Te taha whānau emphasises the link between health and the social context. The whānau, or extended family, is a core Māori collective. It is a primary support system for Māori people, physically, culturally and emotionally. The health of the individual is closely linked to the functioning of the whānau. As well, the whānau provides a sense of identity and purpose for the individual.

Generally, the view of health expressed in Māori models of health is holistic in nature consistent with the theme of interconnectedness. Individuals are located within the family context, emphasis is placed on continuity between the past and the present, there is recognition of determinants of health (spiritual, cultural, social and biological) and good health is viewed as a balance between interacting variables. Health is viewed as of instrumental value in that the ultimate aim is for Māori to achieve control over their own development in order to provide opportunities for Māori to achieve their potential.

There is concern for ensuring access to cultural resources (such as land, elders as the repositories of cultural knowledge and language) and a secure Māori identity is central to good health. In comparison to Western understandings of health, Māori concepts of health place a greater emphasis on holism, and are distinct in placing a premium on a spiritual dimension and on cultural integrity. These are features that are common with other indigenous peoples' understandings of health (Alderete, 1999).

The main criticism of Ngā Pou Mana and the Māori models of health are that they do not take account of the diverse realities of Māori and, in particular, that there are substantial numbers of Māori people who are alienated from their tribal base. It seems that the implication of Māori understandings of health for those Māori who do not have access to Māori resources, such as tribal land and kinship networks, is that they cannot expect to achieve good health. The critical point, however, is more to do with the form that good health might take. Māori models of health together express what it is to achieve an ideal of good health as Māori. Critical to achieving good health as Māori is access to Māori resources and thereby a secure Māori identity. Without access to Māori resources, it is not possible to achieve a secure Māori identity and, therefore, to be well "as Māori". However, that does not exclude individuals from achieving good health as measured by other standards, for example according to the World Health Organization definition of health.

A key point of difference between Māori concepts of health and Western understandings is the emphasis on the link between culture and health. Recognition of Māori identity as a key element of Māori health can be considered as a criterion for Māori health practice (as opposed to generic health practice that happens to involve Māori individuals as patients). A philosophy underlying Māori health practice is therefore "for Māori to be healthy as Māori".

E mahi ana i te tirohanga kaupapa Māori: Operationalising a Māori paradigm and philosophy in practice

Tipu Ora is one of the longest standing Māori health initiatives, established in 1991 by the Māori health organisation the Women's Health League, and provided mainly in the Rotorua district in the central North Island of New Zealand (Ratima, 1999). Tipu Ora aims to improve the health and wellbeing of children and to improve understanding of and access to child health services through appropriate health education and support programs. In practice, the scope of the program is broader as reflected in its mission statement "for Māori to be healthy and Māori".

The service has registered around 2000 caregivers and 2000 children aged under five years. The intervention is delivered by kaitiaki (Māori community health workers). Kaitiaki are required to have well-developed community networks, proven child-rearing skills and the capacity to understand and work within the realities of consumers (while some have a nursing background this is not a pre-requisite). The service is based on children's age-related health education and family support needs.

The Tipu Ora initiative locates itself within a Māori paradigm and its services are founded on a Māori concept of health. This approach does not, however, exclude the use of the range of contemporary methods and tools, but rather influences the ways in which they are applied in order to ensure that they are acceptable to Māori communities. Further, the service is required to meet high quality standards in both technical and cultural terms to enable the provision of enhanced services for Māori. Examples of the ways in which the themes of a Māori paradigm are operationalised within the Tipu Ora service are discussed below.

The principle of interconnectedness has implications at a number of levels. A Māori holistic concept of health underpins the service and health is placed within the context of the wider Māori development. Therefore links between health and wider social, cultural, economic and political factors are recognised. This is reflected in the broad range of support functions carried out by kaitiaki including advice on financial management, assistance in seeking employment, facilitating access to a range of social support agencies and assisting families in securing accommodation.

Māori potential as a principle is expressed in the overall mission of Tipu Ora, that is for Māori to be healthy and Māori. Expressed another way, the intervention aims to achieve positive health outcomes for Māori, and thereby greater opportunities for Māori to fulfil their own potential as Māori.

The principle of control requires that meaningful Māori input, participation and control will be a priority. The Tipu Ora program is a Māori driven, managed and delivered intervention. In supporting this principle, a focus on Māori workforce development has been important given the under-representation of Māori in the health workforce generally. Tipu Ora has recently begun providing Māori health workforce training. The principle of control is further operationalised by the requirement that when applying for positions with the program, kaitiaki must be endorsed by iwi (Māori tribes) and that the Tipu Ora Board includes members who are active in iwi/tribal affairs.

As a principle, collectivity requires that there is recognition of and meaningful roles for Māori collectives (for example whānau/extended family and iwi/tribal groups) in the service. The service does not have a solely individual focus, but rather works with and through whānau structures and seeks to strengthen those structures. For example, young mothers are often recruited through whānau networks and kaitiaki proactively seek to strengthen links between caregivers and their whānau in order to strengthen the support base. Whānau and iwi networks are also used as an informal mechanism through which health information can be disseminated. Requiring the endorsement of kaitiaki by iwi also ensures that kaitiaki have credibility with Māori collectives and therefore within the local community.

The principle of Māori identity implies that Māori participation in the Tipu Ora service should not compromise the expression of Māori cultural identity, but rather Māori identity should be reaffirmed by the service. Put another way, at a minimum practice should be culturally safe, and ideally affirm culturally identity. Tipu Ora services are delivered in Māori domains, including homes, marae (Māori community centres) and kohanga reo (Māori preschool centres). Further, kaitiaki are required to have Māori cultural competencies that enable them to work effectively with Māori. The competencies may include Māori language skills, networks, understanding of Māori process and links to Māori collectives.

Ngā whakataunga mō te mahi i te kōpaki tangata whenua: Implications for practice in indigenous contexts

Competent health practitioners should have the capacity to practice effectively within indigenous contexts, that is, in the places where indigenous peoples gather and give free expression to their cultural preferences. This would include homes, indigenous-specific health centres and indigenous peoples' communities. The themes identified as underlying a Māori worldview and a Māori philosophy for practice provide a simple framework that may have broader application when practising within other indigenous contexts.

At a minimum, practitioners should have some understanding of the congeries of historical, social, economic, political and cultural determinants that have shaped, and continue to shape, the health status of indigenous peoples. Practitioners should also have an awareness of the holistic concepts of health that underpin indigenous peoples' understandings of wellness, while balancing an appreciation that, like other groups, indigenous peoples are diverse. While for some, a consumer's appreciation and accommodation of their spiritual beliefs will be critical, for others it may be less important.

Consistent with indigenous peoples' calls for greater control over their own affairs, including health, practitioners should not only be open to, but proactively seek, opportunities to support indigenous peoples' control over their own health — both at individual and institutional levels. There are important roles for mainstream practitioners to play in supporting this type of approach. While in some countries, it may seem unrealistic for indigenous peoples to control their own health development, the New Zealand Māori experience suggests otherwise. It is a realistic long-term goal that will require staged and well-resourced measures, and there are models that have been operationalised in countries like New Zealand that are likely to be transportable.

While health practitioners may consider improved health outcomes for individuals or groups as an endpoint to effective health services, for indigenous peoples it is likely to be considered differently. Instead, there are broader indigenous development goals, to which the health sector is one contributor. Positive health outcomes for indigenous peoples are more likely to be viewed as an important contributor to their aspirations to participate equitably in society and to achieve their own potential rather than as an endpoint. Health practitioners should bear these distinctions in mind, as a way to understand better the meaning of their practice within indigenous contexts, particularly when working with indigenous institutions. As an example, when justifying to indigenous institutions why resources and attention should focus on health issues rather than say on an economic initiative, it is useful to make direct links between health benefits and broader development goals.

Indigenous peoples' collectives are the hub of indigenous communities and represent a potential mechanism to enhance the effectiveness of health practitioners' efforts. Indigenous peoples' groups are able to provide, among other things, cultural expertise to inform acceptable and effective practice, an access point to communities, informal networks to disseminate health information, and are able to add community credibility to interventions. Health practitioners working in indigenous contexts should have mutually beneficial links with indigenous collectives. From a practitioner's perspective, the links potentially facilitate enhanced practice and community input while from the perspective of indigenous peoples' collectives, these links better ensure the servicing of their communities in appropriate ways consistent with broader goals.

The mix of competencies required to work within indigenous contexts are not only technical, but also cultural. This does not mean that all practitioners must have an in-depth understanding of the cultures of indigenous peoples, but rather that there is a sufficient level of awareness and willingness to take an open-minded approach, to listen to the expressed preferences of indigenous peoples, and under the guidance of indigenous peoples with cultural expertise, to utilise contemporary methods and tools in ways that are acceptable to indigenous communities. While as a bare minimum, indigenous peoples should not have to compromise their cultural identity in order to receive health services, ideally interventions will affirm that identity.

Kōrero whakakapi: Concluding comment

Practice in indigenous contexts should meet not only high technical standards, but also high cultural standards, in order to provide a service that is enhanced to meet the requirements of indigenous communities and thereby reduce disparities. A Māori paradigm and philosophy that underlies Māori-specific health practice provides a framework that is likely to have wider application and may be transportable to guide practice that is responsive to the needs and aspirations of other indigenous peoples. The value of the paradigm and philosophy in guiding work in other indigenous contexts and the way in which it may be operationalised can only be determined by indigenous peoples in their own communities.

Rārangi Pukapuka: References

Ajwani, S., Blakely, T., Robson, B., Tobias, M. & Bonne, M. (2003). *Decades of disparity ethnic mortality trends in New Zealand 1980–1999*. Wellington: Ministry of Health.

Alderete, E. (1999). *The health of indigenous peoples*. Geneva: World Health Organization.

Barlow, C. (1994). *Tikanga whakaaro: Key concepts in Māori culture*. Auckland: Oxford University Press.

Bishop, R. (1994). Initiating empowering research? *New Zealand Journal of Educational Studies, 29*(1), 175–188.

Buck, P. (1950). *The coming of the Māori*. Wellington: Māori Purposes Fund Board: Whitcombe & Tombs.

Centre for Human Rights. (1997). Human rights: The rights of indigenous peoples fact sheet no. 9 (rev.1). Geneva: Centre for Human Rights.

Cooper-Patrick, L., Gallo, J., Gonzales, J., Vu, H., Powe, N. R., Nelson, C., et al (1999). Race, gender, and partnership in the patient–physician relationship. *Journal of the American Medical Association, 282*(6), 583–589.

Cram, F. (1995). Ethics and cross-cultural research (unpublished paper).

Cunningham, C. (1998). *A framework for addressing Māori knowledge in research, science and technology.* Paper presented at the Te Oru Rangahau Māori Research and Development Conference, Palmerston North.

Daes, E.-I.A. (1996). *Working paper by the Chairperson-Rapporteur, Mrs Erica-Irene A. Daes on the concept of "indigenous people".* Geneva: Economic and Social Council.

Durie, A. (1998). *Me tipu ake te pono: Māori research, ethicality and development.* Paper presented at the Te Oru Rangahau Māori Research and Development Conference, Palmerston North.

Durie, M. (1998a). *Whaiora: Māori health development* (2nd ed.). Auckland: Oxford University Press.

Durie, M. H. (1996). *Characteristics of Māori health research.* Paper presented at the Hui Whakapiripiri, Hongoeka.

Durie, M. H. (1998b, July). *Te Oru Rangahau — concluding remarks.* Paper presented at the Te Oru Rangahau Māori Research and Development Conference, Palmerston North, New Zealand.

Glover, M. (1997). Kaupapa Māori health research: A developing discipline, a paper presented to Hui Whakatipu, Whaiora Marae, Otara, 10–11 December 1997.

Gluckman, L. K. (1976). *Tangiwai: A medical history of 19th century New Zealand.* Christchurch: Whitcoulls Limited.

Health Workforce Advisory Committee. (2002). *The New Zealand health workforce a stocktake of issues and capacity 2001.* Wellington: The Health Workforce Advisory Committee.

Henare, M. (1988). Ngā tikanga me nga ritenga o te ao Māori: Standards and foundations of Maori society. In R. C. o. S. Policy (Ed.), *The April Report* (Vol. III, pp 24–232). Wellington.

Irwin, K. (1994). Māori research methods and processes: An exploration. *Sites, 28,* 25–43.

Kressin, N. & Petersen, L. (2001). Racial differences in the use of invasive cardiovascular procedures review of the literature and prescription for future research. *Annals of internal medicine, 135*(5), 352–366.

Loomis, T. M. (2000). Indigenous populations and sustainable development: Building on indigenous approaches to holistic, self-determined development. *World Development, 28*(5), 893–910.

Macdonald, C. (1973). *Medicines of the Māori.* Auckland: William Collins.

Mayberry, R., Mili, F. & E, E. O. (2000). Racial and Ethnic Differences in Access to Medical Care. *Med Care Res Rev, 57 (suppl 1),* 108–145.

Ministry of Health. (1999). *Our health, our future: Hauora pakari, koiora roa.* Wellington: Ministry of Health.

Pōmare, E., Keefe-Ormsby, V., Ormsby, C., Pearce, N., Reid, P., Robson, B., et al (1995). *Hauora: Māori standards of health III — a study of the years 1970–1991.* Wellington: Te Rōpū Rangahau Hauora a Eru Pōmare / Eru Pōmare Māori Health Research Centre.

Poole, I. (1991). *Te iwi Māori: A New Zealand population past, present & projected.* Auckland: Auckland University Press.

Puketapu, B. T. T. (2000). *Māori organisation and contemporary Māori development.* Unpublished PhD, Massey, Palmerston North.

Ratima, M. (2003). A Māori inquiry paradigm a health research perspective. *He Pukenga Korero, 7*(2), 9–15.

Ratima, M. M. (1999). *The Tipu Ora model: A Māori-centered approach to health promotion.* Palmerston North: Massey University.

Royal, T. A. C. (1992). *Te haurapa: An introduction to researching tribal histories and traditions.* Wellington: Bridget Williams Books Limited.

Te Awekotuku, N. (1991). *He tikanga whakāro.* Wellington: Manatu Māori.

Te Puni Kōkiri. (1998). *Progress towards closing social and economic gaps between Māori and non-Māori, a report to the Minister of Māori Affairs.* Wellington: Te Puni Kōkiri.

Tuhiwai Smith, L. (1996). *Nga aho o te kakahu mātauranga: The multiple layers of struggle by Māori in education. Unpublished doctoral thesis,* University of Auckland, Auckland.

Young, E. (1995). *Third world in the first: Development and indigenous peoples.* London: Routledge.

CHAPTER FIFTEEN

Occupation as a Cross-cultural Construct

Michael K. Iwama

Culture
Cultural relativism
Context
Collectivism
Amae

Chapter Profile

In the chapter preceding this one, attention was focused on indigenous constructions of knowledge and how these can inform and influence practice by health professionals. In this chapter, occupation as a foundational concept in occupational therapy is examined with respect to its cross-cultural saliency. The chapter commences with an exploration of familiar (Western) constructions of occupation and its genesis to date before comparing these constructions with those of a different cultural (Japanese) origin. Overall, the objective of the chapter is to stimulate critical awareness of the complexity of occupation and that it cannot be assumed to be "given" in cross-cultural contexts. The chapter concludes with some reflections on the future directions for the profession of occupational therapy if it is to realise the true power and utility of occupation with respect to the populations it serves in diverse environments.

Introduction

Do the complex meanings and essential ties to human wellbeing ascribed to the concept of occupation in our own social experience carry the same veracity when taken into *other* cultural contexts? As occupational therapists continue to participate in a renaissance of the concept of "occupation" (Whiteford, Townsend & Hocking, 2000), this may be an appropriate juncture to examine whether the meanings that have been attributed to the experience of human agency, evident in the profession's developing epistemology and theory, really are as universally powerful to explain occupation's appropriateness and beneficence for all. Many may wonder why it is necessary to examine such a fundamental tenet of our profession critically — the meaning of occupation and the notions of fulfilment and wellbeing that are associated with it. In other words, is it really worth our effort to question the very nature and the rightness of occupational therapy? Yet others, many of whom are among our own clients and professional colleagues, may point out that these same assumptions and tenets of our profession do not resonate similarly in their lives, often seeming as if they were cast in some unfamiliar context of meanings. If such incongruities do exist, and there is a will for our membership to direct this profession toward a culturally inclusive and meaningful service for all, we may need to reconsider our ideology, knowledge, theories and practice.

Understanding the cross-cultural applicability of the core concept of the profession of occupational therapy holds profound implications for its current practice, research and the future outlook. In this chapter, a familiar Western social construction of occupation is critically examined. Occupation is visited in the social and cultural contexts in which it had been constructed and fostered to its current forms and meanings. This mainstream Western construction of occupation is then juxtaposed onto a vastly differing set of social and cultural conditions to clarify its cross-cultural potential and implications. By doing so, occupational therapists should be able to appreciate the profound significance of culture. How occupational therapists the world over regard and conceptualise occupation in different social and cultural contexts will determine to a large extent how universal our profession's core concept is and perhaps then how meaningful and inclusive the idea of occupational therapy will be for all.

Culture, context and the ascription of meaning

Culture forms the basis to this contextual examination of occupation. Culture, however, remains a slippery construct, taking on a variety of definitions and meanings depending on how it has been socially and historically situated, and by whom. At times, culture is treated synonymously with race and ethnicity; a restrictive, static and often stereotypic embodiment of individual identity and being. Similarly, in its application to collectives, culture can represent larger modal behaviour patterns and social tendencies of groups of people who are often reduced to simple, categorical depictions of the *other*. This perspective of culture can sometimes be observed in our own practice contexts when a client's "culture", or remarkable behaviour patterns ascribed to his or her ethnicity, is understood to be the reason or cause for non-compliance to therapy. Often, being judged as "non-compliant" to a set treatment regimen is synonymous with being "unco-operative"; an attitude looked upon unfavourably by health professionals who believe they are offering treatment with noble intentions. The connection between a particular attitude or behaviour pattern and an unyielding, static descriptor ascribed to the client can often result in a stereotypical attribution of a problematic behaviour.

Such occurrences have compelled occupational therapists and medical social scientists to foster the development of "cultural competence" in practitioners. Skills of being able sensitively to regard culture primarily as a client's embodiment is a central concern in such an approach. Unfortunately, this can result in centring the problem squarely on the individual, thereby shifting cause away from the broader social context that might better explain the subject's particular conduct and behaviour.

In a former era, perhaps removed by just a few decades, culture was viewed by some to be synonymous with "civilisation", referring to a class or level of enlightenment enabling one or a privileged group to judge rationally what was good, true and beautiful (Bourdieu, 1984) in the surrounding world relative to their own social norms. For example, a person who listened to classical music, read classical literature, attended the theatre and ballet, dressed impeccably in the latest fashions and imbibed the finest spirits, and so on, may have embodied the qualities required to be seen as having culture. Unfortunately, such constructions of culture can result in unfavourable judgment and designation of "other" people to less privileged categories, having been disadvantaged by standards constructed in foreign, unfamiliar and incongruent contexts. This attitude toward culture was well demonstrated in anthropological studies of a former era when social scientists from Northern places studied and depicted their other Southern subjects as lacking in refinement, undeveloped and subsequently in desperate need of cultivation. Descriptors such as "primitive", "dirty" and "simple", which held negative and pejorative values, were often applied by researchers to describe and depict the researched. The occupation and colonisation of foreign lands by the more powerful and technologically advanced nations were often justified by this need to cultivate the *other*. Thus, the regard for culture in this particular construction could lead to a raceological (Gilroy, 1993) effect in which people from one particular reference group classify and develop certain static and often subordinating definitions of the other.

A more benign but equally demeaning effect can be found in the adjectives developed within a framework of Western social norms when used to describe peculiar behavioural and occupational patterns of the other. What might be deemed normal in one particular context can be interpreted as "abnormal" when evaluated through the cultural lens raised from another context. For example, such descriptors as "irrational", "dependent" and "selfless" can represent negative value-laden descriptors for persons abiding in a Western social context.

Connected to these previous perspectives on culture but situated perhaps a layer deeper in the Western social experience, is a regard for culture as simply a complex interplay of meanings that shape the collective lives of people. Such a viewpoint of culture is consistent with what is often referred to in the postmodern genre of social science discourse as a position of cultural relativism (Whiteford & Wilcock, 2000). Briefly, unlike the universalism associated with views and constructions of truth in the modernist era, cultural relativists would take the view that truth is relative to each individual within their environment, based upon the prevailing discourse of his or her society (Winch, 1964). By environment, the social context is of primary concern. This view is consistent with Berger and Luckmann's (1966) treatise on the sociology of knowledge, that humans socially construct their realities. Such a view is radical when taken as a rejection of the line of epistemology handed down to us through the enlightenment thinkers that essentially regarded truth as singularly universal (and therefore not variable according to social context), separate to the knower and knowable through persistence and systematic (scientific) enquiry.

When such a powerful system of explanation has pervaded virtually all aspects of currently-accepted knowledge production, even within occupational therapy, we can often overlook or even dismiss alternative experiences and different but equally valid constructions of reality and truth. Asia and her sub-continents, for example, which make up more than half of the world's population, have their own systems and traditions of ethics, religion, politics and aesthetics, forged over millennia, that diverge substantially from the social contexts that supported the enlightenment of 18th century Europe. To accept that such aberrations of epistemology and ontology exist depending on different spheres of experience and place requires occupational therapists to rethink the veracity and universal applicability of their current constructions of truth, including the universality of the concept of occupation and the meanings of occupational therapy. This is a necessary position to take if we really are sincere about making our profession and its epistemology and practice culturally inclusive (Iwama, 2003).

Culturally relevant occupational therapy is a challenging notion to consider for obvious reasons. Rather than an intention to cultivate the other to our own cultural constructions of reality, we may need to consider cultivating occupational therapy and its current ideology to suit our clients' diverse worlds of meanings. For the balance of the chapter, occupation as a cross-cultural concept will be examined from a vantage of cultural relativism.

The context of occupation

Now we can appreciate culture not only as a trait or a feature embodied in the identities of ourselves and our clients, but rather as a social process by which our shared experiences and interpretations of truth (and therefore our values and valuing of objects and phenomena around us) support ascription and associations of meaning within occupational therapy. To illustrate this point, an example is offered utilising the mandarin orange and the meanings constructed and associated with this citrus fruit originating from Japan, in the context of shared meanings in two separate cultural situations. In Western countries, this delectable fruit, orange in colour and usually about 10 cm in diameter, floods the produce section of grocery stores during the months of November through to January. Usually this fruit can be bought by the box and subsequently finds its way into school lunches and onto snack tables. In Western countries where the fruit is imported, it is not uncommon for consumers to associate this fruit with Christmas. Some may regard the mandarin orange as a harbinger of the Yuletide season, conjuring thoughts and sentimental memories about the celebration of the birth of Christ among devout Christians. According to the regard for culture stated earlier, these collective experiences comprise meanings associated with and ascribed to this fruit by a large number of people situated in Western social contexts.

Two Japanese students studying abroad at a Western university, when encountering the same object, may associate a different set of meanings and cognitions with it. In their shared experiences with the *mikan*, as it is called in their homeland, there is little chance of this object being associated with the celebration of the birth of Jesus Christ. The contexts of experiences they have shared in another geographical and temporal location have imbued the same object with different meanings and realities. Rather, the *mikan* may conjure sentimental memories for their homes and families. In the warmth of an oceanic summer, they are feeling the warmth of the *kotatsu* — a common heating table used in homes in the Japanese winter. These tables are similar in size to a coffee table in Western homes, but each incorporates a central heating element and a blanket that goes around the circumference of the table to retain its warmth. Upon entering the winter-cooled room, all will head directly toward the *kotatsu* and sit with their legs crossed under the enveloping blanket. The family may be gathered there, each appearing to be engaged in some meaningful *occupation*: father watching the baseball game on the television; mother performing some embroidery; sister doing her schoolwork; and brother reading a magazine. There is usually a plate or bowl in the centre of the *kotatsu* filled with *mikan*. The fragrance of the peel in the air can be appreciated by anyone entering the room.

The object is the same but there are different spheres of experience associated with it that contribute to its distinct meanings. The two Japanese may, despite being strangers to each other, exchange a knowing glance to one another to convey their mutual appreciation for a commonly ascribed meaning to the object and its associated phenomena. The smell of peeled mandarin orange might even spur pangs of homesickness. Both individuals have referred the phenomena to a common context of experience and meanings. So, in one context, the mandarin orange announces the coming of Christmas and, in another context, the same object conjures feelings of family and belonging.

Instead of a physical object that acquires certain meanings from the surrounding social context, we might now consider what occurs when we examine how phenomena or human actions in the world are ascribed or imbued with certain values and meanings from a specific, surrounding social context and then transferred into another context. If we were to insert a social phenomenon, such as "human action" into a similar comparison between two different shared social spheres of experience, a similar contrast of associated meanings as was demonstrated with the concept of the *mikan* would be apparent. Some similarities in meaning may exist. For example, both Easterners and Westerners may understand that this delectable fruit is consumed during the months of November through to January. In this day of multi-media internet exchanges, telecommunications, television and accessible air travel, the mechanisms for shared experience transcending geographical distance are greater than ever before. However, for the cultural relativist, the respective social contexts that surround and give value to the concept of interest are believed to be substantially unique and different enough to yield varying, yet still valid, interpretations of the observed phenomenon.

The concept of occupation was purposely avoided in this illustration of culturally-situated ascription of meaning to phenomena of human action. That is because occupation, as it has been explained and treated in occupational therapy professional discourse to date, has already been richly imbued with culturally-situated meanings. Current definitions of occupations demonstrate a valuing that is particularly reflective of Western experience and worldviews. To an outsider — a person who has constructed his or her perceptions and views of the world through a different set of traditions, religious and philosophical tenets, beliefs of what is true, worth knowing and worth doing — our current definitions of occupation look particularly individual-centred and rational. Such a worldview appears to construct self and nature as separate, discrete entities that reflect a kind of divinely set order. A future temporal orientation is often associated with this view combined with an assumption that humans are subsequently *occupational* beings who are naturally imbued with a will and right to exert control over nature and its circumstances.

What is it about the construction of occupational therapy's core concept, then, that makes its transference into foreign settings so challenging and often problematic to others? A large part of the answer, if the relativists' argument is followed here, is found in and explained by differences in the social contexts that support the specific meanings attributed to the concept of meaningful human action, or "human occupation". The concept of occupation, with its rich associated meanings, never did exist in a similar social frame nor currently exists in the lexicons of many non-Western nations and cultural groups. In Japan, for example, occupation has been termed *sagyou* — a Japanese word approximating tedious, laborious work in English. Though the same system of written characters are used in the various dialects of Chinese, occupational therapists in China, Hong Kong, Taiwan and Singapore, for example, use different characters/symbols or words for "occupational therapy" (Sinclair, 2003). The problem is not simply one of language in which the other merely needs to find better words to represent an *occupation* that was believed to exist universally despite issues of culture. Rather, it may be that specific shared social contexts that give rise to the naming of objects and ascription of meaning to phenomena are unique to time and place. These social contexts, as a group, may not have valued meanings of individual actions in a similar manner to the modal Westerner's particular existential, rational and individual-oriented understandings of *occupation*.

Divergent contexts of occupational therapy

The cross-cultural utility of occupation, or any other construct carrying social or behavioural dimensions, has yet to penetrate the academic discourse in occupational therapy significantly. People abiding within a common worldview that assumes a singular truth and the possibility of rational, universal explanations (a feature of grand theories) of phenomena may not have realized or ceded much credence to alternative worldviews and spheres of human experience. Such alternative views of the world are often dismissed as irrational and simply "wrong", although science and its rationalistic procedures offer us glimpses of its existence and potential problem. From an empirical vantage, issues of construct validity and generalisability of research outcomes to populations outside of those represented by the research sample (external validity) inform us that aberrations from certain norms can and do exist. Researchers, conscious of such threats to the reliability of a certain instrument or data, go to extraordinary lengths to institute the required rigour to minimise these effects of what is related often times to *culture*.

An alternate vantage affords opportunities, through the exercise of comparing and contrasting, to recognise the familiar and to clarify what had previously lain hidden in the tacit and shared assumptions situated within Western social and cultural forms. For example, many readers will have been surprised and unsettled by these observations of normal Western experience depicted as extraordinary. When occupation is viewed from an alternate cultural point of reference and interpretation of reality and meaning — one like Japan's which has been frequently described in the social scientific literature as polytheistic (Johnson, 1993), naturalistic (Lebra, 1976), collectivist (Hendry, 1987), interdependent (Doi, 1973), hierarchical in social structure (Nakane, 1970) and temporally oriented to the present (Iwama, 2001) — the universal explanatory power of occupation along its original meanings is threatened.

Few single concepts are generalisable to an entire ethnic population. There is some danger in developing stereotypes of groups under these kinds of comparisons. However, some modal social patterns observed in both Western and Japanese settings are used here briefly for the purpose of highlighting the implications of social context on meanings within and between cultural groups.

Perceptions of self and environment and inadequacies of dualisms — A case vignette

During a lecture on occupation that was delivered a few years ago by a North American occupational therapist teaching occupational therapy theory to undergraduate students in Japan, a young student took exception to the professor's explanation of occupation. The foreign professor explained occupation as the bridge between the self and the environment. "Through our actions on the world around us, we occupy our environment, and in turn we derive a sense of being ..." The student countered that the notion that we occupy our environs through purposeful and meaningful action was offensive to him as well as to most of his classmates. From his perspective, the student viewed and experienced the world in a different way to his teacher who was, no doubt, reiterating his understandings of occupation from his experiences and knowledge acquired through his acculturation into a culture of occupational therapy and Western life. The student's question in reply to the professor's assertion was: "How does one act to occupy anything that one already occupies?" From his view of the world, a cosmology supported by Eastern philosophies like Buddhism and ethical systems like

Confucianism, there was no strong sense of the centralised agent self or a separate and distinct environment to subjugate as one's own. The predominantly Euro-Western intellectual tradition of rationalism that separates, delineates and categorises the universe into separate discrete elements, handed down through the preceding centuries since at least the enlightenment era, was not adequate to explain particular Japanese and Asian views of self, universe and the meaning of human being and existence. Neither would such knowledge adequately represent truth for aboriginal societies, nor any other social group outside of Euro-Western social experience in the world.

Instead of the vestiges of Cartesian dualism serving to explain the centralised self and man's quest to control his circumstances, there exists an alternate sense of reality that places self, others and nature into one inseparable, holistic entity. In such a naturalistic regard for the world and truth, there is no need to occupy anything through agency; you are already *there* and it is already a part of you. This is not unlike the decentralisation of the self that post-structural scholars have incorporated in their critique of "centrisms" that have pervaded theological and philosophical discourses of the West. Even Jacques Derrida (as cited in Ivy, 1987) acknowledged that decentralisation was already a basic element of the Japanese worldview as observed in Mahayana and the radically acentric Zen Buddhism.

Non-existent also is the attitude of stewardship over, or utilitarian need to control, an environment or set of circumstances situated outside of and set in opposition to the self. Japanese people, like other non-Western situated people, may tend to hold a "me in the world" rather than "me against the world" attitude that is consistent with subject-object dualisms. This may have a bearing on how the modal Japanese person may regard certain motivations for action in the world — especially pertaining to the perception, valuing and response to challenges encountered in daily living. Does one "take the bull by the horns" or "break through barriers" rather than evade confrontation with the bull or find some way to slip around those barriers?

Once the effects of a centrally positioned transcendent, single God, truth or a primal self have been rendered powerless or inconsequential, other social structural changes and features can be observed to coincide. Single, universal explanations of truth give way to the possibility of multiple truths and socially-situated interpretations of reality. Gone is the single, privileged perch from which all phenomena can be viewed, valued and judged so that a situation-based ethic (Lebra, 1976) supersedes any stable, static, singular point of reference. In the case of the Japanese, social, truth, discernment of right and wrong or any other process of valuing, is dependent on the conditions of the social frame. In contrast, in Western rationally ordered social contexts, matters of right and wrong are often reflected back to an internally held singular set of beliefs, morals and ethics. Judgement or subsequent personal action is less swayed or influenced by the social frame. In Japan, this social frame, to which one commits one's loyalty, is referred to as *ba* (Nakane, 1970). It can be roughly translated into English as "place" or "situation", and represents an essential reference point from which all things are valued and judged. The collectivism of the Japanese social frame that has been frequently referred to is supported by the particular emphasis and embedding of the self in nature, which encompasses the social. If personal agency or occupation purportedly forms a basis or ethos to the Western individual, "belonging" (Lebra) would be its counterpart in the collectivist Japanese social context.

The coincidence of a decentralised self and temporal orientation to the present is worthy of some consideration. Both contribute to a context for the assembly and performance of human occupation in some non-Western settings. When the spectre of rational self-determinism is lessened and the tendency to reflect all matters to the self loses much of its primacy, temporal orientation toward the future gives way to the consciousness of the here and now. In the Japanese experience, resignation of future matters to *unme* or fate is a common practice. Collective will and collectively held future objectives seem to hold greater potency in guiding and influencing individual action. What the individual wants to do is strongly modified by the interests of the collective over any strong narcissistic drive. The notion of "becoming" (Hasselkus, 2002) through "doing" is typically lost to the modal Japanese person, whose sensation of personal agency and time are configured according to a different social context and structure than the one in which the Western notion of occupation emerged.

Amae: Normal Japanese dependency as a context for human agency

There are many other concepts or points of comparison within the Japanese social frame as reported in the social scientific literature that could be employed to examine how the Western concept of culture crosses cultural boundaries of meaning. For the purpose of concluding this chapter, the Japanese idea of *amae* is introduced as a final concept of comparison to elucidate further the profound effect of context on meaning. Amae is derived from the Japanese word for "sweetness" and is frequently used to describe a necessary, adaptive aspect of Japanese social relations.

Though the construct of dependency in social relationships can be observed in most societies, social scientists specialising on Japan appear to have incorporated the concept of *amae* into their interpretations and descriptions of dependent behaviour patterns in Japanese society. Some may go as far as to regard *amae* as a unique form of dependence that sets Japanese society apart from other modern, industrial societies (Hendry, 1995). Doi articulated this behaviour pattern over 30 years ago in his publication titled "Amae no Kouzou" (the structure of dependence) (Kodansha, 1973). Since then, *amae* as a concept has found its way into the lexicon of social scientific research in Japan and it seems that no comprehensive work concerning the Japanese *social* can forego mention of this ubiquitous term.

Doi (1973) defines *amae* as: "the need of an individual to be loved and cherished; the prerogative to presume and depend upon the benevolence of another" (p 165). In this way, *amae* is seen to be both a noun (as a concept to describe a pattern of behaviour) and as a verb (to symbolise a behaviour of seeking the indulgence of another). Doi states "… that *amae* is, first and foremost an emotion, an *emotion* which partakes of the nature of a drive and something instinctive as its base" (p 166) (my italics) and that "in its most characteristic form, [*amae*] represents an attempt to draw close to the other person" (p 167). Doi likens *amae* to:

> ... the craving of a new born child for close contact with its mother, and in the broader sense, the desire to deny the fact of separation that is an inevitable part of human existence, and to obliterate the pain that this separation involves (p 169).

It takes some effort for Western adults (especially men, perhaps because of the lack of experience of mothering) to recall emotions that were associated with childhood — of the intimacy of infant-parent relationship. This may be due to most Westerners having been socialised strongly toward developing independence and an identity that is separate from others. It is thus unusual for the average Westerner to imagine that most Japanese, as Doi would have us believe, do not frustrate the "drive to dependence" (p 169) but rather prolong it throughout their lives — even well into adulthood.

In present Japanese society, the existing value pattern that supports vertically structured collectivism affords much leeway for *amae* behaviour. In fact, it could be argued that life in modern Japan would be extremely difficult to navigate without demonstrating some aspect of *amae* behaviour or its associated language. *Amae*, or "Japanese interdependency" holds profound consequences for how Japanese people construct meaning in human action. Not only are states of dependence tolerated, but actually expected as part of a pattern of normal, adaptive behaviour in Japanese social contexts of meaning. This aspect of Japanese social relations stands in direct opposition to the Western value of independence, self-efficacy and self-determinism, so strongly and tacitly advocated and established in matters pertaining to the Western social construction of occupation.

Implications of emerging cultural relativistic views

Through these limited descriptions of the Japanese social context that contrast sharply in many instances with the spheres of experience in which the concept of occupation has been traditionally and conventionally enacted and interpreted, the cross-cultural viability of occupation has been examined. Much of how the reader interprets the relativist argument put forward here depends on the reader's particular view of reality and truth. If your regard for truth happens to be singular, external to the self and universally applicable across cultural boundaries, then there should be little here to compel you to alter the message of occupation and occupational therapy to people situated outside of mainstream Western social experience.

Much of the current discourse on culture in occupational therapy has centred on competency and sensitivity of practitioners toward clients and the cultural features and practices they are seen to embody, more than the cultural construction of occupational therapy itself and the implications this holds when contemplating issues of meaning and inclusion in our clients' lives. From the vantage of the other, some glaring questions require our attention. With whose cultural norms do we view our clients — especially those clients who fall outside of our conceptions of the normal? Do our current epistemologies, ideologies, theories and practices in occupational therapy truly abide within the lived realities of those we serve? To what extent do occupational therapists situated outside of the mainstream social spheres of experience participate in our knowledge production and discourse? These are all formidable concerns for those who consume and contribute to the product contained in the pages of our professional journals, textbooks and professional policy manuals. In our zeal to assist and perhaps cultivate the other, we may have unwittingly assumed that our particular view of truth and reality — what is considered to be good, true and beautiful — was universally adequate. This, despite such profound differences between our and their explanations of reality, truth, and what is worth knowing and what is worth doing.

The current social construction of and ideology around occupation within occupational therapy discourse are readily appreciable in contemporary occupational therapy conceptual models as well as in the profession's persuasive literature. Recent literary contributions have helped to advance occupation as a universal construct but historically placed in modern American (referring to the important contributions of figures like Adolf Meyer, as cited in Yerxa, 1998), or even further still into Medieval English beginnings (Wilcock, 2002). This construction and situation of occupational therapy's "occupation" in Western traditions and locations can be interpreted as a boon for occupational therapists situated in the West whose professional legitimacy is further reified through information that affirms that occupational therapy is indeed theirs. To many who are privileged to identify with similar origins, this is perhaps simply a statement of the obvious. However, this reclamation of occupational therapy into Western culture does little to support non-Western occupational therapists in reconciling the meaning of the concept of occupation into their own professional and clients' collective spheres of meaning; into their own particular cultural contexts. There is a subtle proclamation of power and authority in statements of ownership — of having propriety to a profession's history, traditions, epistemology and truth. That authoritative power is further canonised when coded into an exclusive set of concepts and language that favour a particular social and cultural context. Occupational therapists and their clients located in contexts differing markedly from the West's must find ways to reconcile an alien lexicon, theoretical materials that reflect a different experience and appreciation of lived reality and a historical record that is interesting but ultimately someone else's. The challenge now stands for the profession to acknowledge its exclusive leanings and to find and incorporate ways to expand its social vision to make its enterprise truly relevant and just to varying contexts.

Conclusion

Some of the conundrums of constructions of *occupation* across cultural boundaries have been raised in this chapter. As occupational therapy moves further into a post-modernistic discourse and turns its concerns toward a more inclusive mandate, these challenges carry the potential to become more of a primary issue. How occupational therapists view social context for determining the meaning and power of occupation from a cultural perspective will determine occupational therapy's utility and potential meaningfully to touch people's lives in truly useful ways.

References

Berger, P. & Luckmann, T. (1966). *The social construction of reality; a treatise on the sociology of knowledge*. New York: Anchor Books.

Bourdieu, P. (1984). *Distinction: A social critique on the judgement of taste*. London: Routledge.

Doi, T. (1973). *The anatomy of dependence*. Tokyo: Kodansha International.

Gilroy, P. (1993). *The Black Atlantic: Modernity and Double Consciousness*. London: Verso.

Hasselkus, B. (2002). *The meaning of everyday occupation*, Thorofare: Slack Inc.

Hendry, J. (1987). *Understanding Japanese society* (2nd ed.). London: Routledge.

Ivy, M. (1987). Critical texts and mass artefacts: The consumption of knowledge in post-modern Japan. *South Atlantic Quarterly, 87*(3).

Iwama, M. (2003). The issue is: Toward culturally relevant epistemologies in occupational therapy. *American Journal of Occupational Therapy, 57*, 582–588.

Johnson, F. (1993). *Dependency and Japanese socialization: Psychoanalytic and anthropological investigations into amae*. New York: New York University Press.

Lebra, T. (1976). *Japanese patterns of behavior*. Honolulu: University of Hawaii Press.

Nakane, C. (1970). *Tate shakai no ningen kankei* [Human relations in a vertical society]. Tokyo: Kodansha.

Sinclair, K. (September 2003). *Conference Proceedings. WFOT Presidential address*. Paper presented at Third Asia Pacific Occupational Therapy Congress, Singapore. 15–18.

Whiteford, G., Townsend, E. & Hocking, C. (2000). Reflections on a renaissance of occupation. *Canadian Journal of Occupational Therapy, 67*, 61–69.

Whiteford, G. & Wilcock, A. (2000). Cultural Relativism: Occupation and independence reconsidered. *Canadian Journal of Occupational Therapy, 67*, 324–336.

Wilcock, A. (2002). *Occupation for Health — Volume I; A Journey from Self Health to Prescription, 'a history of occupational therapy from the earliest times to the end of the nineteenth century and a source book of writings'*. London: British Association of Occupational Therapists.

Winch, P. (1964). Understanding a Primitive Society. *American Philosophical Quarterly, 1*(4), 307–324.

Yerxa, E. J. (1998). Health and the human spirit for occupation. *American Journal of Occupational Therapy, 52*(6), 412–418.

CHAPTER SIXTEEN

Sustainable Practice in Resource-poor Environments

Heather Jensen
Yvonne Thomas

Occupation
Culture
Community development
Sustainability
Resource-poor communities

Chapter Profile

This chapter identifies and explores the major issues encountered by health professionals working in developing countries where resources are scarce, services are minimal and community awareness of disability is informed by differing belief systems. Increasing opportunities for professionals to work in resource-poor communities highlight the need for consideration of theories of community development and sustainable programs. In this chapter, readers are provided with a case example of the experience of a professional group of staff and students, in this instance occupational therapists, working on an island in Papua New Guinea. The description of the experience explores the salient issues of access, individual and community needs and cultural differences relating to communication, occupation and the meaning of disability. Specific case vignettes are included to illustrate these issues more powerfully. Analysis is provided by relating the experience to theories of culture, occupation, primary health care and sustainability. The chapter concludes with consideration of the importance of reflection on practice and the benefit of the experience to working in any culture, including one's own.

Introduction

Despite increasing numbers of allied health professionals crossing international boundaries to practise in many resource-poor countries, there is remarkably little literature published on the subject. The authors of this chapter were fortunate to experience working in Misima, a small island of Papua New Guinea. The opportunity arose while employed in an Australian university and included three separate trips to the island, together with groups of occupational therapy students. Some aspects of the experience are described in order to provide a context for the challenges faced. Relevant theory has been integrated when applicable. Some case studies have been included to illustrate particular issues. The challenges encountered are relevant to health professionals considering working with people in other cultures and in places where there is limited health care for people with disabilities.

Practice in resource-poor settings

Increased opportunities for overseas travel, as well as a growing network of aid organisations employing health professionals, have resulted in many allied health professionals working with people in resource-poor environments. The challenges of working with people who have few of the benefits taken for granted in Western society are great, and can seem overwhelming when health professionals perceive their skills in terms of meeting the needs of individuals with disabilities. Issues such as limited basic health care, housing, employment and education provide additional challenges for people with disabilities and those working with them to improve their ability to do what they want and need to do with their lives. Cultural differences and attitudes to people with disabilities may also adversely affect their position in society. A further challenge exists to ensure that any benefits to the individual and community as a result of intervention can be sustained in the long term. Health professionals taking up opportunities to work in these countries need to consider not just the individual but also their potential to influence social policies and support professions' social vision (Townsend, 1993).

Disability

Seven to ten per cent of the world's population is estimated to have a disability and two thirds of these live in resource-poor countries. Lower rates of disability may be reported in these countries due to differential identification of disability as well as higher mortality rates. These may be offset by an increased risk of disability due to increased incidence of trauma, such as land mines, increased infections, such as malaria, and limitations in health-care systems (Boddington, 1999). It is estimated that only 2 per cent of people with disabilities living in resource-poor countries have access to assistance (World Federation of Occupational Therapists (WFOT), 2003). In part, this is because many live in small communities and do not have access to services that are available in larger communities (WHO/DAR & IAFO, 2003).

People may experience physical disability (for example, amputations from injury by land mines or cerebral palsy), psychological conditions (for example, depression or schizophrenia) or intellectual deficits resulting from congenital conditions or acquired brain injury. There is considerable inequality of women in many of these communities both when they have a disability and as carers of people with disabilities (WFOT, 2003).

Disability may not be identified in many communities because it is primarily a social construct that has developed in Western societies since the industrial revolution when it became necessary to sell one's labour. Prior to this, people with disability had a "lowly but legitimate position in society" (Arriotti, 1999, p 217). People in communities without a developed labour market, such as Misima, may not have developed "disability" as a concept and people are only seen to have disabilities when identified by health or rehabilitation service providers. These "professionals" have often classified disability using the medical model, which means that the problem lies within the person as a result of trauma or pathology and consequent intervention involves medical and other treatment. The social model of disability, on the other hand, views disability as a result of society not providing sufficient supports for the integration of all people into the community. The way to reduce disability is through political action for human rights.

The International Classification of Functioning, Disability and Health (WHO, 2001) combines these two models and classifies people with health-related problems, including disability, on the basis of impairment, activity and participation restrictions. Impairments are identified when a person's body structures and functions mean he or she is unable to function at a level expected in the normal population. Activities refer to tasks the person wishes to do and participation is being involved in a life situation.

People need to be able to participate in occupations that are meaningful and important to them and their community for good health (Kramer, Hinosjosa & Royeen, 2003). Occupational deprivation exists in Western countries for people who do not have a disability and the plight of unemployed people, prisoners and refugees is well documented (Whiteford, 2000). In resource-poor countries, people who have been displaced from normal living due to severe physical and mental illness or disability continue to be excluded from engaging in occupations and roles that are valued by society (Yeoman, 1998). Society may facilitate or inhibit people with a particular impairment from being able to do certain activities and engage in certain occupational aspects of their lives. Thus, each person's situation is seen as a complex interplay between the health condition, the individual and the environment.

Sustainable practice

Sustainable development is a concept derived from concerns about the global environment where any development must operate within the parameters of available resources and the productive potential of the ecosystem, without compromising the ability of future generations to meet their own needs (O'Connor-Fleming & Parker, 2001). Given the close relationship between environment and health, public health practice has begun to incorporate the social, political and economic reality for people in their policies.

Primary health care was declared by the World Health Organization (WHO), in its 1979 Alma Ata Declaration, as the way in which all people could achieve socially and economically productive lives. WHO recognised that inequities in health are embedded in the way a society works — politically, culturally and socially. The way in which communities and the people in them can achieve lasting improvement in the quality of their lives is through the principles of equity, social justice, community participation and empowerment, and intersectoral collaboration (O'Connor-Fleming & Parker, 2001).

Community Based Rehabilitation (CBR) is a community development strategy based on the principles of primary health care, which aims to provide rehabilitation, equalisation of opportunities and social integration of all children and adults with disabilities. It is implemented through the combined efforts of people with disabilities themselves, their families and communities, and the appropriate health, education, vocational and social services (ILO, UNESCO and WHO joint position paper 1994 cited in WHO and Swedish Organizations of Disabled Persons International Aid Association, 2002). The core ingredients of CBR are being community based, rehabilitation focus, and cultural compatibility and utilisation of local resources (IDDC, 2002). These elements are explored below.

Community based

Being community based means that, wherever possible, the locus of control must remain with people with disabilities and their families working within the community rather than in large institutions. Intervention must be at both an individual level and at a community level, which is in keeping with the ICF already outlined. Health professionals must not only have knowledge about disability and the individual's needs and interests but also use socio-political skills within the community (WFOT, 2003).

Workers involved in any community development, including CBR, need to establish an equal partnership with community organisations as well as individual members of the community. Sustainability of any program can only be developed if there is active participation from community members and the recognition and utilisation of expertise already present in the community. The agenda needs to be led by the community including less powerful members such as people with disabilities (and their carers) who may have less access to resources, such as education, and land than others. Community development requires advocacy on behalf of people with disabilities to raise the awareness of the community about the particular needs of this disadvantaged group so that they can have greater access to resources. The entire community needs to benefit from any action. Over time, building the capacity of individuals and organisations within the community to take responsibility for continuing the aims of the program ensures that gains are sustained. This will require a longer time frame than other ways of introducing change into communities (Hobbs, McDonough & O'Callaghan, 2002).

Rehabilitation

Rehabilitation has been criticised by people with disabilities as emphasising the medical rather than social aspects of disability with the focus on overcoming impairment rather than increasing participation in community activities. The social inclusion aspects of rehabilitation need to be emphasised to overcome this perception by people with disabilities for community based rehabilitation to be seen to be effective (IDDC, 2002). Health promotion and prevention of disease and deformity can also be a focus.

Cultural compatibility

Cultural compatibility means responding flexibly, in order to build on formal and informal traditions already in the community (IDDC, 2002). Health professionals are required to work in a wide variety of cultural contexts and must recognise and value different cultural groups. Learning to be culturally sensitive and safe requires that practitioners have an awareness of their own cultural influences and develop the ability to step outside Western assumptions about family structures, living situations and gender relationships, (Hocking & Whiteford, 1995; Jungersen, 2002). Concepts such as independence and productivity should be recognised as Western values (Franscisco & Carlson, 2002) that may not be relevant to people whose beliefs differ from those of this dominant paradigm. Effective intervention must be culturally relevant to the individual and their community and requires a socio-political overview of practice, including a critical awareness of the structures and processes by which people are marginalised in their society (WFOT, 2003).

Local resources

Utilising local resources is an important way to ensure the sustainability of any intervention since any equipment created is cheap, adaptable and replaceable. People with disabilities and their community can also be actively involved in the design and manufacture of equipment. While health professionals may provide some ideas and examples, utilising and acknowledging local skills and expertise is more empowering for the community.

The Misima Project

The following section gives an overview of a project undertaken by the authors together with a group of occupational therapy students during 2000 and 2001. This project provides one example of practice in a resource-poor environment and a context for further analysis and application of issues outlined above.

Misima is an island of about 12 000 people in Milne Bay Province, which serves as a regional centre for the Louisiade Archipelago, Papua New Guinea. It has a mountainous centre and most people live in villages around the coast. Roads are present only around the eastern half of the island with the rest of the villages being serviced by foot tracks and boats. Misima Mines Ltd commenced a mining operation on the island in 1994. The social impact of the mine caused rapid population growth as opportunities for employment grew, with improvements in health, education and housing facilities. The economic growth resulting from the mine also created increased land costs, consumption and dependence on imported food as well as increased alcohol consumption (Misima Mines, 1998).

The Community Development and Education section of the mine sponsored the project, as it was seen as potentially contributing to their goal to "leave behind a better future" for the people of Misima (Placer Dome Asia Pacific, 2001, p 5). The mine generously provided flights and accommodation to the staff and students who worked voluntarily in this project. During the project, students worked in the mining environment under the supervision of the Occupational Health and Safety Department, as well as in the community, to improve the quality of life of people with disabilities. A total of twelve students visited Misima over three visits with stays of four to five weeks each time.

The first visit was primarily exploratory to ascertain whether the people of Misima could benefit from the services that occupational therapists had to offer and to plan for future visits. Initially, one of the main projects instigated, with the support of the doctor at the hospital and council members, was to develop a register of people with disabilities living in Misima. Over the three visits, knowledge and understanding of the team and of occupational therapy increased and more people were added to the register. On the second visit, students continued to work with adults and children who were identified with disabilities within the community and to provide further input to staff at the hospital and Education Department. On the third and final visit (due to the imminent closure of the mine), the focus moved to providing more sustainable intervention to families and education of hospital staff and teachers to assist them in working with people with disabilities. An evaluation of the project of the community and health workers was conducted on the last visit from interviews using local community members and written surveys. Students were also interviewed about the impact of the learning gained from the experience.

Misiman culture

Misimans are basically subsistence farmers, who generally work together to produce sufficient food for family groups. Sharing of produce and wealth is part of a culture of communal living and co-operation. Extended kinship relationships are important. The concept of family includes several generations with grandparents being actively involved with the upbringing of children, and family consultation in major decisions being essential. Recognising the importance of the family and upholding the cultural values for discussion and collective decision making made it possible to make a difference to people's lives.

The ability to garden and fish enhances the status of the individual in this community, as does ownership of livestock. The community gardens were usually some distance from the villages which limited opportunities for people with disabilities to contribute actively to their communities. One woman who was unable to walk crawled to her garden daily, regardless of her increasing pain, because this important occupation provided her not only with sustenance but also with status within her community. Women also spend a great deal of time in domestic duties: cooking, cleaning and washing clothes. Men and women worked together to provide housing, largely built from local materials.

The mine provides employment for many people. Other employment includes government work such as within the health and education systems but there is very little employment in the private sector.

Children go to school in the local village, usually from the age of seven years, and then attend primary school from age eleven. Many children walk long distances each day to attend school and frequently it is distance and poor mobility that prevents children with disabilities from attending along with their brothers and sisters.

Appreciation of the cultural beliefs and norms ensure that practice is relevant and appropriate. For instance, in Misima houses are set high so that domestic animals, dogs, chickens and pigs are kept out, resulting in lack of access for people with disabilities, who become housebound as soon as they are too heavy to be lifted. Misiman people bathe regularly throughout the day, using a community tap. Toileting in the house is considered unclean so that incontinence may result in a person being excluded from the family living areas. The solutions to these problems of daily living required a new approach in practice (clearly a commode and shower stool were not the answer). Only through understanding the culture and discussing possible solutions with clients and their families was it possible to ensure workable solutions.

Communication

English is a second language for most Misimans and so communication was at times difficult due to this language barrier. Western professionals rely on verbal skills to inform and instruct clients. However, over time the team was able to develop a range of appropriate communication skills. Some basic Misiman was learnt and body language and pictures were used to communicate effectively. However, the use of an interpreter was essential to develop effective communication.

Selection of an interpreter should be considered carefully in terms of knowledge base, gender and acceptability to the whole community. A period of training is essential both to teach the interpreter basic concepts of your practice so that these can be translated and also to learn about the culture and language of the community.

In Misima, the team was fortunate to be introduced to Dominic, who was encouraged by the church where he worked to act as interpreter. Dominic had cerebral palsy, and his personal experience of disability made him well suited to this position. His own story is presented later as a case study. However, his affiliation with one of the two main churches presented difficulties on some occasions, which necessitated using alternative interpreters who were not associated with this church. Also, on some occasions, it was more appropriate to use a female interpreter.

Adhering to local protocols when visiting villages communicated respect for the Misiman culture. Each village group had an elected council member who held community meetings to discuss important issues. The team and interpreter would meet with the council members to ensure they were aware of the group's activities. On several occasions, the team was invited to speak at the village meeting and the council members' support resulted in positive community action for an individual with a disability.

Disability

Through interactions with people with disabilities and their families, it became clear that they attributed different causes for disability than those accepted by Western medicine. While people had access to education and information from the media, their understanding of illness and disability remained culturally influenced. It appeared that people had quite different understandings of how their bodies worked. For example, they believed that the spine was one bone, people with chronic disabilities could be cured by blood transfusions and they did not distinguish between the nervous and circulatory systems. It was therefore important to provide necessary health information so that people could manage their conditions within the context of their existing beliefs.

In many cases, diagnoses were not available and decisions regarding intervention were based on narrative and pragmatic reasoning rather than scientific reasoning (Schell, 2003). The history of the client's condition was often impossible to determine and frequently told using a mixture of circumstantial, religious and "magical" events that were believed to be causative. Often, peoples' stories about how they developed an illness involved a lengthy narrative about the days leading up to the incident. Spiritual beliefs, both Christian and otherwise, also provided an important role in explanations of causality and recovery. People of the Milne Bay Province are renowned for their strong belief and involvement in sorcery and this may be seen as a source of illness or disability, even if is not publicly acknowledged (Lipscomb, McKinnon & Murray, 1998). Christianity is very strong on the island with most people being involved in one of the two major churches present. People we met attributed recovery from illness to prayer and divine intervention.

People who develop disorders or are injured as adults seemed to be well accepted by the community, perhaps because they have already demonstrated the skills to contribute to the community and have developed necessary relationships within the family structure. Being born with a disability results in loss of opportunity to contribute, and although family members provided care, they seldom encouraged participation in the community. There appeared to be a degree of shame for the family associated with them.

Towards sustainability in Misima

Conducting three visits separate visits to Misima enabled the team to reflect on the value of the project and assess its effectiveness. Through the evaluation process, the focus of interventions was seen to be on achieving sustainable changes for individuals and for the community. Four aspects of practice instigated during the

Misima project are described below and are discussed in relation to the concepts of sustainability and capacity building.

Partner organisations

As women were usually the ones who cared for people with disabilities, the most obvious non-government community organisation to work with was the Women's Association which was active throughout the island. They also had a well-established program of workshops on issues such as health and development of small business running throughout the villages. An educational session presented to the annual general meeting of the Women's Association included information about back care for carers and promoted inclusion of children with disabilities in schooling and other aspects of community life. While the Women's Association was an ideal group to foster the development of a community based rehabilitation program, this proved to be difficult to implement because of conflict within the organisation on the last two visits of the occupational therapy team. This highlights major disadvantages the team faced by not being there for a longer period of time, as not only would conflict within the Association eventually have been resolved, but also further raising of awareness by the team could have been achieved within each village. As already emphasised, time is an important factor in building capacity within a community and this was not available for this project. There were only three visits to Misima by the team and it is therefore uncertain whether some of the apparent gains of people with disabilities outlined above were, in fact, sustainable in the longer term. Evaluation found that people in Misima found the visits useful and there was evidence of some changes in the awareness about disability within the community. Further evaluation after the end of the project was needed to ascertain whether there was any long-term benefit. Unfortunately, this has not been possible to date.

Back care education

With the support of the Occupational Health and Safety Department, the team identified a back care education program to be an appropriate project within the mine. The majority of the mine employees were local people who lived with their families in the villages of Misima. By conducting health education and promotion for the mine employees, it would be possible to improve health and safety not only within the mines but also to impact on community health. Education sessions were developed and conducted for mineworkers on all three visits by the students. The sessions were aimed at ensuring workers maintained safe habits at the mine as well as continuing these good habits when at home. Presentations were made to work teams allowing a focus on problem solving of awkward tasks to ensure injury prevention at work and at home.

Many of the male mine employees lift and carry heavy loads including canoes, outboard motors, house building materials and food, such as pigs and large bunches of bananas, as part of their home responsibilities. Women carry heavy loads in baskets on their heads. The students therefore included in the program alternative methods to carry out these activities in a safer manner. Exercises that helped maintain a healthy back were taught and practised, and good sleeping positions were discussed. Handouts with culturally appropriate illustrations were provided to all workers to take home and share with other family members.

The occupational therapy students became closely associated with good back care practices and took every opportunity to promote back care in the Misiman community. There was evidence to suggest that this increased awareness resulted in earlier reporting of back injury at the mine clinic and feedback from the community demonstrated that information was being passed on to family members. Similar programs were conducted with community groups such as the Women's Association and to carers who were frequently lifting relatives with disabilities. The advantage of this health promotion program was its benefit to the whole community and its simplicity. Within the mine, the information and resources were provided for future use by the occupational health and safety staff, and could be passed on to all community members.

Working with people with disabilities

Council members, health workers and local people identified to the occupational therapy team a number of children and adults with physical and cognitive disabilities, during each visit. The team was able to provide interventions for rehabilitation, advice and ideas for family members to enable them to care for people with a disability more effectively, by providing easier ways for toileting, lifting and managing difficult behaviours. During the visits, the team also worked directly with patients in the hospital, providing a rehabilitation focus and following up those with permanent disabilities resulting from injuries.

Like other occupational therapists working in developing countries, the lack of resources available for intervention presented an initial problem. Preparation for this project included gathering resources that would be helpful for implementing treatment including elasticised bandaging material, foam pipe insulation material and thermoplastic splinting material, together with references from books and catalogues. Familiarity with service delivery models in Western countries, where resources and funding are available to meet client needs, limited our concept of effective occupational therapy. Over the course of the three visits, it became evident that a change in the focus was necessary from delivering services to individuals and their families, to providing information to families and assisting them to find solutions that were sustainable. It was essential that families who were responsible for ongoing care were empowered to continue to provide occupational therapy to their relatives. Time was spent with families discussing possible solutions to problems and providing information and pictures of easily constructed equipment for future use. This equipment was then more likely to be appropriate and used, and the family could fix any breakdowns.

Funding for rehabilitation in the community was not available and health workers had little knowledge in this area, leaving people to manage as best they could in the community. Ideally, a community based rehabilitation program would have been effective in Misima but could not be implemented due to the time constraints of the project and the limitations of any suitable partner organisation.

However, the evaluations demonstrated that hospital staff and health workers reported greater awareness of the needs of people with disability which may mean that the longer-term needs of people with chronic conditions are considered in the future before discharge back to the community.

The incidence of children with disability in Misima was not high and they were well cared for by their families. If a child could not perform a particular task at the expected age (for example, drinking from a cup) then he or she might not be given the opportunity again. Therefore, the occupational therapy team worked with these families by advising on appropriate seating and feeding techniques as well as exercises and other forms of stimulation, which promoted the children's development and decreased the possibility of future deformity. Sometimes, involvement was only one visit but for some people, a number of visits were provided in order to give as much assistance as possible. Some people were visited over the three trips by the occupational therapy team.

The evaluation of the project found that a major impact was to increase the community awareness of people with disabilities and thereby reduce the shame involved in having a child with a disability. The involvement of the occupational therapy team with young children and their families resulted in better outcomes for the children with disabilities such as being taken out into the community whereas prior to the visit they were housebound.

CASE STUDY

Genevieve's story

"Genevieve" was the granddaughter of one of the council members and the only child of a young couple whose father worked at the mine. She was two-years-old and appeared to have cerebral palsy, with low tone. She spent most of her time, apart from feeding, lying on her back in the main room of the house as she did not have enough muscle strength to sit, or even hold her head up. The initial interventions with Genevieve aimed to increase muscle strength. The team provided a covered foam wedge and taught Genevieve's mother, through demonstration, to position the child in a prone position to weight bear through her arms and to encourage head control and neck extension using an overhead frame with toys suspended at eye level.

During the next visit, Genevieve was followed up and little progress was observed. The foam wedge was not being used and Genevieve was still lying on her back for the majority of the day. A new approach was therefore taken with a focus on encouraging community access and a supported sitting posture. The family had already purchased a stroller, which did not provide

Genevieve's story — *continued*

her with sufficient support to sit upright. This was adapted by the team and her family using plywood and foam.

The team demonstrated how the stroller could be adapted and provided some of the materials; however, the resources of the family were used to cut and attach the board and cover the foam. The adapted stroller was much more successful and it was soon reported to the team that Genevieve had been taken out into the community in the stroller which had previously not happened. The adapted stroller made feeding easier for her mother and enabled Genevieve to play with objects on the attached tray as well as interact with others in her environment.

Community education

In addition to providing health promotion programs and individual rehabilitation, the group maintained the focus on educating local people in the community, especially those who could influence future policies. Talking at villages meetings and with local council members ensured that there was widespread understanding of the services that we could provide, both to individuals and to the community as a whole. Moreover, the talks presented the concept that people with disabilities had rights and the potential to contribute to the community. Teachers and health workers were actively sought out and involved in finding solutions for individuals. The Women's Association was identified as influential especially in child rearing practices, and so the chairperson was included where possible on our visits.

Through visits to the villages and schools, it became clear that children with disabilities were frequently excluded from educational opportunities, as well as other normal childhood activities. Older children were frequently housebound and deprived of social interaction and stimulation — both physical and intellectual. Liaison with the Education Department and school teachers identified a need for a consistent sign language program due to a significant number of deaf children in some parts of the community. It was perhaps easier for the community to identify the problems in relation to deaf children who were physically capable of attending school, but with whom teachers had difficulties communicating directly. Sign language was identified as one way in which the whole community, including school peers, could encourage inclusion in the community.

With the support of the Education Department, the occupational therapy team facilitated a one-day workshop for all elementary teachers on the island. During the workshop, the team was able to promote the concept of inclusion in schools for children with disabilities to the majority of teachers. The workshop included training in sign language, teaching strategies for children with learning disabilities, as well as information on the concept of inclusion of children with disabilities.

Dominic, our interpreter, was involved in the planning of this workshop and offered to talk about his own experience of being excluded from school as a child. Dominic's story was later written and illustrated so that he could continue to educate people about the importance of providing educational opportunities to children with disabilities. Evaluation of the workshop indicated that teachers now felt more confident to include children with disabilities in their classroom activities.

CASE STUDY

Dominic's story

Dominic worked with the occupational therapy team during each of the three visits. He was in his early twenties and employed by the church. Although he had not been born in Misima, he was well known to the community. Dominic was well suited to the role of interpreter as he spoke a number of local languages and English fluently. He also had a disability himself, having been born with cerebral palsy, and he generously shared with us his own remarkable story.

During his childhood Dominic had been unable to walk. His father worked away from home and his mother had frequently left him alone in the house to attend the gardens. He had not attended school due to his disability, until a visiting doctor came to see him at home when he was 10-years-old. The doctor told him and his mother that he must learn to walk, and he was given a stick to practise standing and strengthen his legs. After this, Dominic, with the help of his family, taught himself to walk. He remembers going outside for the first time and being afraid of everything that he had not previously experienced. He started elementary school at the age of 14 years and was often laughed at by the other younger students. However, he was a good student and worked hard. Among his other accomplishments, Dominic learnt to ride a bike one handed and he played volleyball with the young people at the church. He is now an active community member engaged in sport, church and other social activities.

While working with the team, it became apparent that Dominic had learnt a great deal about the way the team worked with people during our visits. His genuine interest in helping people and his willingness to learn encouraged the team to explain to him some basic principles which he could continue to pass on to people in the community. At the end of the final trip, all the accumulated resources were passed on to Dominic including a copy of *Disabled Village Children* by David Werner (1987), which he could use with clients and families to follow up on our input. Limited time, however, resulted in lack of in-depth and ongoing training, which meant that Dominic has limited skills in working with people with disabilities.

Reflection as a tool for personal enquiry and professional development

Profound learning transpires when living and working in another culture. This necessitates a high level of self-reflection which is rarely discussed in the professional literature. Reflection was first described by Dewey as the "active, persistent and careful consideration of any belief or supposed form of knowledge in the light of the grounds that support it and the further conclusion to which it tends" (Dewey, as cited in Brown & Ryan, 2003, p 9). The process of reflection on practice is transformative. It allows practitioners to reassess their knowledge and understanding, to consider the relevance and worth of their action (Brown & Ryan) and to change both personally and professionally (Denshire, 2002). Through reflection on the Misima experience, there has been an opportunity to learn about the relevance of providing sustainable and culturally appropriate occupational therapy that is transferable to practice anywhere.

During the Misima project, the occupational therapy team used reflection to ensure that the interventions provided would be sustainable in the community. Despite a belief in community education and development, the team initially focused on addressing individual needs and providing equipment and strategies to encourage independence. Three separate factors challenged us to "think outside of the square". First, our own observations that interventions were generally not continued by families between our visits clearly indicated that we had not empowered the carers by our actions. Secondly, the imminent closure of the mine, including the airport and the accommodation, meant an end to occupational therapy access to Misima and therefore a focus on sustainable intervention was necessary. Lastly and thankfully we were challenged by the manager of the Community Services Department at the mine to review our service delivery. He indicated that what we were doing had more to do with making us "feel good" than ensuring people's needs were met in the longer term.

Living and working within another culture highlights the prejudicial assumptions underpinning practice in Western cultures, and resulted in enhanced cultural competence and professional growth. Issues of personal prejudice, previously unrecognised, were highlighted and tested in this kind of experience, where the dominant paradigms of the culture is not shared by Western ideologies. In addition, professional values and principles may conflict with local cultural beliefs, such as the value placed on independence and productivity. This can contribute to professional ethnocentricity reinforced by the perception of expertise and the concept that "our way is the right way". Examining these thoughts through ongoing discussion and self-reflection, both verbal and written, ensured a broadening of our perception to include different beliefs and understanding especially in relation to our focus on health and occupation.

As a result of the reflection process, some personal attributes were identified that facilitated working well in this setting. These included being flexible, innovative, an effective team player, having a willingness to learn, having patience to get to know the community before trying to intervene in too great a way and an enjoyment of the privilege of being allowing into people's lives. This confirms findings from occupational therapists working in indigenous communities in Australia (Jensen, 1999). Finally, a willingness to engage in self-exploratory reflection and openness to other viewpoints ensures personal and professional development that contributes to the success of any interventions.

These skills are directly transferable to working more effectively in any society. The students involved in this project had no difficulty in identifying how the experience has influenced their professional practice following graduation. The opportunity to work in a resource-poor environment encouraged both students and staff to feel confident in providing culturally compatible interventions for all future clients.

Conclusion

Working in resource-poor environments necessitates a long-term perspective, which includes community development and community capacity building. Allied health professionals with skills in both health education and promotion are suited to this role, and should work with existing community organisations to ensure ongoing ownership and maintenance of programs. Adopting the core ingredients for community based rehabilitation is recommended to ensure sustainable practice; being community based, culturally compatible, social inclusion of people with disabilities and using local resources. In order to work in this way, health professionals must be willing to learn about the cultural and political systems of the community and advocate for the rights of people who are occupationally disadvantaged.

The concept of rehabilitation, criticised for emphasising the medical model and focusing on treatment of individual deficits, must be expanded to promote community awareness and inclusion of people with disabilities. Health professionals have a responsibility to ensure that interventions aim to address disadvantage and engage in socio-political action that supports the rights of people with disabilities. Self-reflection and discourse with other professionals proved to be essential in evaluating assumptions and interventions, and ensuring that practice was both culturally compatible and sustainable.

References

Algado, S. S., Mehta, N., Kronenberg, F., Cockburn, L. & Kirsh, B. (2002). Occupational therapy intervention with children survivors of war. *Canadian Journal of Occupational Therapy, 69*(4), 205–217.

Arriotti, L. (1999). Social construction of Anungu disability. *Australian Journal of Rural Health, 7,* 216–222.

Boddington, M., (1999). Sustainability of prosthetic and orthotic programmes in the low income world: The case of Mozambique. *Journal of Mine Action, 3*(3), 1–6. Retrieved 5 December 2003 from http://maic.jamu.edu/journal/3.3/focus/power.htm

Brown, G. & Ryan, S. (2003). Enhancing reflective abilities: Interweaving reflection into practice. In G. Brown, S. Esdaile & S. Ryan (Eds), *Becoming an advanced health care practitioner,* pp 118–144. Edinburgh: Butterworth-Heinemann.

Clemson, L. & Martin, R. (1996). Usage and effectiveness of rails, bathing and toileting aids. *Occupational Therapy in Health Care, 10*(1), 41–59.

Denshire, S. (2002). Reflections on the confluences of personal and professional. *Australian Occupational Therapy Journal, 49*, 212–216.

Franscisco, I. & Carlson, G. (2002). Occupational therapy and people with intellectual disability from culturally diverse backgrounds. *Australian Occupational Therapy Journal, 49*, 200–211.

Hawe, P., King, L., Noort, M., Jordens, C. & Lloyd, B. (1999). *Indicators to help with capacity building in health promotion.* Sydney: Australian Centre for Health Promotion.

Hobbs, L., McDonough, S. & O'Callaghan, A. (2002). *Life after injury: A rehabilitation manual for the injured and their helpers.* Penang: Third World Network

Hocking, C. & Whiteford, G. (1995). Multiculturalism in occupational therapy: A time for reflection on core values. *Australian Occupational Therapy Journal, 42*, 172–175.

International Development and Disability Consortium (IDDC). (2002). Reflection paper on CBR by IDDC CBR Task group. Retrieved 15 January 2003 from http://www.iddc.org.uk/dis_dev/strategies/cbr.shtml

Jensen, H. (1998). Best Practice for Occupational Therapy intervention when working with Australian Aboriginal People. Proceedings from 12th International Congress of the World Federation of Occupational Therapy Conference, Montreal. *Sharing a Global Perspective.* Montreal: World Federation of Occupational Therapy.

Jungersen, K. (2002). Cultural safety: Kawa whakaruruhau — An occupational therapy perspective. *New Zealand Journal of Occupational Therapy, 49*(1), 4–9.

Kronenburg, F. (2003) Draft position paper on Community Based Rehabilitation for the International Consultation on reviewing CBR. World Federation of Occupational Therapy. Retrieved 10 January 2004 from http://www.wfot.org.au/Articles/CBRcomment.pdf

Lipscomb, A., McKinnon, R. & Murray, J., (1998). *Papua New Guinea.* 6th ed. Melbourne: Lonely Planet Publications.

McMurray, A. (1999). *Community health and wellness: A socioecological approach.* Sydney: Mosby.

Misima Mines. (1998). *The Misima Social Impact Study.* Unpublished report.

O'Connor-Fleming, M. & Parker, E. (2001). *Health promotion: Principles and practice in the Australian context.* (2nd ed.). Sydney: Allen & Unwin.

Placer Dome Asia Pacific. (2001). Misima Mine sustainability report 2001: Towards a sustainable future. Retrieved 5 December 2003 from http://www.placerdome.com/sustainability/downloads/reports/2001/misima.pdf

Schell, B. (2003). Clinical reasoning: The basis of practice. In E. B. Crepeau, E. S. Cohn & B. Schell (Eds), *Willard and Spackman's Occupational Therapy.* (10th ed.), pp 131–139. Philadelphia: Lippincott.

Townsend, E. (1993). Occupational Therapy's social vision. *Canadian Journal of Occupational Therapy, 60*, 174–184.

Werner, D. (1987). *Disabled Village Children: A guide for community health workers, rehabilitation workers and families.* Berkley: The Hesperian Foundation.

Whiteford, G. (2000). Occupational deprivation: Global challenge in the new millennium. *British Journal of Occupational Therapy, 63*(5), 200–204.

World Federation of Occupational Therapists. (2003). Draft position paper on community based rehabilitation (CBR) for the international consultation on reviewing CBR. Retrieved 15 January 2004 from http://www.wfot.org.au/Articles/websitefinal%20draft-guidelines9.8.pdf

World Health Organization. (2001). *International classification of functioning, disability and health.* Geneva: WHO.

World Health Organization Disability and Rehabilitation and Italian Association Amico di Raoul Follereau, *Equal Opportunities for all: Promoting Community Based Rehabilitation (CBR) among urban poor populations.* Retrieved 10 January 2004 from http://www.who.int/ncd/disability/cbr-slums.pdf

World Health Organization and Swedish Organizations of Disabled Persons International Aid Association. (2002). Community Based Rehabilitation as we have experienced it ... voices of people with disabilities part 1. Retrieved 10 January 2004 from http://www.who.int/ncd/disability/cbr-part1.pdf

Yeoman, S. (1998). Occupation and disability: A role for occupational therapists in developing countries. *British Journal of Occupational Therapy, 61*(11), 523–527.

The Political and Economic Context of Practice

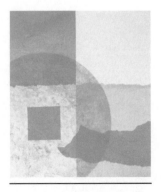

CHAPTER SEVENTEEN

Economy as Context: Evaluating Occupation Focused Services

Paul Brown

Valerie Wright-St Clair

Michael Law

KEY WORDS

Occupational participation

Outcome measures

Quality of life

Occupational outcomes

Cost measures

Best practice

Chapter Profile

The economic context and realities of health and disability services are frequently forgotten or invisible in the everyday practice world. However, occupation focused practitioners ought to be concerned with the economic outcomes of their work with clients, in terms of delivering both individual and public benefits. The purpose of this chapter is to help practitioners understand how to interpret outcomes evidence from published studies and to measure the success of their interventions. Two types of measures — outcome measures that demonstrate the positive or negative consequences for the client, and cost measures reflecting the financial implications of the intervention — are discussed. Qualitative evidence such as clients' lived experiences and practice wisdom are considered important and integral to comprehensive understandings about practice outcomes. However, given the ground swell of literature interpreting what constitutes valued evidence, this chapter primarily limits itself to considering measurements of consequence and cost. While the discussion centres on occupation focused practice, occupational therapy is used as a case example in illustrating the complexities of measuring outcomes and interpreting quality of life for clients.

Introduction

Human engagement in occupation is integral to everyday living as people of all ages plan, structure and use their time doing the things they need and want to do. Human occupation can be thought of as a conduit, as it is through doing that people serve their own and others' essential needs for survival, explore and develop their capacities for thinking and doing, interact with others and adapt to changing life contexts (Wilcock, 1998). Through the natural rhythm of the day, the seasons and the lifespan, people continually face the demands of their changing spiritual, embodied and contextual lifeworlds. Meanings about the self and things are constructed, and the potential for recovery can be unlocked, through human engagement in occupation (Pierce, 2001). Following this line of thought, health and disability services ought to be fundamentally about preventing or removing barriers to people's participation in occupations and communities. Even though Western health systems seem preoccupied with a mechanistic view of the human body and mind, few health practitioners would oppose the notion that, as a consequence of seeking professional help, people are enabled more readily to meet the everyday, or the exceptional, life demands they face. That is, implicitly or explicitly, health and disability services ought to be occupation focused.

If changes in people's ability to do, or their personally held experiences of, everyday occupations are indicators of wellness or recovery from adverse events, then an assessment of occupational participation is a useful outcome measure of health and disability interventions. While people's engagement in occupations can be observed and categorised by health practitioners, any interpretation of the personally held meanings is necessarily an inexact science (Pierce, 2001). For the purposes of this chapter, occupations are categorised as being "everything people do to occupy themselves, including looking after themselves (self-care), enjoying life (leisure), and contributing to the social and economic fabric of their communities (productivity)" (Canadian Association of Occupational Therapists CAOT, 1997, p 3).

Providing occupation focused services

Occupation focused services within the health and disability sectors are typically aimed at enabling people or groups to increase participation in, and gain control over, their everyday lives when their usual occupations are interrupted. Life interruptions may be an effect of disability, physical or psychosocial development, ageing, social disadvantage or ill-health (CAOT, 1997). Unlike clinically focused health goals, such as saving or extending life, occupation focused goals aim to help people make a life worth living. Occupation focused services may seek to instil hope for a better future, to reduce the burden of illness or disability on the everyday, to help people make new meaning of their experiences and to enable people to craft enriched, occupationally satisfying lives. In other words, the goal is to enhance people's occupational performance.

To achieve this goal, occupation focused services engage with persons, places, structures and systems to develop interventions that overcome or minimise the barriers preventing people from engaging in the occupations of their everyday lives (Law & Baum, 2001). For the health practitioner, developing an intervention involves a number of stages. First, the practitioner must correctly identify the occupational performance issue and its potential sources. This involves working in partnership with the client in order to develop one or more hypotheses as to the cause of the occupational performance concerns. Secondly, the occupation focused practitioner seeks to understand what the client hopes to be able to do as a consequence of the intervention. The consultation may involve interactional, observational and interpretive methods of inquiry to explore and understand the client's meaning of occupation within a chosen context. This goal is to identify the areas of quality of life that are most important to the client.

The practitioner then develops and implements one or more interventions, discussing with the client the purpose of each intervention and how it may move the client toward his or her goals. Contextually focused interventions include removing barriers to, or enhancing the environmental facilitators of, people's participation in occupations through modifying the physical, attitudinal or socio-cultural environments. It may also involve interacting with groups, communities, organisations or governments to refocus their purpose, policies, resources and structures or to develop the organisational capabilities for enabling people's participation in occupations. Interventions focused on positively influencing the personal or intrinsic factors underpinning occupational performance include assessing, developing, restoring or preserving the person's capacity for doing. The interventions may include a focus on body structures and function, performance capabilities as they relate to skilful effective and satisfying performance and prescribing and educating people in the use of assistive technologies that enable occupational performance (WHO, 2002).

Considering the consequences

Once an intervention is agreed upon and implemented, the practitioner must identify whether the intervention is successful or not. The practitioner might survey clients to see how satisfied they were with the service and measure changes in occupational performance. Or the practitioner might use a more general quality of life measure to ascertain how the intervention has affected their lives in areas such as leisure, productivity and self-care. The choice of measure is essential for allowing the practitioner and client to identify what worked and why, and what areas require additional attention.

Within an economic context, there are several roles for outcomes research (Robertson & Colborn, 2000). First, the practitioner must consider previous research when developing interventions. Knowledge from previous studies on what worked and why is relevant to developing an effective intervention. Effectiveness means the intervention achieves what it was intended to achieve. The practitioner must consider this information in light of his or her own practice and the client's goals and desires. This is especially true when the interventions differ significantly in the areas of the quality of life that are impacted and when there is a trade-off between improvements in one area (for example, the person making new meaning of changes to their body structure and function) over another (for example, the person's ability to access and participate in community life). In these cases, the practitioner must be able to understand the importance the client places on the various aspects of quality of life in order to help them select the intervention that is best for them.

Secondly, the therapist needs to understand how to determine whether the implementation of the intervention has been successful. Given the multitude of factors that contribute to developing interventions, measuring the success is challenging. Law and Baum (2001) interpret occupational performance as reflecting the person's "dynamic experience of engaging in daily occupations within the environment" (p 9). They suggest that occupation focused practitioners integrate three dimensions of information when working to promote occupational performance: the person's expectations and goals (the occupational dimensions, needs, expectations and aspirations related to self-care, leisure and productivity); extrinsic or contextual dimensions (such as the socio-cultural, economic and political influences); and individual abilities (such as physical, cognitive and psychosocial strengths or limitations).

The purpose of this chapter is to help practitioners understand how to interpret evidence from published studies and measure the success of their interventions. We focus upon two types of measures: (a) *outcomes measures* that demonstrate the positive or negative consequences for the client; and (b) *cost measures* reflecting the financial implications of the intervention. The rationale for measuring outcomes is straightforward. In order to assess the impact to the client's quality of life, the practitioner needs to measure the relevant impact of the intervention. That is, it allows the practitioner to answer the question: "Did the intervention improve the client's quality of life?" Measuring costs allows the therapist to addresses a different question: "Is the intervention good value for money?" This question is of interest to the funder of the service, be it the client, the government or a third party payee (such as an insurance company).

Given the climate of rising costs and fiscal scrutiny, payers increasingly require evidence that a proposed procedure is more beneficial and less costly than no intervention or an alternative intervention. Our aim is to help practitioners and service managers consider knowledgeable choices based on evidence and to understand the rationale (or lack thereof) behind purchaser's funding decisions.

Introducing outcome evaluations

Suppose an individual comes to the practitioner complaining of an inability to work a full day because of back pain. The practitioner speaks with the client to learn more about the person, his occupations, how the pain is impacting upon engagement in occupations and about how different occupations or environmental conditions influence the experience of pain. For example, the practitioner identifies extended periods of time working at the computer as a key influence and identifies the person's patterns of use and positioning at the workstation as causative factors. The practitioner, the client and the employer discuss the preferred intervention of altering the workstation and providing the client with strategies to minimise the intrusiveness of pain in the everyday work occupations. The practitioner explains the intervention to the client and employer and collaborates in setting realistic goals. The intervention proceeds over a number of weeks. At the end of this time, the client is not satisfied with the results and the practitioner is left to wonder what went wrong.

Intervention is not properly implemented

There are a number of reasons why the intervention might have failed to satisfy the client. Suppose the proper procedure called for the practitioner to discuss the problem with the client, identify the potential sources of the problem, identify the intervention options (using clinical judgement, professional reasoning and support resources), discuss the options with the client and then adapt and implement the chosen intervention. One reason the intervention might go awry is if this procedure was not administered properly. For instance, there may have been communication differences between the client and the therapist (for example, a language barrier). Or the practitioner might have incorrectly understood the client's preferences and goals, or failed to ask the client relevant information about other possible causes. A problem might have occurred during the implementation of the intervention, such as a delay in correctly identifying the causative factors or a failure to provide adequate instruction to the client. Thus, the intervention might have been ineffective due to a failure to follow the appropriate *procedures* or administer the intervention appropriately.

One way to detect problems such as described above is through a *process evaluation*. The purpose of a process evaluation is to determine whether the appropriate steps were followed at each stage. A process evaluation does not examine the outcomes from the intervention (for example, longer time working pain-free or improved quality of life), but focuses upon whether the appropriate steps were followed. This might involve assessing the adequacy of the consultation, the procedure the practitioner went through to research and develop the intervention options and how the intervention was implemented.

Intervention is not effective

A process evaluation can identify problems at the practice and implementation levels that are likely to limit the effectiveness of the intervention. Yet interventions can fail to achieve the desired effects even if the procedure is appropriate. A second possibility is that the *intervention* might have been ineffective. For instance, perhaps the new chair and keyboard were poorly designed, incorrectly adjusted or were not associated with the cause of the pain. Or perhaps the presence of a third factor, such as a longstanding susceptibility to back pain or a previous injury, was the true cause of the pain and thus limited the success of the intervention.

The purpose of an *outcome evaluation* is to examine whether the practitioner was successful in meeting the goals of the intervention. This might include improvements in occupational performance, a decrease in disabling back pain, timeliness in returning to work or improvements in quality of life. These *outcome measures* are the yardsticks the therapist uses to assess the impact on the client's quality of life.

A common way to assess the effectiveness of a procedure is to compare the person's occupational performance or quality of life before intervention with the quality of life after intervention. The implicit assumption is that the change in outcomes can be attributed to the intervention. Yet care must be taken when interpreting these types of results. The "before-after" comparison with an individual client can lead to inappropriate conclusions because it is not possible to know how well the client might have done had no intervention been given or had an alternative intervention been used. Perhaps the intervention actually delayed recovery. A stronger interpretation of effectiveness would come from assessing the effectiveness for clients given the chosen intervention with other clients who are given no intervention or the standard care (see Figure 17.1).

Figure 17.1 illustrates a comparison of both measurement outcomes and costs of intervention for clients in an "intervention" group receiving the preferred intervention (for example, as proposed above) with those for clients in the "standard care" group receiving the usual intervention. Pre-intervention evaluation, such as clients' occupational performance, time with disabling back pain or quality of life, provides the baseline measurement. Repeat of the evaluations after intervention with both groups constitutes the follow-up measurement.

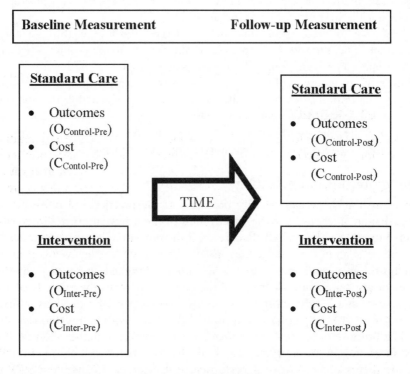

Figure 17.1 Overview of Intervention and Evaluation

Intervention was not appropriate

The problems in interpreting the effectiveness of practice could be avoided through using interventions for which there is good evidence of effectiveness (for example, published guidelines on the characteristics of enhancing occupational performance within workplace environments). Having the choice of interventions informed by sound evidence is undoubtedly a good practice. However, using an intervention that is demonstrated as effective in an intervention study does not necessarily guarantee it will work well for each client or produce client satisfaction. The discussion in chapter three provides a comprehensive and critical look at this argument. For an intervention to result in increased client satisfaction, the intervention must improve quality of life in areas the client cares about. That is, the "effectiveness" must align with the client's wishes and aspirations. If not, then the intervention might have improved aspects of life for which the client cared little while ignoring the aspects the client wanted addressed.

Thus, a third possibility presents as to why the person might not be satisfied. That is, the intervention did not enable participation in occupations of choice, or it did not address valued aspects of quality of life. Occupation focused practice may be categorised across three aspects of life: self-care, leisure and productivity. These are broad categories, and thus the challenge facing the practitioner is to identify those aspects and occupations that are important to the person in his or her environment, the interventions likely to enhance those occupations, set realistic goals and then support the person in his or her efforts to achieve these goals.

From the practitioner's perspective, the key to monitoring whether the intervention leads to increased client satisfaction is to choose outcome measures that reflect the aspects of quality of life that are important to the person. This is not as straightforward as it might appear, as will be discussed in the next section.

What to measure: Outcomes

Outcome assessments focus upon the consequences (both positive and negative) of interventions. However, as mentioned in the previous section, interventions can be ineffective because the strategies used did not improve outcomes, or because the intervention was not implemented appropriately. Outcome assessments are actually measuring the results of both the implementation *and* the effectiveness of the intervention. For this reason, most published studies of the effectiveness of interventions involve closely monitored randomised controlled trials, thereby ensuring the implementation is the same under the baseline and intervention conditions. Studies that express the results of interventions purely in outcome terms implicitly assume that either the processes under both conditions were identical or that any differences in processes between the baseline and intervention conditions did not affect the outcomes. There are numerous guides outlining best practice for practitioners and thus this chapter does not go into the principles associated with developing an appropriate process for implementing interventions. Instead, the discussion focuses upon *how* to measure outcomes and whether the outcomes are appropriate.

The choice of an outcome measure is not straightforward. Interventions typically impact on a number of aspects of a person's life, ranging from changes in body structures, function and performance capabilities to levels of participation in everyday occupations (personal, domestic, vocational, educational, leisure, social and civic) (WHO, 2002), and to spiritual aspects of the person. Spiritual in this sense refers to the "personal philosophy of meaning that informs life choices and the meanings we give to and derive from our every-day lives" (Whalley Hammell, 2003, p 82). An appropriate outcome measure will allow the practitioner to evaluate the effectiveness of the intervention *and* the impact the intervention has on the client's quality of life. These are not always the same thing. For instance, in the case illustration given, the intervention (modification of the physical work environment) was intended to enable the person's participation in his vocational occupation through reducing the strain placed on the back muscles, thus reducing the pain associated with sitting at the workstation. One type of outcome measure is a physical assessment, such as intensity and duration of pain, the assumption being that reductions in muscular strain will lead to less disruption to occupations due to pain. But the client undoubtedly does not care about the strain on the back per se, but rather the limitations in occupational participation and the reduced quality of life that results. Thus, at the other end of the assessment scale are measures that assess the impact on the quality of life directly.

As shown in Figure 17.2, the outcomes from interventions can be divided into three major categories: functional measures, occupational measures and indicators of overall quality of life.

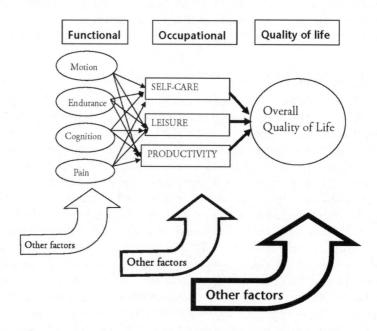

Figure 17.2 Overview of outcome assessments

Functional assessments

Functional measures are defined as a "systematic attempt to measure objectively the level at which a person is functioning in a variety of areas" (Lawton, as cited in Granger, 1998, p 235). Functional measures focus upon identifying the physical and cognitive performance capacities as they apply to daily living. For instance, consider the example of the practitioner seeing the person who is unable to work a full day because of disabling back pain. The practitioner wants to assess the effectiveness of the intervention by comparing scores on an outcome measure pre- and post-intervention. Seeking a suitable measure, the therapist chooses the Oswestry Low Back Pain Disability Questionnaire (Fairbanks, Couper, Davies & O'Brien, 1980; Hudson-Cook, Tomes-Nicholson & Breen, 1989). The measure assesses the extent to which a person's functional level is restricted by back pain. The questionnaire consists of ten sections representing numerous aspects where daily activities are affected by back pain. The client fills out the questionnaire, indicating the statement that most closely applies to him at the present time. There are five statements for each, with a score of 1 given to the response indicating no pain and 5 for maximum pain. For instance, under the category of "lifting", a score of 1 is given if the client chooses the statement "I can lift heavy weights without extra pain" and a score of 5 if the client chooses "I cannot lift or carry anything at all." The final score is expressed as a ratio (cumulative score divided by 50) where 100 per cent represents total limitation due to pain (referred to as the Oswestry Disability Index or ODI).

The measure can be used to assess the client's improvement. It could be conducted with the client pre- and post-intervention, with the reduction in the overall percentage representing the decrease in overall functional limitation due to pain. For instance, suppose the person rated his limitation due to pain on each of the scales prior to the intervention, leading to a total score of 20 (or 40 per cent; Pre Intervention column in Table 17.1). After the intervention, the ODI decreases to a score of 16 (or 32 per cent: Post Intervention column in Table 17.1). Thus, as a result of the intervention, there has been a decrease in the limitations due to pain (as measured by the ODI) by 8 per cent (40 per cent − 32 per cent).

The advantage of a functional measure such as the ODI is that it specifically addresses aspects of life impacted by pain. As such, the measure may be used to interpret improvements in functions as a result of decreased pain resulting from the interventions. However, these types of measures are subject to limitations. For instance, there is an implicit assumption that each of the functional categories is of equal importance to the individual. Calculation of the ODI requires adding up the scores on each category rather than weighting some areas (such as sitting) more importantly than others (such as social life). However, it is more likely that individuals will differ in the importance they place on the categories based on their values and occupations of choice.

Furthermore, there is no assurance that the functional categories included in the survey (for example sleeping and lifting) *are* important to the client. Significant areas of concern (such as playing rugby) might not be included. This is especially

Category	Max Score Possible	Pre-Intervention	Post-Intervention
Pain Intensity	5	2	2
Personal Care	5	2	2
Lifting	5	3	2
Walking	5	2	2
Sitting	5	4	2
Standing	5	1	1
Sleeping	5	2	2
Sex life	5	1	1
Social life	5	1	1
Travelling	5	2	1
Total score	50	20	16

Table 17.1 Example of Oswestry Low Back Pain Disability Questionnaire

Fairbanks, J. C. T., Couper, J., Davies, J. B., O'Brien, J. P. (1980). The Oswestry Low Back Pain Disability Questionnaire. *Physiotherapy, 66*, 271–273.

relevant since areas such as leisure and productivity are only indirectly included and must be inferred from other questions.

The possibility that the measure fails to reflect the appropriate categories or the client's preferences can lead to inappropriate interventions. For instance, if the client placed a great emphasis on being pain-free, then the intervention might involve more strategies to change the subjective experience or meaning of pain. In this case, the measure should ideally reflect the person's preferences else the practitioner risks choosing an inappropriate intervention. Furthermore, the failure to reflect the areas the client sees as important can lead the practitioner mistakenly to conclude the intervention is a success. If the success of the measure is determined by the client's responses, then the practitioner viewing an improved ODI ratio might overlook the fact that the improvements were in areas that the person did not greatly value.

Occupational assessments

The limitations of the above types of functional measure can be overcome by using an outcome measure that reflects the person's preferences and allows identification of important occupations. There are a number of measures developed specifically for evaluating occupational performance (for discussions of measuring occupational performance in occupational therapy practice see Law, Baum & Dunn, 2001; Letts & Bosch, 2001; Baum & Law, 1997; de Clive-Lowe, 1996; Simeonsson et al, 2003; Ellenburg, 1986). An example of such a measure is the Canadian Occupational Performance Measure (COPM) (Law et al, 1998). The COPM measures outcomes in the three areas of interest to occupational therapists: self-care, productivity and leisure. There are three subcategories in each area (see Table 17.2). Clients are first asked to identify daily activities they *want to do, need to do or are expected to do*. The client is asked to identify which of these activities are difficult for them to do now to their satisfaction. This provides a verbal understanding of the areas of concern to the client. The client is then asked to indicate on a scale of 1 to 10 the importance of each activity. This provides the practitioner with information on the areas seen as most important to the person.

After having gone through this process for each of the three occupational categories, the client is asked to identify the five most important problems. The client rates his current performance and satisfaction with performance on each of the five areas (see Table 17.3). An average score is calculated for both performance and satisfaction. When reassessed after the intervention, this allows the practitioner to identify the change in performance and satisfaction for each of the five identified areas.

The COPM has the advantage of directly measuring areas relevant to occupational therapy interventions. Furthermore, because the measure assesses the importance the client places on each area, it allows the practitioner to design interventions to meet the person's specific goals and desires. This can help ensure the intervention is appropriate and that the practitioner is able to determine whether the intervention has met the client's needs.

However, the disadvantage of using a global measure such as the COPM is that there are numerous other factors relevant to the outcomes that are not being measured. For instance, in the sample shown in Table 17.3, the person's score for playing rugby decreased between the initial assessment and the reassessment. This might have been because the intervention resulted in an unintended side effect (fatigue) or it could be because there was some external influence (such as a change in position on the rugby field) that impaired performance. There are numerous other factors that can influence the performance and satisfaction with the areas other than those affected by the intervention.

Moving from a specific to a global measure increases the likelihood that the important aspects of the quality of life will be included, but it increases the risk that other factors will intervene, thereby masking any benefits from the intervention. That is, the influence of other factors becomes more significant as we move from a functional to a global outcome measure (as shown in Figure 17.2). This limits the ability of the practitioner to determine the exact impact of the intervention.

Category	Description	Importance
1a. **Self-Care**		
- Personal care	**Ability to dress myself without pain**	6
- Functional mobility	Ability to sit up in bed without pain	5
- Community Management	Drive to work in car	9
1b. **Productivity**		
- Paid/Unpaid work	Working at workstation without pain	8
- Household management	Gardening	3
- Play/School	Not applicable	0
1c. **Leisure**		
- Quiet recreation	Sitting and reading books	3
- Active recreation	Playing rugby	7
- Socialization	Conversations in the café with friends	6

Table 17.2 Categories included in the Canadian Occupational Performance Measure (Published with permission from Law et al., 1998)

Law, M., Baptiste, S.,Carswell, A., Mc Coll, M., Polatajko, H., & Pollock, N. (1998). *Canadian Occupational Performance Measure* (3rd ed.). Toronto, Canada: CAOT Publications.

Global Quality of Life Scale

Although a measure such as the COPM includes a number of dimensions related to quality of life, there are other aspects that are not touched upon or are only dealt with to a limited degree. Global quality of life scales reduce the likelihood that important areas will not be included in the measurement.

Currently, the most commonly used global quality of life measure is the MOS 36 — Item Short-Form Health Survey (SF–36) (Ware & Sherbourne, 1992). As the name implies, the SF–36 includes 36 questions spanning seven dimensions: physical functions, role limitations due to the physical problem, bodily pain, social functioning, mental health, role limitations due to emotional problems, vitality and general health perceptions. The SF–36 is a generic indicator of health that is commonly used to assess the health of populations. Because of its

Occupational performance problems	Initial assessment		Reassessment	
	Performance	Satisfaction	Performance	Satisfaction
1. Drive in car to work	4 *	1	5	3
2. Work at workstation without pain	5	6	7	7
3. Play rugby	2	5	1	4
4. Conversations in café	8	8	10	10
5. Ability to dress without pain	8	9	8	9
Scoring:	Performance score 1	Satisfaction score 1	Performance score 2	Satisfaction score 2
Total Score	5.4 **	5.8	6.2	6.8
Change in Performance Score	= 6.2 – 5.4	= 0.8		
Change in Satisfaction Score	= 6.8 – 5.8	= 1.0		

* Rated on a scale of 1 to 10
** Average of scores in colum

Table 17.3 Sample Scoring with Canadian Occupational Performance Measure (Law et al., 1998)

widespread use, there are published summaries of SF–36 scores for a variety of sub-populations (see Brazier et al, 1992).

Table 17.4 shows several questions from the SF–36, including two questions dealing specifically with pain (numbers 7 and 8). Compared with a specific pain index such as the ODI, the SF–36 does not explore the depth or the limitations due to pain. However, the measure does tap into a number of other areas of quality of life, including the emotional and mental aspects of health. The practitioner can identify the aspects of quality of life that are troubling to the client by administering the questionnaire as part of the consultation process. Having chosen

1. In general, would you say your health is: (circle one)

   Excellent 1
   Very Good 2
   Good 3
   Fair 4
   Poor 5

3. The following items are about activities you might do during a typical day. Does you health now limit you in these activities? If so, how much?

Activities	Yes, limited a lot	Yes, limited a little	No, not limited at all
A. Vigorous activities such as running, lifting heavy objects, participating in strenuous sports			
B. Moderate activities, such as moving a table, pushing a vacuum cleaner, bowling or playing golf			
C. Lifting or carrying groceries			
Etc.			

7. How much bodily pain have you had during the past 4 weeks?

   None 1
   Very Mild 2
   Mild 3
   Moderate 4
   Severe 5
   Very Severe 6

8. During the past 4 weeks, how much did pain interfere with your normal work (including both work outside the home and housework)?

   Not at all 1
   A little bit 2
   Moderately 3
   Quite a bit 4
   Extremely 5

Table 17.4 Selected questions from SF–36 (Ware & Sherbourne, 1992)

the intervention that best meets the client's needs, the success of the intervention could be ascertained by comparing SF–36 scores at the conclusion with those at the start of the intervention.

Although the SF–36 incorporates a wider range of dimensions pertinent to quality of life than the COPM, it is not without its limitations. First, there is a wide range of other factors that influence health and thus there is no assurance that any improvements in areas such as sense of vitality resulted from the intervention. While these differences might be discernible in published studies where large samples are used, practitioners assessing an individual client cannot be as confident.

A second criticism of the SF–36 is that, unlike the COPM, it does not incorporate the person's views on importance of the dimensions of quality of life. When scoring, the SF–36 is either scored on a scale of 1 to 100 (perfect health) with each category being assigned the same weight, or by applying an alternative weighting system with differential but predetermined weights. Like the ODI, evaluating the success of the intervention using the SF–36 scores alone might lead to the misleading conclusion that the client's quality of life is improved when really the improvements were in dimensions that are not highly valued.

There are other quality of life measures that attempt to the incorporate client's values. For instance, the EuroQol 5–D (EuroQol Group, 1990) asks about the client's quality of life on five categories (mobility, self-care, usual activities, pain/discomfort and anxiety/depression). Unlike the SF–36, the measure attempts to incorporate the level of importance the client places on each of these areas. This resulting score (ranging from 0, worst possible health state to 1, best possible health state) can be used to identify the change in quality of life pre- and post-intervention. In addition, the EuroQol can be used to calculate another quality of life measure, the QALY (Quality Adjusted Life Years). See EuroQol (1990) for a discussion.

What to measure: Costs

The inclusion of "cost" as an outcome measure is unlikely to create a sense of excitement among practitioners. After all, practitioners, especially those in private practice, are all familiar with the financial implications of running a business. But *cost* as used here does not just refer to the reimbursement that is paid to the therapist for his or her services. Rather, cost refers to the total *societal* cost associated with service provision. This includes not only the direct cost of care to the client by the practitioner and other health professionals (for example, primary care providers, pharmaceuticals and hospital), but also the indirect costs to clients and their caregivers.

There are a number of reasons why it is important to focus on the costs of care. First, financial aspects are a major area of concern to the person and their family. The cost of care and the income loss associated with occupational performance problems, injury or disability can be substantial. In addition, the practitioner must ensure that the intervention he or she is providing does not merely shift the health-care costs to another sector. This might happen if the intervention resulted in more visits to the general practitioner or hospitalisation.

Secondly, the funders of health care often make decisions based on the "value for money" the service provides. For occupation focused practitioners to be recognised and funded, they need to demonstrate that the services are cost effective. Indeed, one of the strengths of occupational therapy is that it can help people avoid other types of medical costs and get back to productive occupations faster. Demonstrating that savings in other areas more than make up for the cost of the services strengthens the practitioner's case for the regular inclusion of occupation focused therapies. There is a growing body of evidence indicating the effectiveness of occupation focused practice in enhancing people's participation in the everyday tasks of living (Law, Pollock & Stewart, 2004). While not all the studies have included measurement of cost outcomes, it is surely the next step in outcomes focused research.

And finally, costs provide another metric to compare various interventions. Often two interventions have similar outcomes but one has significantly lower costs. If the choice was made on effectiveness alone, the practitioner might find he or she had opted for a more expensive intervention. Costs provide another way of comparing interventions.

Categories of costs

There are two categories of costs relevant to an intervention. *Direct costs* are those expenses directly associated with health care. This would include visits to the practitioner, equipment that is purchased as a result of the occupational performance problem, concern or issue or attendances at a group program. *Indirect costs* are other costs associated with care. These might include lost wages from missing work, caregiver or home help costs, costs of transportation to and from the health providers and other expenses that arise due to the performance problem.

The basic principle guiding costing methods is simple: identify the number of "units" of resources used by the client (for example, number of practitioner visits, cost of assistive technologies used, number of group attendances) and then apply a price or cost to each unit (for example, $45 per practitioner visit, $95 per workstation adaptation, $550 per day at pain clinic). Comparing the costs before the intervention and after will provide an indication of the total societal cost associated with the treatment.

There are numerous guides to costing interventions, and the interested reader is directed there for specific details on costing methods (Drummond, O'Brien, Stoddart & Torrance, 1997; Watson Landry & Mathews, 1998). However, to illustrate the principles of how to cost an intervention, let's return to the example of the client with the disabling back pain. Suppose at the time of the initial consultation (pre-intervention), the practitioner asks the client about his health care and other expenses during the past three weeks. Note that it is important to define the time period over which resource usage will be compared. In this case, three weeks prior to the start of the intervention and three weeks prior to the end of the intervention are assessed. This time period will capture any therapies and interventions the individual used prior to the current service as well as the cost of the intervention itself (for example, occupational therapy and the new equipment).

	Price or cost per unit	Pre Intervention (Previous 3 weeks prior to intervention)		Post Intervention (Previous 3 weeks prior to conclusion of intervention)	
		Units	Cost	Units	Cost
Number of days missed work	$240 per day	12	$2880	4	$960
Hospitalisations	$550 per day	0	$0	0	$0
Medications	$100 (15 to client, $85 to funder) $25 (to client) $120 ($15 to client, $105 to funder)	1 prescription of antibiotics 3 over the counter pain relief	$100 $75	1 over the counter pain relief 1 anti-inflammatory drug	$0 $25 $120
Health care visits – GP (1 hour) – Occ Therapist (1 hours) – Other (1 hour) (massage therapy)	$45 per visit $75 per visit $25 per visit	3 0 2	$135 $0 $50	1 3 1	$45 $225 $25
Caregivers trips with client to: – GP (1 hour) – Occ Therapist (1 ½ hours) – Other (1 hour)	$25 per hour caregivers time	3 0 0	$75 $0 $0	1 3 0	$25 $75 $0
Distance travelled to health care visits – GP – Occ Therapist – Other	$.75 per km	3 @ 5 km 2 @ 10 km	$11.25	1 @ 5 km 3 @ 15 km 1 @ 10 km	$3.75 $33.75 $7.50
Other costs associated with back pain – Keyboard – Chair	$125 $350	0 0	$0 $0	1 1	$125 $350
TOTAL COST			$3343.25		$2020

Table 17.5 Cost of care

Table 17.5 shows the resource usage, prices and total costs for the pre- and post-intervention periods. In the hypothetical example, prior to the occupational therapy sessions, the individual missed 12 days of work, was not hospitalised, visited his general practitioner (GP) three times and a massage therapist twice. For the GP visits, the person had to be accompanied by a caregiver, but was able to drive himself the 10 km to the massage therapist. There were a number of medications taken during those weeks, including one prescription of anti-inflammatory medication and three bottles of over-the-counter medication for pain.

The table also shows the unit prices for each of these items. There are a couple of points to note regarding the prices. First, the cost of a working day ($240) can be calculated by taking 1/260 (number of work days in a year including holidays and vacation days) of the individual's yearly salary of $62,400. Secondly, even if the client only pays a $15 co-payment for prescription medication (with the government or insurance paying the remainder), the analysis should include the full price of the medication. This reflects the cost to society (not just the individual) of the medication. Thirdly, caregiver's time is not based upon his or her lost wages (as was done with the client), but rather the price associated with having an attendant accompany the individual to the practitioner's office. This reflects the value of the service the caregiver is providing in terms of transport. And fourthly, the cost of transport is calculated using a standard rate per kilometre travelled.

It is worth noting what costs are *not* included in the analysis. Cost of food and clothing, for instance, are not shown. Nor are the costs of housing or rent, entertainment and electricity. There are two reasons for the omission. First, the point of the analysis is to identify the costs directly associated with the intervention. If there is no reason to suspect that the intervention will alter an expense (such as rent or telephone), then it does not need to be included. Secondly, only relevant costs and sizable costs are included. Small, insignificant or discretional costs are not included.

Using the procedure, the total cost prior to intervention is calculated to be $3343.25. In contrast, the total cost in the three weeks prior to the end of intervention is only $2020. The intervention (occupational therapy visits, anti-inflammatory medication, new keyboard and chair) cost $930.75. However, this expenditure was more than made up by the reduction in missed work.

Could the practitioner state that the intervention therefore saved society $1323.25 ($3343.25 − $2020)? Yes, but with many caveats attached. As with the comparison of outcomes, the problem with an individual client, pre-/post-intervention comparison such as this is that the practitioner can never be sure what the expenditure would have been like without the intervention. Perhaps the performance problem would have cleared up by itself and the intervention actually only prolonged the problem. In this case, there might have been no days of worked missed (rather than 4) and the cost over the three week, post-intervention period might have been greatly reduced. Or perhaps the performance problem would have gotten much worse, requiring hospitalisation and an operation. The cost over the three-week period might have been significantly higher ($6000?), meaning that the intervention actually saved society $3980 ($6000 − $2020). Without a proper control group, it is difficult to make definitive statements regarding causality.

Does that mean the comparison is of little value? No, provided the intervention was developed using sound evidence of effectiveness. If there is good evidence that the intervention does not lead to adverse side effects, then there is little chance that the health-care costs might actually have arisen as a result of the intervention. The estimate provides a reasonable measure of the success of the intervention. Furthermore, the information is useful for monitoring the impact on the client (regardless of the cause). The analysis can identify areas where the person is spending significant resources, perhaps unnecessarily. Monitoring and reducing the use of other healthcare resources will help prevent a shifting of costs from one sector to another.

Putting it all together

There are a number of reasons why people might be satisfied or dissatisfied with the health interventions they receive. For instance, the intervention might not have been implemented correctly, the interventions might have been ineffective (for example, outcomes were no better and possibly worse than no intervention or an alternative intervention) or the intervention targeted occupations that were of little concern to the person. The result can be a dissatisfied client and a frustrated practitioner.

The point of this chapter was to discuss how research on costs and consequences of interventions might assist the occupation focused practitioner. Our message is that the practitioner should ensure there are processes (either formal or informal) in place to monitor whether procedures are properly implemented. This is hardly a new or startling conclusion, but it needs to be emphasised. Without quality monitoring, there is no way of knowing whether or not the interventions are right for the person. But the main message of the chapter is that interventions should be chosen based on good evidence, and that the evidence should include both the costs and the consequences of the intervention.

The practitioner who develops a unique and idiosyncratic intervention will not be able to say with confidence, in relation to the measures discussed, whether it was successful (there will be no comparison group). However, when an intervention has good evidence and the intervention fits with understandings of who the person is and his or her valued occupations, the practitioner can employ the measures used in the published studies to assess the impact of the procedures on his or her clients and their occupational performance.

Even if an intervention has good evidence of effectiveness, the practitioner will need to be sure it is targeting the areas that are pertinent to the person and his or her lifeworld. When choosing the intervention, the practitioner needs to be aware of the outcome measures that were included in the studies, whether the outcomes measure change in areas important to the person and whether the intervention is likely to improve the important areas. As the discussion of outcomes highlighted, the trade-off the practitioner must make when choosing is between using specific, functional performance measures and global, quality of life indicators. Functional measures have the advantage of measuring the areas targeted by the interventions in depth. Thus, changes in the pre- and post-measurements can be reasonably attributed to the intervention. However, the areas they target (for example, ability to raise arm above head) may not be areas the person cares about. Global assessments such as the SF–36, on the other hand, measure a wider range of factors pertinent to quality of life. But because there are many factors that can influence quality of life, it is often difficult to detect changes that result from a specific intervention. They are blunt assessments in contrast.

What do researchers commonly use in practice?

Table 17.6 shows a selected summary of studies in the area. The first part of the table (Table 17.6a) summarises the outcome measures used in the various studies. Most studies use a combination of functional and global assessment measures. This allows the researchers to detect changes at each level. The second part of the table (17.6b) shows the cost measures commonly included. While there is wide variation between studies, several include quite comprehensive assessments of costs.

Study	Outcome Measures Utilised
Feldman, Latimer and Davidson (1996)	General Health Status ADL and IADL Questions Depression (CES-D) Hours of home care pre and post intervention Drug-category based severity measure
Dennis (1988)	Total cost for two Occupational Therapy Departments (those with assistants versus those without)
Clancy (1997)	Disability duration
Hay, Labree, Luo, Clark, Carlson, Mandel, Zemke, Jackson and Azen (2002)	SF36 Functional status questionnaire LSI-Z Center for Epidemiological Studies depression scale Medical outcomes study health perception scale
Przybylski, Dumont, Watkins, Warren, Beaulne and Lier (1996)	Functional Independence Measure Functional Assessment Measures Clinical Outcome Variables Scale
Severns, Oerlemans, Weegels, van 't Hof, Oostendorp and Goris (1999)	Impairment-level Sum Score (ISS) Modified Greentest Sickness Impact Profile (SIP)

Table 17.6a Outcome measures used in (selected) cost effectiveness studies

Study	Outcome Measures Utilised
Shalik (1987)	Time spent by student treating patients independently (valued at cost facility charges) Completion of administrative work Performing clerical or aid duties (minimum wage)
Johnston and Miller (1986)	Functional status at admission and discharge Average length of stay
Gladman, Whynes and Lincoln (1994)	Functional ability Perceived health status Cost comparison, as no significant differences were found in these outcomes
Edwards, Law, Worth and Baptiste (1995)	Time spent entering data Accuracy
Oerlemans, Oostendorp, Theo de Boo, van der Laan, Severens and Goris (2000)	Impairment level sum score (ISS) Severity of disability and handicap Radbound Skills Questionnaire Modified Greentest Radbound Dexterity Test
Goldstein, Gort, Guyatt and Feeny (1997)	Chronic Respiratory Questionnaire (CRQ)
Beech, Rudd, Tilling and Wolfe (1999)	Impairment Motricity index Mini-mental state examination Frenchay aphasia screening test Disability Modified Barthel Index Score Rivermead Activities of Daily living score Hospital anxiety and depression score 5-meter timed walk Caregiver Stress and patient and caregiver satisfaction Caregiver strain index Pound questionnaires
Trahey (1991)	Treatment outcome based on case note review – Task performance relative to activities of daily living

Table 17.6a Outcome measures used in (selected) cost effectiveness studies — *continued*

Study	Costs that have been Described
Feldman, Latimer and Davidson (1996)	Face to face interviews – Use of community services (i.e. senior centres) Billing and Payroll data – Collected weekly – Hourly use of home care per client Medicaid Claims data – Home care – Other medical costs – Pharmaceutical costs by drug category
Dennis (1988)	Salary data from AOTA member survey Estimate of supply costs
Clancy (1997)	Lower back pain medical costs to insurance
Clark, Carlson, Jackson and Mandel (2003)	Telephone Interview – Use of health care services
Hay, Labree, Luo, Clark, Carlson, Mandel, Zemke, Jackson and Azen (2002)	Cost of occupational therapy programme – Salary and occ. therapy travel costs Salary for Active control group Health Care expenditure – Physician office visits, home visits by health professionals hospital outpatient and inpatient – Costed through use of Medicare 1995 unadjusted payment schedule and DRG schedule – Annual costs calculated from average of months
Przybylski, Dumont, Watkins, Warren, Beaulne and Lier (1996)	Salary of occupational therapist and physical therapist, compared between two levels of staffing (1:200 and 1:50), based on Alberta 1993/94 paid hourly rates Hourly rates of direct care nurses and degree of contact

Table 17.6b Cost measures included in (selected) cost effectiveness studies

Study	Costs that have been Described
Severns, Oerlemans, Weegels, van 't Hof, Oostendorp and Goris (1999)	Medical Costs – Adjuvant Therapy (OT, PT, Control) – Hospital (inpatient and outpatient) – Practitioners (GP, Psychotherapy, Manual Therapy, Natural Healer, Other Alternative) – Specific treatments (sympathetic block) – Home help (nursing, nonmedical, family or friends) Non-medical Costs – Travel costs (car, taxi, public transit, non-motor) – Out of pocket costs as reported by respondent Lost productivity Costs – Absence from work (paid and unpaid labour)
Shalik (1996)	Time spent by supervisor and other professional staff in teaching the fieldwork placement (valued at clinic rate) Provision of room and board, stipends
Johnston and Miller (1986)	Cost of occupational therapy and physical therapy treatment based on hours per day, charges and overall length of stay Not clear in article if this is based on salary or resource cost (pre-post evaluation technique)
Gladman, Whynes and Lincoln (1994)	Program Cost – Gross employment cost of the therapists plus vehicle running costs Health-based rehabilitation costs – Hospital costs – Ambulance transportation charges No significant differences in those receiving meal programs, day centres, community care assistants, admission to hospital or outpatient care departments
Edwards, Law, Worth and Baptiste (1995)	Cost of occupational therapy and data entry salary levels

Table 17.6b Cost measures included in (selected) cost effectiveness studies
— *continued*

Study	Costs that have been Described
Oerlemans, Oostendorp, Theo de Boo, van der Laan, Severens and Goris (2000)	Health care resources related to the intervention (not specified) – Nonmedical Costs – Productivity Costs • Missed employment
Goldstein, Gort, Guyatt and Feeny (1997)	Care costs – Respiratory rehabilitation – Standard care protocol Hospitalization and Physician costs – Using provincial fee levels Pharmaceutical Costs – Provincial formulary and diary of costs Direct services – Physiotherapy – Occupational Therapy – Home care provision – Includes direct salary and indirect capital costs Other costs – Cost of assistive devices (walkers, etc.) – Transportation costs
Beech, Rudd, Tilling and Wolfe (1999)	Hospital Costs – Calculated by costs of staff on different wards, ward consumables and overheads – Unit costs of tests provided Intervention costs – Salary cost of occupational therapist, physical therapist and speech language therapist and overheads Medical care costs – Physician costs (midpoint salary incl. overhead) Community Services – Meals on Wheels, home help, district nurses, lunch club, day hospitals
Trahey (1991)	Average personnel costs calculated from department records covering the duration of the study

Table 17.6b Cost measures included in (selected) cost effectiveness studies
— *continued*

Hopefully the practice of including comprehensive outcome and cost measures will increase in the future.

Conclusion

Finally, we end with a note regarding qualitative methods of inquiry. The chapter has focused upon quantitative measurement of costs and consequences. Yet the importance of qualitative methods should not be understated. Qualitative methods provide a source of detailed information regarding the lived experience and desires of the person. The areas of concern might be reflected in the quantitative measures. However, if they are not, and if the qualitative data reveals understandings about the person that is not represented in the quantitative measures, then the latter may be inappropriate. Thus, qualitative studies have a vital role to play in occupation focused research. At the very least, they provide an interpretation of the relevance and accuracy of the quantitative measures and the extent to which the measures reflect the values, wishes and aspirations of the person.

References

Baum, C. & Law, M. (1997). Occupational therapy practice: Focusing on occupational performance. *American Journal of Occupational Therapy, 51*(4), 279–288.

Beech, R., Rudd, A., Tilling, K. & Wolfe, C. (1999). Economic consequences of early inpatient discharge to community-based rehabilitation for stroke in an inner-London teaching hospital. *Stroke, 30*(4), 729–735.

Brazier, J. E., Harper, R., Jones, N. M., O'Cathain, A., Thomas, K. J., Usherwood, T. & Westlake, L. (1992). Validating the SF–36 health survey questionnaire: New outcome measure for primary care. *British Medical Journal, 305*, 160–164.

Canadian Association of Occupational Therapists. (1997). *Enabling occupation: An occupational therapy perspective.* Ottawa.

Clancy, E. (1997). Cost-benefit of low back pain intervention using a classification test. *Journal of Occupational Rehabilitation, 7*(3), 155–166.

Clark, F., Carlson, M., Jackson, J. & Mandel, D. (2003). Lifestyle design improves health and is cost-effective. *Occupational Therapy Practice, January 27*, 9–13.

De Clive-Lowe, S. (1996). Outcome measurement, cost-effectiveness analysis and clinical audit: The importance of standardised assessment to occupational therapists in meeting these new demands. *British Journal of Occupational Therapy, 59*(8), August, 357–362.

Dennis, M. (1988). Calculating cost-effectiveness with the certified occupational therapy assistant. *Occupational Therapy in Health Care, 5*(2/3), 37–46.

Drummond, M., O'Brien, B., Stoddart, G. & Torrance, G. (1997). *Methods for the economic evaluation of health care programmes* (2nd ed.). Oxford: Oxford University Press.

Edwards, M., Law, M., Worth, B. & Baptiste, S. (1995). Evaluation of the cost effectiveness of therapist computerized entry of occupational therapy workload measurement data. *Canadian Journal of Occupational Therapy, 62*(2), 95–99.

Ellenburg, D. (1996). Outcomes research: The history, debate and implications for the field of occupational therapy. *American Journal of Occupational Therapy, 50*(6), 435–441.

EuroQol Group. (1990). EuroQol: A new facility for the measurement of health-related quality of life. *Health Policy, 16*, 199–208.

Fairbanks, J. C. T., Couper, J., Davies, J. B. & O'Brien, J. P. (1980). The Oswestry Low Back Pain Disability Questionnaire. *Physiotherapy, 66*, 271–273.

Feldman, P., Latimer, E. & Davidson, H. (1996). Medicare-funded home care for the frail elderly and disabled: Evaluating the cost savings and outcomes of a service delivery reform. *Health Services Research, 31*(4), 489–508.

Gladman, J., Whynes, D. & Lincoln, N. (1994). Cost comparison of domiciliary and hospital-based stroke rehabilitation. *Age and Ageing, 23*, 241–245.

Goldstein, R., Gort, E., Guyatt, G. & Feeny, D. (1997). Economic analysis of respiratory rehabilitation. *CHEST, 112*, 370–379.

Granger, C. (1998). Emerging science of functional assessment: Our tool for outcomes analysis. *Archives of Physical and Medical Rehabilitation, 79*, 235–240.

Hay, J., LaBree, L., Luo, R., Clark, F., Carlson, M., Mandel, D., Zemke, R., Jackson, J. & Azen, S. (2002). Cost-effectiveness of preventive occupational therapy for independent-living older adults. *Journal of the American Geriatrics Society, 50*(8), 1381–1388.

Hudson-Cook, N., Tomes-Nicholson, K. & Breen, A. A. (1989) A revised Oswestry disability questionnaire. (pp 187–204). In M. O. Roland & J. R. Jenner (Eds), *Back pain: New approaches to rehabilitation and education.* New York: Manchester University Press.

Johnston, M. & Miller, L. (1986). Cost-effectiveness of the Medicare three-hour regulation. *Archives of Physical and Medical Rehabilitation, 67*, 581–585.

Law, M., Baptiste, S.,Carswell, A., McColl, M., Polatajko, H. & Pollock, N. (1998). *Canadian Occupational Performance Measure* (3rd ed.). Toronto: CAOT Publications.

Law, M. & Baum, C. (2001). Measurement in occupational therapy. In M. Law, C. Baum & W. Dunn (Eds), *Measuring occupational performance: Supporting best practice in occupational therapy*, pp 3–20. Thorofare: Slack Inc.

Law, M., Baum, C. & Dunn, W. (2001). *Measuring occupational performance: Supporting best practice in occupational therapy.* Thorofare: Slack Inc.

Law, M., Pollock, N. & Stewart, D. (2004). Evidence-based occupational therapy: Concepts and strategies. New Zealand Journal of Occupational Therapy, *51*(1), 14–22.

Letts, L. & Bosch, J. (2001). Measuring occupational performance in basic activities of daily living. In M. Law, C. Baum & W. Dunn (Eds), *Measuring occupational performance: Supporting best practice in occupational therapy*, pp 121–133. Thorofare: Slack Inc.

Oerlermans, H., Oostendorp, R., de Boo, T., van der Lann, L., Severns, J. & Goris, J. (2000). Adjuvant physical therapy versus occupational therapy in patients with reflex sympathetic dystrophy/complex regional pain syndrome type I. *Archives of Physical Medical Rehabilitation, 81*, 49–56.

Pierce, D. (2001). Untangling occupation and activity. *American Journal of Occupational Therapy, 55*, 138–146.

Przybylski, B., Dumont, E., Watkins, M., Warren, S., Beaulne, A. & Lier, D. (1996). Outcomes of enhanced physical and occupational therapy service in a nursing home setting. *Archives of Physical Medical Rehabilitation, 77*, 554–561.

Robertson, S. & Colborn A. (2000). Can we improve outcomes research by expanding research methods? *American Journal of Occupational Therapy, 54*(5), 541–543.

Severns, J., Oerlemans, H., Antonius, P, Weegls, J., van't Hof, M., Oostendorp, R. & Goris R. (1999). Cost-effectiveness analysis of adjuvant physical or occupational therapy for patients with reflex sympathetic dystrophy. *Archives of Physical and Medical Rehabilitation, 80*, 1038–1043.

Shalik, L. (1987). Cost–benefit analysis of Level II fieldwork in occupational therapy. *American Journal of Occupational Therapy, 41*(10), 638–645.

Simeonsson, R. J., Leonardi, M., Lollars, D., Bjorck-Akesson, E., Hollenwerger, J. & Marinuzzi, A. (2003). Applying the International Classification of Functioning, Disability and Health (ICF) to measure childhood disability. *Disability and Rehabilitation, 25*, 602–610.

Trahey, P. (1991) A comparison of the cost-effectiveness of two types of occupational therapy services. *American Journal of Occupational Therapy, 45*(5), 397–400.

Ware, J. & Sherbourne, C. (1992). The MOS 36 item Short-Form Health Survey (SF–36). I: Conceptual framework and item selection. *Medical Care, 30*, 473–481.

Watson Landry, D. & Mathews, M. (1998). Economic evaluation of occupational therapy: Where are we at? *Canadian Journal of Occupational Therapy, 65*(3), 160–167.

Whalley Hammell, K. (2003). Intrinsicality: Reflections on meaning and mandates. In M. A. McColl (Ed.), *Spirituality and occupational therapy.* Ottawa, Ontario: CAOT Publications.

Wilcock, A. (1998). *An occupational perspective of health.* Thorofare: Slack Inc.

World Health Organization. (2002). *International classification of functioning, disability and health.* Geneva: WHO.

CHAPTER EIGHTEEN

Understanding Work in Society

David O'Halloran

Ev Innes

Work

Theories of work

Occupational rehabilitation

Work-related rehabilitation

Occupational science

Work-related assessments

Chapter Profile

Work is hard to define absolutely and agreement about what work is, cannot be assumed. The motivation to work depends on a combination of intrinsic and extrinsic factors, the relative importance of which is variable. This chapter discusses notions of work and how understandings and management approaches to work have changed over time. Work can be seen as having two aspects — being a job (point in time) and career (lifetime). Theories of work may be about jobs or careers or both and understanding the distinction is helpful. Work-related rehabilitation theory and practice can vary depending on the pre-existence of a relationship between the worker and a workplace. Vocational rehabilitation presumes no relationship; occupational rehabilitation presumes a relationship. The chapter goes on to consider how occupational therapists' perspective on health is at variance with the political responsibility for work and what this means for the complex process of assessing the ability of a person for work.

Introduction

> Everyday we are reminded that, for everybody, work is a defining feature of human existence. It is the means of sustaining life and of meeting basic needs. But it is also an activity through which individuals affirm their own identity, both to themselves and to those around them. It is crucial to individual choice, to the welfare of families and to the stability of societies.
>
> (Somavia, 2001, pp 5–6)

Work is one of the most general words for describing purposive human effort. Frequently, work is defined by contrasting it to another occupational description, or in terms of what it is not — "play", "unpaid activity", "unemployment" or "recreation" to name a few. However, each comparison creates assumptions about the nature of work that do not hold up to close scrutiny. A comparison with play suggests that work is not fun, which is not necessarily true. In addition, many traditional aboriginal cultures have no such distinction. The comparison to unpaid activity places an exaggerated importance on extrinsic rewards and loses the significance of the intrinsic value of work, whereas the contrast to recreation suggests an obligation or pressure, and is more in keeping with a view that work is a burden. Furthermore, the contrast between work and other occupations creates a distinction that cannot be precisely delineated in many situations, such as seemingly paradoxical yet commonplace concepts as *working for the dole* or a *recreation professional.*

Despite the difficulty in describing work, it is widely seen as different to other occupations. This distinction develops early in life and is well established for children as early as six years of age, who can hold clear, unambiguous and individual views about what constitutes work versus self-care, play or rest (Chapparo & Hooper, 2002).

Why work? Theoretical perspectives

Differences and overlaps exist between social, economic and psychological theorists regarding the purpose of work. Particularly in the case of economic and social theories, the perspective of historical moment, class or gender adds the complication of relativity to exploring the meaning of work.

One of the earliest economic theories proposed by Adam Smith (1776) in *The Wealth of Nations* suggested that work is a disutility and rested upon an assumption that work is done for an external reward. In the 18th century world of Adam Smith though, much work was indeed burdensome and slavery was common. Even so, Smith's theory is the foundation of much that is contemporarily labelled as economic rationalism, which maintains the assumption of work needing an economic value in order for it to be considered as work. Many authors, particularly feminist authors (for example Mitter & Rowbotham, 1995; Rose, 1994), have challenged these notions. It is argued that the work of a woman who gives birth, feeds and cares for her child, and the work of all those who only produce for their subsistence (such as those who live in a tribal or peasant society) are considered unproductive because they do not produce money directly. However, many authors, notably Marx and Polanyi (Humphreys, 1969), have maintained the focus on external rewards by calling for economic systems, often utopian, that somehow reward people fairly for this work.

Intrinsic value of work

However, not all theorists agreed that work rests on an external reward. Psychological theorists (for example Deci, 1975; Maslow, 1954) particularly have explored the intrinsic value of work, although it is argued that since the 1980s, the intrinsic value of work has been less explored than it was in the earlier part of the 20th century. It is postulated that the drive to increase the number of jobs over the past 20 years has deflected attention from the intrinsic value of work. Nowadays, discussion about quality employment means limiting hours or ensuring parental leave; in short, being away from work (McQueen, 2001).

The work of Frederick Taylor at the beginning of the 20th century attempted to study, analyse and describe work. He believed that the most efficient way of performing a job was determined by subdividing it into the smallest possible units of time and motion. One of Taylor's basic tenets has been largely overlooked, yet it alludes to the intrinsic nature of work. He felt strongly that doing a job well was a motivating phenomenon including getting elemental motions correct (Nelson, 1980). Yet he was realistic about the informing nature of money and so urged that the best workers should also receive pay commensurate with their efforts without any upper limit to earnings — another tenet of Taylor's that is often ignored. It is standard practice for management writers to criticise Taylor. It is widely believed that: Taylor was solely interested in efficiency, that is, in reducing costs and increasing output; he believed workers responded only to financial incentives; he invented the assembly line; and he wanted to put all power in the hands of management. Drucker (1981) believes all these interpretations are false. Taylor, for example, had no knowledge of the assembly line which was a creation of Henry Ford. He also foresaw the matrix management style, wanting to eliminate "the boss" whom he saw as counter productive. Taylor believed that performing work in an efficient manner was far more motivating than inefficient useless motions.

Elton Mayo's Hawthorne studies or experiments in the 1920s and 1930s (Stuart-Kotze, 2004) came as welcome relief for the dehumanising effects of the misapplication of scientific management. This theory asserted that it was the role of management to facilitate human relationships and it spawned the human resources movement still prevalent today. The success of this theory has often been attributed to the recognition that harmonious social relationships and feelings of belongingness motivate workers, now called "employees". The human relations movement did very little however to address a fundamental mistake in the application of Taylorism, namely ignoring the motivating effect of the work. However, it did establish a social context for workers to perform their work, which had largely disappeared at the commencement of the industrial revolution.

Content theories of work

The "neo human relations" theorists, Maslow (1954), Herzberg (1959) and McGregor (1960), attempted to explain motivation to work in terms of factors that initiate employee behaviour. They are called content theories because they define what is doing the motivating. Although Maslow is perhaps best known for the Need Hierarchy, for at least two decades during the middle of the 20th century, his work about the nature of human motivation was integral to the work of Herzberg and McGregor.

Herbert's Motivation-Hygiene theory at least places some focus on the work itself. Herzberg identified that there are two distinct entities — job satisfaction, which leads to motivation and job dissatisfaction or hygiene factors, which do not motivate. Emery and Phillips' (1976) influential study on the nature of work in Australia concluded, in line with Herzberg's theory, that bad working conditions can be a potent source of dissatisfaction but very good conditions do not do much to create motivation.

McGregor's Theory X, Theory Y, takes the emphasis off the work and places it on the attributes of the worker, suggesting that individuals have a strong motivation mostly for achievement, power or affiliation. Content theories serve a useful purpose in focusing a manager's attention on employee needs and their satisfaction. However, they are limited by their inability to explain the underlying dynamics of motivation and behaviours workers will choose in order to satisfy their needs.

The psychologist, R. W. White's (1959) theories on motivation originally postulated the concept of competence for a theory of intrinsic motivation, asserting that we have a biological urge to feel competent and be self-determining. Consequently, the reward is not internal to the self but internal to the nervous system. White's theory echoed Taylor's belief in the motivating effect of doing a job well. Likewise, Herzberg's (1959) motivators are listed as concepts such as challenge, responsibility, personal achievement, internal recognition and growth and learning which are consistent with the intrinsic motivation described by White.

Rewards for work

Clearly, however, work does involve an external reward, even where there is an intrinsic reward. Csikszentmihalyi's (1975) study of surgeons and musicians for example met his criteria for engaging in an intrinsically satisfying activity/ occupation, which he termed "flow". However, particularly in the case of surgeons, substantial extrinsic rewards are present in the form of income and status. The distinction between intrinsic and extrinsic rewards is difficult to determine in this instance. Lane (1991; 2000) identifies this type of problem not as a scientific question at all, but rather a philosophical one. Lane's work echoes the earlier work of Deci (1975) who argued that rewarding intrinsically satisfying activities actually interferes with the level of satisfaction reported. Paying people to do work they enjoy not only detracts from that enjoyment, but can also reduce effort, degrade quality, decrease work commitment and may even increase premature mortality. In fact, rewarding enjoyable activities in one experiment reported by Lane (1991) reduced the reported satisfaction of the activity below that of a boring task, while conversely, rewarding a boring task raised the enjoyment ratings reported for it. However, pay can be interpreted as both information and control. When pay is interpreted as the former, intrinsic motivation need not be compromised, such as in the case of a performance bonus for a highly successful worker who has multiple sources of evidence that affirm his or her positive self-image. The track record for the introduction of performance-based pay systems, which would support Lane's proposal, is very mixed in both Australia and the United States of America (Harrington, 1998; Waite & Stites-Doe, 2000). It is entirely possible that some performance-based pay systems could still be interpreted as control as Deci argues, if people are vulnerable to the illusion of control, they will interpret acts as controlling even if they have to distort the facts to do so. For example, a performance bonus might be interpreted as too meagre if the recipient is of the belief that their supervisor actually has a low opinion of them while ignoring the fact that it is still a performance bonus.

Occupational science and work

The field of occupational science is much younger than the bodies of knowledge underpinning economics, sociology and psychology. Occupational science is founded upon the belief that humans are occupational beings and have a biological drive to engage in occupation (Wilcock, 1998). Occupational science's focus is on individual experience and the multiple dimensions of its context. Therefore, research into other occupations such as play, or into the impact of changed life circumstances such as disability on the occupational being of humans, may have some explanatory worth for the study of work. Motivation theories that have tried to analyse work as extrinsically driven fail to recognise the intrinsic nature of work. On the other hand, theories that consider the content of work without the context do not have sufficient explanatory power for individual differences.

Responsibility for work

Differences and overlaps occur in government policy and administration of work-related matters. For the general population, work is usually considered with a *labour* orientation, while occupational therapy's concern generally has a *health* orientation. Indeed, within the international system, occupational therapy's purview is predominantly consistent with that of the World Health Organization (WHO). The taxonomy predominantly used by occupational therapists is the "International Classification of Functioning, Disability and Health" (ICF), which was introduced by the WHO (2001). On the other hand, work, including the administration of work and disability policies and international conventions on vocational rehabilitation, is predominantly the concern of the International Labour Organisation (ILO). These distinctions are also amplified at national and state/provincial levels. Occupational therapists predominantly work within the health sector, while matters such as workers' compensation are administered by employment or workplace relations sectors and vocational rehabilitation falls into the domain of social security or community service sectors (O'Halloran, 2002).

As the focus of this chapter is to inform the practice of work-related rehabilitation, a predominantly labour orientation will be taken when considering this area. Although occupational therapists think of productivity as more than just paid employment, there is a strong societal imperative to focus on this aspect of productivity. In addition, when considering work-related rehabilitation, the emphasis is definitely on the concept of work as paid employment, or at least the contribution/production of goods, services and knowledge to support the individual, family or community/society.

The ICF taxonomy is useful for occupational therapists to consider an individual's difficulty engaging in work/employment as a restriction in participation, due to current health concerns resulting in activity limitations and/or body system impairments (Gibson & Strong, 2003). Occupational therapy models, such as the Occupational Performance Model (Australia) (Chapparo & Ranka, 1997), however, are concerned with a client and the client's performance needs and/or desires that may or may not be related to an ICD-10 classification (Ranka, 2003). So while the ICF is based on a person's health condition in terms of a disorder or disease, the Occupational Performance Model (Australia) views people as having occupational performance needs or desires that are not necessarily related to disruptions in health (Ranka).

Jobs and careers

Within the world of work-related literature, two terms frequently appear, namely "career" and "job". Distinctions are seldom drawn between the two and more confusingly still, the terms are sometimes used interchangeably. In this chapter, these two terms will be used to mean two distinct concepts that relate to work.

The word career comes from the French *carriere*, and originally from the Latin *carrus* to mean carry and means: "(a) a general course of action or progress of a person through life, as in some profession, in some moral or intellectual action, or (b) an occupation, profession etc followed as one's lifework" (*The Macquarie Dictionary*, 1997, p 274). The word job on the other hand means among other things: "(a) a piece of work; an individual piece of work done in the routine of one's occupation or trade; or (b) a piece of work of defined character undertaken for a fixed price. The etymology of the word job is uncertain" (*The Macquarie Dictionary*, p 947).

For the occupational therapist, the distinction is important. The onset of changed circumstances for example may have deleterious effects on either a career or a job or both. Therefore it is important to understand the difference and the interaction between one's job and one's career. However, even within these broad concepts, confusion exists. For example, Innes and Straker (1998) discuss the confusion of job-related terms in work-related assessments created by the limited specificity of assessments to assess items that are relevant to the context and functional level of the client.

In an effort to work our way through this confusion, two models are presented (see Table 18.1), one for careers and one for jobs.

	Temporal orientation	Contextual orientation	Intrinsic factors	Extrinsic factors
Job	Point in time	Determined by context	Satisfiers Hygiene	Monetary Outputs
Career	Lifetime	Determines context	Value Worth	Status

Table 18.1 Comparative characteristics of jobs and careers

Jobs

In a number of countries, such as Australian, Canada and the United States of America, there are dictionaries of jobs (Australian Bureau of Statistics, 1997; Human Resources Development Canada, 2001; U.S. Department of Labor Employment & Training, 1991a, 1991b). These volumes invariably define jobs in terms of their title, duties, tasks and educational/training requirements. In some cases, there is also consideration of the temperaments required to perform the job. Additional companion documents or information may also detail the specific demands of the job on the individual in terms of physical, psychological and cognitive requirements, although physical demands are the most commonly detailed (for example, Field & Field, 1992; Human Resources Development Canada, 2003; U.S. Department of Labor Employment & Training, 1991c). Environmental conditions in which the job is performed may also be provided.

While these job definitions tend to be generalisations, and employers develop more specific job descriptions, the emphasis is very much on what the person is required to do when in a particular situation, rather than on what the individual wishes to gain from the position. That is, the emphasis of formal job descriptions and definitions is focused on the output produced as the result of work, in terms of goods or services, rather than intrinsic motivators or the individual's reasons to work.

The focus when examining jobs, therefore, is on what people need to do in the here and now to fit into a job and whether the fit is in terms of what duties and tasks the person is required to perform or the environment in which the job is undertaken. When analysing jobs, there is frequently a hierarchy commencing with the job title, followed by the duties to be performed, the tasks that comprise the duties, the sub-tasks or task elements that make up the tasks, and finally the elemental components that are required for the sub-tasks (U.S. Department of Labor Employment & Training, 1991c). This is all then put in the context of the environmental demands or constraints of the job. The educational/training/experience requirements are identified, as are the temperaments that suit the job.

While today there is some consideration given to the career development opportunities for individuals within large organisations, there remains an emphasis on how the job will contribute to meeting the organisation's mission. Any focus on jobs is also fixed to a particular point in time, rather than careers, which are on a continuum that develops over time.

Careers

Career counselling or career planning are processes that have been present in some form or another since the beginning of the 20th century when Frank Parsons first wrote about matching people with jobs on the basis of concern for and work with youth making the transition from school to work (Super, Savickas, & Super, 1996). In the last few decades, economic and organisational restructuring has meant significant changes to the concept of career. People change their employing organisations frequently but also organisations themselves restructure and have different employee requirements.

Brousseau, Driver, Eneroth and Larsson (1996) have argued for a pluralistic model of career experience as a means of integrating the diverse and changing needs of individuals and organisations. Their model presented here identifies four fundamentally different patterns of career experience. The concepts differ in terms of direction and frequency of movement within and across different types of jobs over time. The four concepts can be combined in various ways to form hybrid concepts that in turn can be used to describe many different patterns of career experience. These are: (a) linear career; (b) expert career; (c) spiral career; and (d) transitory career. The defining characteristics of these careers are described below and outlined in Table 18.2.

Linear Career

The focus of a linear career is primarily upon progressive steps upward in a hierarchy to positions of ever-increasing authority and responsibility. This career path is pursued by those seeking the traditional symbols of career success such as a large office, accountability for many staff and power to influence decisions and other people. It is a very traditional model of "starting at the bottom and working one's way to the top".

Expert Career

This type of career reflects a lifelong commitment to developing a high level of skill in a particular field or speciality. Rather than moving up the hierarchy, people on this career path view "getting ahead" as becoming more and more proficient in their area of expertise. The nature of their work is an integral part of their self-identity.

Spiral Career

A spiral career is characterised by periodic shifts between occupational areas, specialities or disciplines. These changes typically occur after a person has been in a field long enough to develop some in-depth competence (that is, 7–10 years). The ideal spiral is from one area (for example, research) into an allied area (for example, new product development). Knowledge and skills acquired in a previous field are used as a lever to developing an entirely new set of knowledge and skills.

Transitory Career

Changes made in a transitory career are most likely to occur every 3–5 years from one field or job to another that is very different or wholly unrelated. People who have these careers are more likely to be seeking variety and independence in life, rather than seeing themselves as actually having a career in the traditional sense.

	Linear	Expert	Spiral	Transitory
Direction of movement	Upward	Little movement	Mainly lateral	Mainly lateral
Duration of stay in one field	Variable	Life	7–10 years	3–5 years
Core career values	Power Achievements	Expertise Security	Personal growth Creativity	Variety Independence
Key competencies	Coordination Competitive-ness Cost efficiency Logistics	Quality Commitment Reliability Technical skills	Creativity Teamwork Skill diversity Lateral coordination	Speed Networking Adaptability Fast learning
Orientation	Profit	Stability	People development	Project focus

Table 18.2 The defining characteristics of career patterns

While few people have a career path that is perfectly described by the one type of these career paths to the exclusion of others, this model presents a useful way of understanding the nature of careers.

Work-related rehabilitation

The literature surrounding work-related rehabilitation uses a variety of terms: vocational rehabilitation, occupational rehabilitation, injury management and disability management. The terms are frequently used interchangeably, however the question of whether or not there is a pre-existing relationship with an employer appears to be a key distinction. While there are many exceptions to this categorisation, vocational rehabilitation literature often does not presume a pre-existing relationship with an employer while occupational rehabilitation, injury and disability management generally presume an existing relationship and frequently have the overlay of workers' compensation.

The bodies of knowledge surrounding vocational rehabilitation and occupational rehabilitation are frequently separated. Even at a government administration and policy level, the two spheres frequently are administered by differing government jurisdictions as has been mentioned previously. There are debates about whether the locus of responsibility for work-related rehabilitation should lie within health, vocational education and training, employment and industrial relations, social security or community care (O'Halloran, 2002). A number of international studies (McAnaney, 2001; Riddell, 2001; Thornton, 1998) have underlined the importance of *joined-up* approaches to disability, employment and benefits policy. In addition, there are debates about which actors should have prime responsibility for the management of national and individual rehabilitation plans, for example should these be managed by professional rehabilitation workers, employers or disabled people?

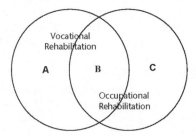

Figure 18.1 Overlap between vocational rehabilitation and occupational
        rehabilitation

The following examples may be useful in terms of practical applications of this continuum.

Area A (Figure 18.1) represents the situation where vocational rehabilitation is the most appropriate approach. For example, a young person with spina bifida who has recently left school and is entering the workforce for the first time (that is, no work history or experience as a worker; no existing relationship with employer).

Area B (Figure 18.1) represents the overlap between vocational and occupational rehabilitation approaches. For example, a person with a psychological injury is re-entering the workforce after an extended period away (that is, no recent/relevant work history or experience as a worker; no pre-existing relationship with future employer).

Area C (Figure 18.1) represents an approach based on occupational rehabilitation. For example, a person with a back injury re-entering workforce after a short period away, or maintaining a position at work, but is having difficulty due to injury/illness (that is, recent work history or experience; still views self as a worker; has an existing relationship with employer).

Vocational rehabilitation

Vocational rehabilitation literature has a predominant focus on the individual's need to choose, get and keep employment and carries no implicit assumption about a pre-existing relationship with an employer. Interest in vocational rehabilitation and employment opportunities for persons with disabilities occurred around the time of World War II, although this was mostly due to social reform charters of Western governments of the 1930s, coupled with the number of people disabled during the war and the need to find trained workers to fill jobs left vacant by mobilised workers (O'Halloran, 2002).

In May 1944, the International Labour Conference adopted a comprehensive Recommendation (No 71) on employment services, including labour market information, vocational guidance and vocational training (International Labour Organization, 1944). One of the groups specifically covered by the Recommendation was disabled workers who, "whatever the origin of their disability, should be provided with full opportunities for rehabilitation, specialized vocational guidance, training and retraining, and employment on useful work" (International Labour Organization, 1944, R71 General Principles, X). The Recommendation provides early examples of a number of concepts such as mainstreaming, equality of opportunity and affirmative action. A specific recommendation on vocational rehabilitation (No 99) was ratified in 1955 (International Labour Organization, 1955). That recommendation defined vocational rehabilitation as "a process which enables disabled persons to secure, retain and advance in suitable employment and thereby further their integration into society" (International Labour Organization, 1955, R99, Definitions 1(a)).

In 1983 the ILO, conscious that significant developments had occurred since 1955 in the understanding of rehabilitation needs, the scope and organisation of rehabilitation services and the law and practice of many countries, decided that new international standards were necessary to ensure equality of opportunity and treatment to all categories of disabled persons, in both rural and urban areas, for employment and integration into the community. Convention No 159 called on the competent authorities to provide and evaluate vocational guidance, vocational training, placement, employment and other related services, using, wherever possible and appropriate, existing services for workers generally, with any necessary adaptations. Convention No 159 entered into force on 20 June 1985. As of March 2004, 75 countries have ratified Convention No 159, including Australia, China, most of the European Union countries (except the United Kingdom) and Japan.

Occupational rehabilitation

Terms such as occupational rehabilitation (National Occupational Health & Safety Commission, 1995a, 1995b; WorkCover NSW, 2000), injury management (Guthrie, 2001; *Workplace Injury Management and Workers Compensation Act 1998*, 1998) and disability management (Currier, Chan, Berven, Aback & Taylor, 2001; Habeck, 1996; National Institute of Disability Management & Research, 2000; Williams & Westmorland, 2002) have a predominant focus on the return of an injured worker to the workplace. That is, these terms are based on an assumption of an existing link between a worker and a workplace and that the person is a worker and sees him or herself in this role. In addition, there is usually a link to workers' compensation. Occupational rehabilitation and injury management are terms more commonly used in Australia, while disability management is a more common term in North America. These terms characterise direct access to the workplace and intervention at the onset of work-related injury or illness.

In addition, occupational rehabilitation tends to be employer-based, in contrast to the individual orientation of vocational rehabilitation practice. There is incr-easing recognition that the most effective occupational rehabilitation programs are workplace-based and involve support, communication, co-ordination and co-operation among the relevant parties (for example, employees, employers, insurers, doctors and rehabilitation providers) (Commonwealth of Australia, 1994). Occupational rehabilitation aims to get formerly injured or ill employees back to work as soon as safely practicable. In so doing, successful rehabilitation programs reduce the costs of work-related injury and illness to both employers and employees. Successful programs also reduce indirect costs such as retraining, disruption to production and labour turnover (Comcare, 2001; Commonwealth of Australia, 1994).

Most occupational rehabilitation schemes demonstrate many of the following principles:

1. Return to work (RTW) activity should commence as soon as possible after injury.

2. The employee's workplace should be the focus of the rehabilitation program.

3. RTW plans are tailored to the employee's needs and are well co-ordinated, accountable and results-oriented.

4. The employee is actively involved in the development of the RTW plan.

5. The employer takes preventative action.

The importance of effective rehabilitation as a means of dramatically reducing compensation costs is reinforced by evidence from one scheme, which suggests that, whereas only about one in five claims extend beyond four weeks, they nevertheless account for approximately 85 per cent of total costs (Australian Cap-ital Territory Government, 1990). Over the last two decades, most jurisdictions in Australia have incorporated provisions relating to rehabilitation into their legislation. However, the schemes vary in their approach and emphasis. The New South Wales, Victorian, Australian Capital Territory and Comcare (federal) schemes emphasise workplace-based programmes and employer involvement in the process (Heads of Workers' Compensation Authorities, 2002). By contrast, Queensland, Tasmania and South Australia place greater emphasis on services provided by external rehabilitation specialists, and a case management approach (Heads of Workers' Compensation Authorities). In addition, Queensland has adopted a program aimed at assisting employers to develop their own workplace-based programs. The Northern Territory requires that employers take reasonable steps to provide rehabilitation and suitable employment (Heads of Workers' Compensation Authorities). The Western Australian system does not expressly require employers to provide rehabilitation, although the workers' compensation authority may require the employer to do so in certain cases (Heads of Workers' Compensation Authorities).

Assessing an individual's ability to work

Both vocational rehabilitation and occupational rehabilitation rely on providing "appropriate, adequate and timely services based on assessed needs" (National Occupational Health & Safety Commission, 1995a, p 1). These assessed needs form the basis for interventions or programs that are relevant and appropriate for the individual, incorporating environmental and temporal aspects. The categories of assessments commonly used to determine an injured, ill or disabled individual's capability to work have been described by Innes and Straker (1998). They see these types of assessments as being hierarchical in nature, with each assessment type incorporated within the one above it (see Figure 18.2).

Vocational assessment

This type of assessment uses multiple measures to determine an individual's ability to fulfil the worker role (that is, whether this person can work) and identifies the most appropriate occupational category by examining physical, cognitive and psychosocial abilities (Innes & Straker, 1998). This assessment approach can address career options and include investigation of interests, temperament, educational/training undertaken and transferable skills from previous work experiences or life skills in general. It is often compiled from information provided by various members of a multi-disciplinary team (for example, occupational therapist, physiotherapist, psychologist and/or rehabilitation counsellor).

Work-related assessment

This assessment approach uses:

> ... multiple measures to determine an individual's ability to perform the work requirements of specific job tasks or activities, an entire job, group of jobs (i.e., occupational category or group), or broadly defined work demands (e.g. sedentary, light, medium, heavy, very heavy).
>
> (Innes & Straker, 1998, p 195)

This group of assessments includes workplace-based assessments, work trials, situational assessment, functional capacity evaluations, work samples and work simulations (Innes & Straker, 1998).

Functional capacity evaluation

This is a one-time evaluation that measures performance of the physical demands and skills usually associated with work (Innes & Straker, 1998). Many commercially available functional capacity evaluations use the United States Department of

Labor's (1991c) physical work demands as a basis for their content. These physical work demands include postural (sitting, standing, walking, kneeling, stooping, crouching) and manual handling (lifting, lowering, pushing, pulling, carrying) aspects, as well as upper limb function (reaching, manual dexterity).

Physical capacity evaluation
This is a one-time evaluation measuring isolated physical attributes, including static and dynamic muscle strength, flexibility, balance, co-ordination, and cardiopulmonary endurance (Innes & Straker, 1998). These aspects are often incorporated into a functional capacity evaluation.

Conceptual basis for work assessments

While these assessment approaches to work may be hierarchical in nature, they are not linked to a conceptual basis. This lack of a conceptual basis has been identified as an area of concern by a number of authors (Gibson & Strong, 2003; Innes & Straker, 1998) and several frameworks have been proposed. Gibson and Strong suggested the use of the WHO ICF framework. They indicate that functional capacity evaluations assess at the activity limitation level. Innes and Straker had previously suggested a framework linking a wide range of work-related assessments, including functional capacity evaluations, with a more detailed conceptualisation that had similarities to the WHO ICF, and linked an individual's performance with levels of job analysis detail. This enables the selection of work assessments relevant to the specific job requirements, as well as the level of detail of the individual's ability. Table 18.3 shows how the different levels of an individual's occupational performance compare to similar levels of work that are considered in job analyses. Table 18.4 presents the definitions of each of these individual and work levels to allow further comparison and understanding of the similarities between these two aspects.

An extension of this framework incorporating vocational assessment and the concept of a career over time, in addition to a job at any point in time, is presented in Figure 18.2.

The purpose of using such a framework is to provide a conceptual basis from which to select and perform relevant and appropriate assessments targeted at an

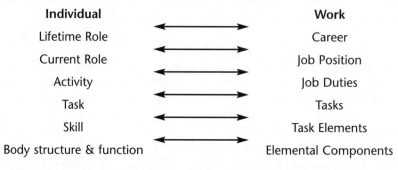

Table 18.3 Comparing levels of individual performance and work

Individual	Work
Lifetime Role — career developed over lifetime; not context dependent.	**Career** — general course of action or progress through life; may be linear, expert, spiral or transitory, or a combination.
Current Role — worker; dependent on context.	**Job Position** — complex of tasks and duties for any individual.
Activities — complex collection of tasks that result in an identifiable whole (for example, making a table).	**Job Duties** — represent major activities involved in the job, and consist of several related tasks.
Tasks — discrete identifiable component that contributes to a whole activity (for example, hammering a nail).	**Tasks** — a discrete unit of work performed by an individual; logical & necessary step of a duty; typically has identifiable beginning and end.
Skill — ability to perform specific physical demands (for example, manual dexterity).	**Task Elements** — smallest step into which it is practical to subdivide any work activity without analysing separate motions, and so on.
Body System — physical, cognitive and psychological aspects of function (for example, strength, balance, colour discrimination).	**Elemental Components** — very specific separate motions or movements (biomechanical aspects); may also include cognitive and psychological variables.

Table 18.4 Definitions of individual performance and work levels

appropriate level. This will assist in answering referral questions received in either vocational or occupational rehabilitation settings.

Conclusion

Occupational therapy has a long history of using work as a therapeutic medium (Harvey-Krefting, 1985; Wilcock, 2001) and has developed a large and unique body of knowledge about the construct of work. The construct in occupational therapy literature largely stresses the experiential nature of work and how the performance of work influences health or how health influences performance. While occupational therapists' health paradigm is at variance with the political responsibility for work, perhaps this paradigm underlies the profession's greatest potential contribution to the advancement of understanding about work.

In the early part of the 21st century, much political attention is being paid to the impact of work on the health of workers. However, official inquiries into this

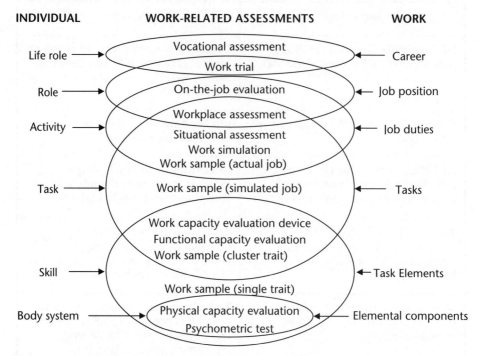

Figure 18.2 Work-related assessments relevant to individual performance and work levels (adapted from Innes & Straker, 1998)

matter usually have an economic, sociological, medical or psychological frame of reference, depending on the commissioning individual or organisation. While these frames of reference are all valid, an occupational science frame of reference may yield new insights, hitherto unknown, to the broader society. In making a contribution from this perspective, work-related rehabilitation practitioners need to ensure a thorough understanding not only of their practice, but also of its theoretical underpinning.

References

Australian Bureau of Statistics. (1997). *Australian standard classification of occupations and ASCO coder* (2nd ed.). Canberra: Commonwealth of Australia.

Australian Capital Territory Government. (1990). *Australian Capital Territory Government submission: Inquiry into aspects of Australian workers' compensation*. Canberra, ACT: Australian Government Publishing Service.

Brousseau, K. R., Driver, M. J., Eneroth, K. & Larsson, R. (1996). Career pandemonium: Realigning organizations and individuals. *Academy of Management Executive, 10*(4), 52–66.

Chapparo, C. & Ranka, J. (1997). *Occupational Performance Model (Australia): Monograph 1* [Electronic version]. Retrieved 31 March 2004 from http://www.occupationalperformance.com

Chapparo, C. J. & Hooper, E. (2002). When is it work? Perceptions of six-year-old children. *WORK, 19*(3), 291–302.

Comcare. (2001). *Rehabilitation: Managing return to work* [Internet]. Commonwealth of Australia. Retrieved 24 March 2004 from http://www.comcare.gov.au/pdf_files/managing_return_to_work.pdf

Commonwealth of Australia. (1994). *Workers' compensation in Australia industry commission inquiry report*. Canberra, ACT: Australian Government Publishing Service.

Csikszentmihalyi, M. (1975). *Beyond boredom and anxiety*. San Francisco: Jossey-Bass Publishers.

Currier, K. F., Chan, F., Berven, N. L., Habeck, R. V. & Taylor, D. W. (2001). Functions and knowledge domains for disability management practice: A Delphi study. *Rehabilitation Counseling Bulletin, 44*(3), 133–143.

Deci, E. L. (1975). *Intrinsic motivation*. New York: Plenum.

Drucker, P. F. (1981). Towards the next economics. In D. Bell & I. Kristol (Eds), *The crisis in economic theory*, pp 1–18. New York: Basic Books.

Emery, F. E. & Phillips, C. (1976). *Living at work*. Canberra, ACT: Australian Government Publishing Service.

Field, J. E. & Field, T. F. (1992). *The classification of jobs* (4th ed.). Athens: Elliott & Fitzpatrick.

Gibson, L. & Strong, J. (2003). A conceptual framework of functional capacity evaluation for occupational therapy in work rehabilitation. *Australian Occupational Therapy Journal, 50*(2), 64–71.

Guthrie, R. (2001). *Report on the implementation of the Labor Party direction statement in relation to workers' compensation* (Report to the Workers' Compensation & Rehabilitation Commission). Perth: Curtin University of Technology.

Habeck, R. V. (1996). Differentiating disability management and rehabilitation. *National Association of Rehabilitation Professionals in the Private Sector (NARPPS) Journal, 11*(2), 8–20.

Harrington, H. J. (1998). Performance improvement: Was W. Edwards Deming wrong? *The TQM Magazine, 10*(4), 230–237.

Harvey-Krefting, L. (1985). The concept of work in occupational therapy: A historical review. *American Journal of Occupational Therapy, 39*, 301–307.

Heads of Workers' Compensation Authorities. (2002). *Comparison of workers' compensation arrangements — Australia and New Zealand*. Melbourne: Victoria WorkCover Authority.

Herzberg, F. (1959). *The motivation to work*. New York: Wiley.

Human Resources Development Canada. (2001). *National occupational classification 2001*. Toronto: Canadian Government Publishing.

Human Resources Development Canada. (2003). *Career handbook* (2nd ed.). Toronto: Canadian Government Publishing.

Humphreys, S. C. (1969). History, economics and anthropology: The work of Karl Polanyi. *History & Theory, 8*(2), 191–202.

Innes, E. & Straker, L. (1998). A clinician's guide to work-related assessments: 2 — Design problems. *Work, 11*(2), 191–206.

International Labour Organization. (1944). *R71 Employment (Transition from War to Peace) Recommendation* [Internet]. Retrieved 31 March 2004 from http://www.ilo.org/ilolex/english/recdisp1.htm

International Labour Organization. (1955). *R99 Vocational Rehabilitation (Disabled) Recommendation* [Internet]. Retrieved 31 March 2004 from http://www.ilo.org/ilolex/english/recdisp1.htm

International Labour Organization. (1983). *C159 Vocational Rehabilitation and Employment (Disabled Persons) Convention* [Internet]. Retrieved 31 March 2004 from http://www.ilo.org/ilolex/english/convdisp1.htm

Lane, R. E. (1991). *The market experience*. Cambridge, NY: Cambridge University Press.

Lane, R. E. (2000). *The loss of happiness in market democracies*. New Haven: Yale University Press.

Maslow, A. H. (1954). *Motivation and personality*. New York: Harper & Bros.

McAnaney, D. (2001, 30 May–1 June). *Early intervention policies and practice: Transnational perspectives on work-based rehabilitation [Keynote Address]*. Paper presented at the Australian Society of Rehabilitation Counsellors Conference, Sydney, NSW.

McGregor, D. (1960). *The human side of enterprise*. New York: McGraw-Hill.

McQueen, H. (2001). *Killing time — alienation theories in an era of chronic under-employment and overwork [ACIRRT Working Paper No. 72]* [Internet]. The University of Sydney. Retrieved 15 March 2004 from http://www.acirrt.com/pubs/WP72.pdf

Mitter, S. & Rowbotham, S. (1995). *Women encounter technology: Changing patterns of employment in the third world*. London: Routledge.

National Institute of Disability Management & Research. (2000). *Code of practice for disability management* [Internet]. Retrieved 8 August 2001 from http://www.nidmar.ca/code/Code_of_Practice_English.pdf

National Occupational Health & Safety Commission. (1995a). *Guidance note for best practice rehabilitation management of occupational injuries and disease [NOHSC:3021(1995)].* Canberra: Australian Government Publishing Service.

National Occupational Health & Safety Commission. (1995b). *Uniform guidelines for accreditation of rehabilitation providers [NOHSC:7032(1995)].* Canberra: Australian Government Publishing Service.

Nelson, D. (1980). *Frederick W. Taylor and the rise of scientific management.* Madison, WI: University of Wisconsin.

O'Halloran, D. (2002). An historical overview of Australia's largest and oldest provider of vocational rehabilitation — CRS Australia. *WORK, 19*(3), 211–218.

Ranka, J. (2003, April). *The International Classification of Function and the Occupational Performance Model (Australia): Positioning therapists to lead change.* Paper presented at the OT AUSTRALIA 22nd National Conference, Melbourne, Vic.

Riddell, S. (2001). *Work preparation and vocational rehabilitation: A literature review.* Glasgow: Strathclyde Centre for Disability Research, University of Glasgow.

Rose, H. (1994). *Love, power and knowledge: Towards a feminist transformation of the sciences.* Oxford: Polity Press.

Smith, A. (1776). *An inquiry into the nature and causes of the wealth of nations* [Electronic version]. Retrieved 24 March 2004 from http://www.adamsmith.org/smith/won-intro.htm

Somavia, J. (2001). *Reducing the decent work deficit: A global challenge* (Report of the Director-General of the ILO International Labour Conference, 89th session). Geneva: International Labour Organization.

Stuart-Kotze, R. (2004). *Elton Mayo and the Hawthorne studies* [Internet]. Retrieved 24 March 2004 from http://www.theworkingmanager.com/articles/detail.asp?ArticleNo=43

Super, D. E., Savickas, M. L. & Super, C. M. (1996). The life-span, life-space approach to careers. In D. Brown & L. Brooks (Eds), *Career choice and development* (3rd ed.), pp 121–178. San Francisco: Jossey-Bass Publishers.

The Macquarie Dictionary. (3rd ed.). (1997). Sydney: The Macquarie Library.

Thornton, P. (1998). *International research project on job retention and return to work strategies for disabled workers.* Geneva: International Labour Organization.

U.S. Department of Labor Employment & Training. (1991a). *Dictionary of occupational titles (Volume I)* (4th rev. ed. Vol. 1). Indianapolis: JIST Works.

U.S. Department of Labor Employment & Training. (1991b). *Dictionary of occupational titles (Volume II)* (4th rev. ed. Vol. 2). Indianapolis: JIST Works.

U.S. Department of Labor Employment & Training. (1991c). *The revised handbook for analyzing jobs.* Indianapolis: JIST Works.

Waite, M. L. & Stites-Doe, S. (2000). Removing performance appraisal and merit pay in the name of quality: An empirical study of employees reactions. *Journal of Quality Management, 5*(2), 187–206.

White, R. W. (1959). Motivation reconsidered: The concept of competence. *Psychological Review, 66,* 297–333.

Wilcock, A. (1998). *An occupational perspective of health.* Thorofare: Slack Inc.

Wilcock, A. (2001). *Occupation for health: A journey from self health to prescription.* London: British Association & College of Occupational Therapy.

Williams, R. M. & Westmorland, M. (2002). Perspectives on workplace disability management: A review of the literature. *WORK, 19*(1), 87–93.

Work Cover NSW. (2000). *Guidelines for employers' return-to-work programs* (Rev. ed.). Sydney: WorkCover NSW.

Workplace Injury Management and Workers Compensation Act 1998, New South Wales (1998).

World Health Organization. (2001). *ICF: International classification of functioning, disability and health.* Geneva: WHO.

CHAPTER NINETEEN

Leisure as Commodity

Bob Neumayer

Clare Wilding

Leisure

Commodification

Health

Occupation

Work

Therapy

Chapter Profile

This chapter discusses issues related to leisure and occupation, which are important since leisure occupations are critically linked to the health and wellbeing of both individuals and communities alike. Compared to other "categories of occupation", such as self-care or work — as we have seen in the previous chapter — it becomes apparent that leisure occupations receive significantly less attention in the health professional literature. This chapter explores the historical evolution of leisure from once being an "ideal" of society, through to more recent times in which it has increasingly become viewed as a "commodity", central to state and national economies. The chapter then discusses the importance of leisure to health and finally posits suggestions as to how health professionals, especially occupational therapists, can incorporate concepts of leisure as part of their everyday practice.

Introduction

"Leisure as a commodity" implies that leisure has increasingly been constructed in contemporary society as an entity that can be bought, sold or traded for profit. Such a development is the result of a complex interaction between numerous factors including the evolution of a more complex relationship between leisure and work. However, while such an increasing treatment of leisure as a commodity arguably has benefits from an economic perspective, it may also result in a net loss of leisure time for individuals and populations alike, and thus have potentially damaging consequences environmentally and socially.

Despite such an apparent increase in its treatment as a commodity in contemporary society, the value and benefits of leisure are so significant that they should be a cornerstone consideration of all health professional practice. However, while the intrinsic health benefits of participation in leisure have been demonstrated through research to date, the current political and social climate may be seen as one which militates against such participation, hence subverting its health-enhancing properties. Indeed, the impacts of economic rationalism with health have increasingly meant that leisure is being "squeezed out" in terms of resources. Accordingly, health professionals (notably occupational therapists) working within a fiscally-constrained health system may use leisure occupations for the purpose of facilitating specific skill development rather than having the time to foster leisure for leisure's sake. Thus, the "true" purpose of leisure may become "distorted" and instead become a mere by-product of intervention. This chapter challenges health professionals to reconsider their attitudes to leisure and the place that it deserves within contemporary health-care settings.

The concluding sections offer suggestions for how the current concept-ualisation and usage of leisure may be altered or improved so that people can participate in occupations that are health-enhancing and ecologically sustainable. The aim is to motivate health professionals to influence current political and social constructions of leisure, in particular, how it is perceived and performed in the community. Through such action, it is hoped that leisure can be conceptualised differently, enabling it to become increasingly valued and valuable as both community-enriching and health-enhancing.

Defining leisure

The study of leisure is an interdisciplinary field (Kelly & Godbey, 1992; Veal & Lynch 2001) and has become the object of much conceptual discussion from many different disciplinary perspectives (Fullagar, 2000). Accordingly, defining the meaning of leisure is a challenging task. Leisure theorists and philosophers have not agreed on a single definition of leisure for centuries. This difficulty of defining leisure can be seen to be a strength because it signifies the complexity of leisure and shows it to be a social phenomenon that cannot be easily dismissed as "just having fun".

Some of the major themes that keep recurring in leisure theory include: freedom of choice; time away from work; activity done for its own sake; and any meaningful experience (Kelly & Godbey, 1992). Leisure is a forum where relationships develop between people and a sense of community is produced. It is the quality of these relationships, no matter how small, that leisure can contribute in a positive and healthy way, helping to create conditions for "the good life".

Leisure is often defined through concepts of time, activity, attitudes, space, freedom and experience. Since each of these terms has different meanings for every individual, there can be no agreed definition. Therefore, for the purpose of this chapter, leisure is defined as the interaction of four major dimensions being time, activity, attitude and freedom. That is, the time to engage freely in a chosen activity that brings value or positive outcomes to the individual. The activity may be any form of occupation that might even include work, but it must be freely chosen and not solely for economic benefit. In this context, leisure should also have positive personal outcomes that enhance wellbeing and health.

Leisure can therefore be described as a general concept that portrays a diverse range of cultural practices and activities (including arts, sports, outdoor pursuits, shopping, bushwalking, travel, hobbies, social interaction and solitary activities such as reading and listening to music, and so on). Leisure per se is not a static entity, but rather definitions of leisure are produced through the social relationships particular to certain historical periods and contexts, as evidenced by the evolution of leisure as a concept.

A brief history of leisure

Providing a brief history of leisure assists in understanding leisure's historical evolution and how its role and value in society changed over time. It is also important to demonstrate how leisure is linked to our health and wellbeing. Contemporary understandings of leisure are formed in part by our past values and beliefs. Throughout history, humans have maintained a desire to participate in leisure activities in various forms and that aspiration continues today. The history of leisure in this chapter will be limited to its development and impact on Western society only, since this informs understanding about how leisure has evolved from an ideal to being viewed increasingly as a commodity. Table 19.1 provides an overview of significant historical time periods in the evolution of leisure and highlights how concepts of leisure have changed over time.

Era	Time Frame	Concept of Leisure
Greek	500 to 300BC	Leisure as the ideal of life. More important than work.
Roman	Pre-industrial revolution	Leisure as activity for political, utilitarian and entertainment outcomes.
Dark and Middle Ages	400 to 1500s AD	Roman Catholic influence with carnival and holy day festivities. Leisure measured cyclically.
Reformation	1500s to 1600s AD	Leisure as potentially evil. Protestant work ethic the new "ideal".
Industrial Revolution	1600s to 1800s AD	Leisure fractured by time. Work to be rewarded by leisure.
Contemporary	1800s to today	Leisure as commodity and product. An item for sale and consumption.

Table 19.1 Historical evolution leisure constructions

Western concepts of leisure began with the Greeks around 400BC. For the Greeks, leisure was valued above all else and it provided the opportunity to debate life's meaning. Leisure was synonymous with the Greeks' concept of *schole* or education. The Greek philosophers adhered to leisure as the ideal of one's life allowing for contemplation and education (Lynch & Veal, 2001). It was a privilege to engage in leisure as one needed to be free from the demand to labour. Thus the ideal was also elitist, since it was dependent upon others' work and precluded most women and slaves from participating in leisure. Yet, despite this limitation, the contribution of ancient Greek thought in the philosophy of leisure and education cannot be dismissed. Sebastian de Grazia's (1962) classical writings about leisure frequently refer to the Greeks since their ideal of leisure was so essential to their society and subsequently to Western civilisation. Aristotle (considered the "father" of leisure) and Plato both argued that leisure was the highest ideal of any society as it represented freedom from labour (de Grazia). The goal of leisure was to be contemplative, and to undertake self-development and intrinsic pleasure through such activities as music and the study of philosophy.

A paradigm shift occurred in leisure's meaning when Roman societal values advocated that leisure activity become oriented towards political and utilitarian outcomes, much to the benefit of Roman society. These ideals were expressed through the creation of Roman baths, stadiums, parks, theatres and gardens. Such examples of leisure were among the first in the development of commodified leisure and its application to entertainment, fun and consumption of goods.

Concepts about leisure took another dramatic turn during the Reformation period, when the Protestant work ethic was increasingly embraced. This religious ideal emphasised that work was more important than leisure. Work was thought to be virtuous, and "idle hands" fell prey to the devil. Leisure was replaced by hard work and its rewards, that is, ultimately earning a place in heaven. The Protestant work ethic has endured in Western civilisation in various forms, and may still be seen as influencing today's concepts of leisure and work.

The arrival of the Industrial Revolution witnessed dramatic social changes, including impacts on individual and community leisure practices. Prior to the Industrial Revolution, many people (largely the peasant classes) experienced leisure as an integral aspect of their daily lives, regulated by the cycles of the seasons. With the arrival of factories and the mass production of goods, people and time were increasingly influenced by the introduction of clocks and work schedules. The move from an agricultural to an industrial economy meant a massive reorganisation of time into measurable, and hence profitable, units. There was a radical shift in the relationship between work and leisure time whereby leisure became moments of fractured time (Cross, 1990). Work and production of goods became increasingly vital to society, culture, economies and governments and leisure became a reward to be engaged in after work. Thus, the Greeks' original meaning and ideal of leisure as more important than work was reversed and it became increasingly difficult to experience leisure for "leisure's sake".

Some health benefits of leisure

Highlighting the connection between leisure and health is not a new undertaking (Veal & Lynch, 2001). The Greek philosophers' notion of sound mind and sound body was strongly linked to active leisure. The Romans engaged in games and music for relaxation and healing, thus recognising the health benefits of leisure.

More recently, however, there is a growing body of literature that describes the benefits of leisure. Driver, Brown and Petersen (1991) edited an entire book dedicated to the benefits of leisure demonstrating that leisure behaviour is not only intrinsically rewarding but carries with it natural benefits, including improved health. Leisure benefits are evidenced by increasing physical activity, assisting family bonding, developing spirituality, enhancing child development, reducing stress and promoting wellbeing. The benefits of leisure have also been addressed in a compilation of papers on leisure and mental health (Compton & Iso-Ahola, 1994).

Research is increasingly identifying leisure activities that contribute to improved health and wellbeing (Brown, Brown & Powers, 2001; Carpenter, 1994). Findings in leisure research illustrate that leisure enhances health by serving as a buffer to the stressful events of one's life (Siegenthaler, 1997). These events can include marriage, divorce, death of loved ones, illness and work. Studies also consistently demonstrate that people who regularly participate in leisure activities that match their interests and personality have an increased sense of wellbeing (Melamed & Meir, 1995).

Occupational therapy research into leisure also demonstrates its benefits. For example, Specht, King, Brown and Foris (2002) interviewed people with spina bifida or cerebral palsy about their experiences of engaging in leisure and found that leisure provided benefits of enjoyment, an opportunity to "prove oneself", friendship and a sense of belonging to a group. It is recommended that a focus on leisure occupations be adopted in occupational therapy because of the health benefits that leisure can afford. Passmore's (2001) research with young people determined that leisure that provides a range of both challenges and demands, and that is social, contributes positively to mental health. Holidays can also be a form of leisure that is fundamental to maintaining health and wellbeing (Luboshitzky & Gaber, 2001). Drummond and Walker (1996) evaluated the effectiveness of group therapy for people who had experienced stroke. They reported that clients whose treatment utilised leisure occupations were significantly more mobile and had more psychological wellbeing than a control group and those in a conventional occupational therapy group.

The benefits of engaging in a preferred leisure activity for a person's wellbeing are considerable. Through leisure one can temporarily escape from the pressures of time and the burden of commitments and responsibilities, and for many, leisure produces relief from stress (Kelly & Godbey, 1992). Leisure can be an asset in dealing with life's demands and assisting a person to develop a more balanced life. The physiological benefits of leisure activities are also numerous and translate into the potential to reduce health-care costs (Veal & Lynch, 2001).

Two important theoretical constructs of leisure that provide health benefits are those of flow and serious leisure. Csikszentmihalyi (1996) developed the concept of flow after researching the way people engaged in their favourite activities, be they work or leisure. This research is important because it demonstrates that leisure is not simply the opposite of work. People engaging in flow are totally immersed in their chosen activity. To experience a complete sense of flow, one has to let go of the desire to master time and instead master the experience. Flow experiences are intrinsically motivated. People engage in these experiences for the love or pleasure that participating in the occupation can provide, and this subsequently enhances health and wellbeing.

Serious leisure (Stebbins, 1996) is leisure occupations that have become central to one's life interests, and are similar to Csikszentmihalyi's notion of flow. Serious leisure activities are those that become self-actualising, self-enriching and re-creative, and enhance one's sense of personal wellbeing. This type of leisure can take the form of sport, hobbies and voluntary activities and produces lasting benefits to the participant. Serious leisure can demand exceptional output from the participant producing feelings of success, accomplishment and flow with improved health outcomes.

The research evidence and theoretical ideas about flow and serious leisure connect leisure to health and thus justify the promotion of leisure by health professionals as a health-enhancing type of occupation. That leisure can be health-sustaining, self-actualising, and re-creative are fundamental concepts which should underpin the efforts of health professionals to enable clients to have greater opportunities to experience meaningful leisure.

The commodification of leisure

While the varied and valued aspects of leisure have been discussed thus far, this section highlights how the commodification of leisure as a product has occurred with various outcomes. Even though employment, production and consumption of goods have provided gains in living standards in Western societies, it could be argued there have been costs to our "leisure lives", the environment and ultimately to people's health and wellbeing.

One contemporary concept of leisure is as a product to be consumed, and as an opportunity to be taken after completion of work. The development of leisure as a commodity arose after the Industrial Revolution produced the need for increased consumption of goods, since businesses needed to sell their products in order to make profits. Hence, the free market and capitalistic society were born, dependent on the mass production and consumption of goods in order to progress. One of the best examples of leisure conceptualised as a product is the current tourism industry, which today is one of the largest industries in the world.

After World War II, mass consumerism reached new heights when ideas of how to work and achieve were replaced with concepts of how to spend and enjoy (Bell, 1996). New forms of leisure evolved, such as holidays, cinemas, sporting events, dancing and shopping. As spending habits became increasingly important to people's lives, shopping developed as a core activity. As people's spending power increased, their desire to purchase goods rose to higher levels. Interestingly, however, for several decades now, leisure time has grown significantly less than in comparison to people's spending power (Roberts, 1999). Thus, although some have significant spending power, they have less time to participate in leisure.

Time, therefore, has also become a commodity in contemporary society. Understanding how time is conceptualised is one of the components that define leisure occupations. The commodification of time refers to how it is valued in terms of money and what can be bought or sold with it. People sell their labour time for wages, and then exchange that money for goods and services to use in their leisure time. They then have "free time", compressed into units, which is spent consuming the goods they have purchased. Leisure consumption therefore becomes a domain through which a certain social status is achieved. This can have potentially negative impacts upon health as there is often a cost to the amount of time people can engage in personal and community relationships.

Economist Staffan Linder's (1970) book entitled, *The Harried Leisure Class*, demonstrates through a cost analysis process that in order to increase people's income constantly, their lives have become proportionately more hectic. Thus, they have sacrificed a more leisurely lifestyle at the expense of economic affluence. In essence, this economic formula states that with economic growth, there has been an increase in hours devoted to productivity and thus a reduction of time for engaging in other meaningful occupations. Even though this book was written over 30 years ago, much of Linder's economic formula would still be accurate today, and for some, there would be even less time available.

Interestingly, while consumption of goods has increased, apparently people have not become any happier (Hamilton, 2003). Though inculcated into a belief system which suggests that consumption of goods will make them happy, such consumer activities actually diminish people's ability to engage in valuable and varied leisure activities and expressions of creativity. It is not, however, a simple case of greed. Rather, it is the cultural power of capital that convinces people of the need to work harder and longer hours (Hamilton). People do so because they believe that a significant income is required in order to maintain a certain lifestyle and that jobs and income are inextricably linked to social status. Thus, one's level of income is connected to one's identity and sense of worth.

Hamilton (2003), along with leisure theorists such as de Grazia (1962), also considers the belief that consumerism will lead to increased happiness levels is problematic, and is largely the responsibility of advertising and marketing schemes which target specific audiences such as young people (Lobo, 1999). One solution is for governments to place major restrictions on advertising agencies and companies with respect to their marketing practices. The difficulty with this solution, however, is that Western governments are quite dependent upon sustained economic growth as a measure of their perceived success, demonstrating positive growth figures in all sectors of the economy. By depending on economic growth as the major indicator for improved lifestyles, there is limited consideration of the comprehensive welfare of a society's citizens and its environment (Hamilton). There is concern that unfettered consumerism could lead people to participate in leisure practices that are potentially health damaging. This might include spending excessive amounts of time in "passive" activities (that can lead to obesity and other related health problems) such as television or computer games, or in "consumptive" leisure, such as extreme shopping.

Interestingly, there is considerable literature (Beder, 2000; de Grazia, 1962; Linder, 1970; Hamilton, 2003; Roberts, 1999) that criticises consumerism and capitalism for interfering with people's pursuit of healthier forms of leisure. Commercialism has been argued to be responsible for making leisure purely a form of amusement and diversion for people's simple desires and wants, while leaving them unfulfilled (Hamilton).

Overall, the effect of viewing leisure as a product is that leisure becomes increasingly inaccessible to all people. To "buy" leisure, one must work increasingly hard in order to raise the necessary funds. Paradoxically, however, this leads to reduced time in which to enjoy and use one's leisure. People who are unable to work due to shortages of suitable employment opportunities or because of disabilities are frequently unable to generate the funds with which to "purchase" their leisure, and although they have plenty of time they cannot afford many leisure products. These people may believe that the only leisure options available to them are to engage in passive leisure pursuits such as watching television. This establishes a frustrating cycle in which the television offers tempting scenes of exotic leisure activities and locations, for example in the form of travel and lifestyle shows, and yet these luxuries are unable to be realised given the financial limitations of living on restricted incomes. Television has also been found to be a popular yet unsatisfying form of leisure (Di Bona, 2000). In addition, Passmore's (2001) research found that engaging in leisure activities that involved solitary activity and which had minimal demands correlated with poor mental health.

Identity and value in work

Much of what has been presented thus far has been critical of Western society's shift to the primacy of the work ethic. Despite much criticism that leisure is frequently considered now to be in opposition to work, it is also closely related to work and cannot be truly disassociated from it (Jamrozik, 1986; Stormann, 1989). Many people's identities are strongly linked to their work which in fact may determine or actually be a part of their leisure. There is considerable agreement that leisure and work are meant to complement each other, not to be in opposition or competition (Stormann). For Stormann, leisure is freedom within work and that is where one's true identity is located. Thus, the purpose of work is not to earn money, but for self-discovery and to find meaning in one's life. Worker autonomy is needed in order for this to happen in addition to a shift from the current focus on labour as purely for production of goods. Unfortunately, Stormann concludes that today our society is still filled with "meaningless work and purposeless leisure" (p 28), meaning many people are not being fulfilled either at work or leisure.

Restoring the balance

It has been argued that the commodification of leisure and time has created a situation in which people might engage in behaviours that are potentially harmful to their health and wellbeing as individuals and as community members. This potential threat should prompt individuals to challenge the social context in which time can be spent in excessive hours of work, which then reduces time available for leisure, self-care and rest occupations. Primarily, people do not need to work more to achieve wellbeing. Rather, current work practices might change in order that people have the opportunity, time and energy to engage in meaningful leisure. A society might develop healthier values where people strive to achieve balance in their lives that elevates quality of life to at least the same level as quantity of production.

There are also an increasing number of people who want more control over their work lives and wish to free up more time for other activities that include leisure. This is evidenced by an increase in part-time work and independent contractors or consultants. These people who choose to do less work are frequently called downshifters (Schor, 1999; McKnight, 2001). Downshifters are described as people who wish to reduce their levels of consumption, and paid work, in exchange for more leisure and balance in their lives. This includes developing a slower paced life, having more time for their children and living daily lives that match their values (Schor, 1999). Downshifters should not be confused with people who can only find part-time employment and are seeking additional work.

Typical constructions of leisure as consumption have been challenged (Kelly, 1991), and many people's core leisure activities are in fact low cost and revolve around social relationships rather than shopping. In this way, when people prioritise their leisure preferences, it has been shown that participating in social activities with others is more important than leisure as consumption (Kelly).

Hamilton (2003) believes that, "the price of abundance has been the disintegration of community and the disintegration of self" (p 214). Aristotle's concept of *eudemonia* is presented as an option, which is meant to capture happiness and wellbeing through the full realisation of human potential. It is believed that in reducing the desire for consumption and paid work, people will pursue meaningful leisure through cultural, educational and community work (Hamilton). By increasing engagement in such activities, people will improve their lives, health and wellbeing. Thus, the focus of life becomes less on economic growth and consumption and more on fulfilment in life through meaningful leisure and community involvement.

Another potential solution may be evident in how some people in communities are beginning to "search" for the once "forgotten" spiritual dimensions of life. Historically, spirituality is strongly linked to pursuits of ideal leisure and is defined by some as "finding the balance" and "becoming centred". People's developing sense of the spiritual may allow them to realign the values that drive their doing. For example, Wilding's (2003) phenomenological investigation of spirituality in people who have mental illness found that participants' spirituality provided meaning to their everyday doings and that the process of engaging in a spiritual journey radically reorganised participants' thinking about what was important for them to do with their lives. Rediscovering the spiritual may result in increasing numbers of people choosing a simpler, more leisurely and more spiritual lifestyle (Ostrow, 2002). In the next section of this chapter, the role that health professionals, specifically occupational therapists, can play in enabling people to move towards such lifestyles, is presented for consideration.

Use of leisure in health professional practice: Occupational therapy examined

Leisure is frequently cited in occupational therapy literature as one of three major categories or types of occupation along with work/productivity and self-care (Canadian Association of Occupational Therapists, 1997; Christiansen & Baum, 1997). From an Australian perspective, Chapparo and Ranka (1997) note that rest occupations provide a fourth major category. Even though leisure is so prominent in a conceptual understanding of human occupation, some therapists claim it is not given any serious attention (Turner, Chapman, McSherry, Krishnagiri & Watts, 2000). Although therapists may state that they value facilitating play and leisure as an outcome of therapy, the professional literature does not support this claim (Primeau, 2003). That this is the case is evidenced through an Australian study of occupational therapists working in adult physical dysfunction settings. The findings of this study reported that leisure/recreation tasks were never/rarely used by most therapists (48.3 per cent), with 39.5 per cent of therapists reporting they sometimes utilised leisure (McEneany, McKenna & Summerville, 2002).

In contrast, other authors report that leisure is facilitated within occupational therapy practice. For example, Craik, Chacksfield and Richards' (1998) survey of occupational therapists working in mental health in the United Kingdom found that various forms of leisure were the most prevalent interventions used by the survey participants. In addition, play/leisure was a common focus of treatment for stage 3 persons with AIDS. A British occupational therapy student questionnaire revealed that leisure activities were frequently seen in mental health and learning disabilities practice settings, but were seldom seen in settings with a physical health focus (Drew & Rugg, 2001).

In other instances, leisure is mentioned in occupational therapy literature but is not focused upon. For example, Unsworth's (1999) survey of people who experienced epilepsy focuses on issues of knowledge of epilepsy and safety from risk of injury during epileptic fits. The survey does ask participants about how home, leisure and work activities might put them at risk of injury. It does not, however, focus on the value or types of leisure the participants engage in or the benefits of such activities. The occupational therapy literature therefore illustrates the range of leisure-related practices: some therapists address leisure needs of clients in their practice; some recognise leisure but do not aim to facilitate it directly; and, finally some therapists choose not to, or are unable to, meet leisure participation needs of their clients.

Leisure as a therapy product

Occupational therapists use all types of occupation, including leisure, as "therapy products". For example, occupational therapists use play and leisure in occupational therapy as "lures or rewards, means, or ends" (Primeau, 2003, p 570). Leisure can be used "as a motivating medium for intervention and exploration" (Hodgson, Lloyd & Schmid, 2001, p 490) and as a relapse-prevention strategy. Leisure can also be used to "help people with mental, cognitive and physical problems in using their spare time and in overcoming the effects of their illness" (Luboshitzky & Gaber, 2001, p 69).

However, there seems to be a philosophical debate that has not been engaged in by many occupational therapists. This is whether leisure should be "used" to achieve therapeutic goals rather than "just" enabling a person to participate in leisure for the "natural" or intrinsic benefits that arise from participation in leisure as posited by Stebbins (1996) and Csikszentmihalyi (1996). The question remains if leisure is used to achieve other goals, albeit valid therapeutic aims, then will the naturally occurring benefits of leisure be lost?

Leisure "squeezed out" of the health system

The problem of addressing leisure in occupational therapy arises because current practice is constrained by numerous societal, political and economic influences. These factors may prevent occupational therapists from being able to facilitate clients' participation in leisure. A principal effect of socioeconomic constraints is that occupational therapists can lose some of their autonomy in decision-making as to how practice might be better conducted. In the worst case scenario, decisions about what should be the focus of occupational therapy treatment with clients is restricted by financial constraints rather than being clients' choices for their therapeutic goals in consultation with the reasoned clinical judgements of therapists. A study into occupational therapists' assessment of leisure found "that some therapists view leisure as a luxury to which they wish they had more time to focus their efforts" (Turner et al, 2000, p 83).

Socioeconomic factors influence the kinds of occupations to which people have access (Sussenberger, 2003). If occupational therapists are to provide "fair and equitable" services, they should be involved in identifying how to access resources to enable their clients to participate in needed and desired occupations. Therapists should document the difference between the "ideal" therapy that could be provided if they were allowed to practice as they saw fit versus the "real" therapy that is constrained by health care and health insurance systems resulting from the economic rationalist approach (Sussenberger).

In addition, economic and quality management tools such as diagnostic related criteria and clinical pathways have meant that clients' assessments and interventions are mapped out for them according to their medical diagnosis rather than by their individualised occupational needs. Such thinking is directly opposed to occupational therapy's valuing of client-centred practice and its philosophical beliefs about the complex and highly individualised nature of ensuring that occupation-focused therapy is tailored to meet the specific and unique needs of each client.

Challenging current notions and "usage" of leisure and occupation

This chapter has demonstrated how society has come to conceive of leisure as a commodity. The Protestant work ethic and the belief that happiness can be obtained by owning more have led to a society where work is more valuable than leisure. The current fiscal rationalist environment coupled with a societal devaluation of leisure have the potential to result in practices in which occupational therapists enable leisure occupations for their clients only after the "real" or "serious" therapy has been completed. For these reasons, it is important to re-visit and re-conceptualise the health profession's understandings of, and engagement with, leisure as a health sustaining pursuit. In particular, occupational therapists as health professionals whose stated philosophical belief is to enhance the health and wellbeing of people through engagement in healthy and satisfying occupations, are well positioned to influence current and future practices as do the specialists in the arena: leisure and recreation therapists. However, the two groups need to overcome a possible lack of understanding and trust between them (Smith, Perry, Neumayer, Potter & Smeal, 1992) in order to work together more collaboratively and to become more politically active in influencing societal trends. The change process might begin by occupational therapists and recreational therapists increasingly working co-operatively, "pooling" their expertise and resources, to design leisure programs which meet diverse needs and are intensely satisfying and meaningful to those who participate in them. While these two professional groups may have a specific agenda to address, in actuality, all health professions need to advocate for the value of leisure as more than a commodity and, accordingly, assist people to live in ways that are health-sustaining and community-building.

Applying concepts of occupational justice to leisure

Occupational justice is premised upon the idea that if society is to be occupationally just, it must enable all people to have the resources to engage in occupations that they need and want to do regardless of disability, socio-cultural position, geographical location, age or gender (Townsend & Wilcock, 2003). When applying the framework of occupational justice, questions are raised about the current economic distinctions of paid and unpaid work and leisure, and challenges arise about whether some occupations (for example, professions and management) should be paid more than other occupations (for example, skilled physical work).

Occupational justice is important to consider since there can be serious health consequences if occupational injustice occurs (Townsend & Wilcock, 2003). Three forms of occupational injustice are cited: occupational deprivation, occupational alienation and occupational imbalance. These states can have significant negative impact upon health and wellbeing, and need to be avoided if people are to work towards becoming healthier and happier.

Some studies have demonstrated how occupationally just or unjust our society is in relation to access to leisure. For example, Hodgson, Lloyd and Schmidt's (2001) qualitative study found that participants experienced barriers to participating in leisure that included mental health, social, transportation and financial issues. A survey of able-bodied children and children with physical disabilities living in England concluded that, "children with physical disabilities have a more restricted play experience than able-bodied children" (Howard, 1996, p 573). Limited opportunities for leisure may result in further injustices, such as limited career opportunities for children with disabilities later in their lives (Howard). Occupational therapists along with other health professionals have a role to play in both exploring and evaluating instances of occupational injustice and in taking actions to prevent such injustices from recurring through advocating for societal change in which leisure occupations can more directly contribute to building healthy individuals and communities.

Conclusion

This chapter has outlined the historical development of leisure and investigated current beliefs about leisure in Western society, that is as a commodity or product for consumption. The net negative impacts of this orientation have been explored from the perspective of individuals, communities and environmental sustainability. Finally, this chapter has posited some suggestions for future synergistic actions by health professionals to re-assert the role and value of leisure as health-sustaining, community-building and as a balance to the increasing demands of work in contemporary society.

References

Beder, S. (2000). *Selling the work ethic: From puritan pulpit to corporate PR.* London: Zed Book Ltd.

Bell, D. (1996). The Protestant ethic, *World Policy Journal,* (13), 61–68.

Brown, L. (1998). The future of growth. In L. Brown et al (Eds), *State of the World.* New York: Worldwatch Institute.

Brown, P. R., Brown, W. J. & Powers, J. P. (2001). Time pressure, satisfaction with leisure and health among Australian women. *Annals of Leisure Research, 4,* 1–18.

Carpenter, G. (1994). Leisure and health during middle adulthood: A case-study. In D. M. Compton & S. E. Iso-Ahola (Eds), *Leisure & Mental Health,* Vol. 1, pp 98–111, Park City: Family Development Resources.

Christiansen, C. & Baum, C. (Eds). (1997). *Occupational Therapy: Enabling function and well-being* (2nd ed.). Thorofare: Slack.

Compton, D. & Iso-Ahola, S. E. (Eds). (1994). *Leisure and mental health.* Park City: Family Development Resources.

Craik, C., Chacksfield, J. D. & Richards, G. (1998). A survey of occupational therapy practitioners in mental health. *British Journal of Occupational Therapy, 61,* 227–234.

Cross, G. (1990). *A Social History of Leisure Since 1600,* State College, PA: Venture.

Csikszentmihalyi, M. (1996). *Creativity: Flow and the psychology of discovery and invention.* New York: HarperCollins Publishers.

De Grazia, S. (1962). *Of Time, Work and Leisure.* New York: Vintage Books.

Di Bona, L (2000). What are the benefits of leisure? An exploration using the leisure satisfaction scale. *British Journal of Occupational Therapy, 63,* 50–58.

Driver, B. L., Brown, P. J. & Peterson, G. L. (Eds). (1991). *Benefits of Leisure.* State College, Pennsylvania: Venture Publishing.

Drew, J. & Rugg, S. (2001). Activity use in occupational therapy: Occupational therapy students' fieldwork experience. *British Journal of Occupational Therapy, 64,* 478–486.

Drummond, A. & Walker, M. (1996). Generalisation of the effects of leisure rehabilitation for stroke patients. *British Journal of Occupational Therapy, 59,* 330–334.

Fullagar, S. (2000). *Introduction to Leisure and Health.* Wagga Wagga: Charles Sturt University Printing Press.

Hamilton, C. (2003). *Growth Fetish.* Sydney: Allen & Unwin.

Hodgson, S., Lloyd, C. & Schmid, T. (2001). The leisure participation of clients with a dual diagnosis. *British Journal of Occupational Therapy, 64,* 487–492.

Howard, L. (1996). A comparison of leisure-time activities between able-bodied children and children with physical disabilities. *British Journal of Occupational Therapy, 59,* 570–574.

Jamrozik, A. (1986). Leisure as a social consumption: Some equity consideration for social policy. In R. Castle, D. E. Lewis & J. Mangan (Eds), *Australian Studies: Work, Leisure and Technology,* pp 155–173. Melbourne: Longman Cheshire.

Kelly, J. R. (1991). Commodification and consciousness: An initial study. *Leisure Studies, 10,* 7–18.

Linder, S. B. (1970). *The Harried Leisure Class.* New York: Columbia University Press.

Lobo, F. (1999). The leisure and work occupations of young people: A review. *Journal of Occupational Science, 6,* 27–33.

Luboshitzky, D. & Gaber L. B. (2001). Holidays and celebrations as a spiritual occupation. *Australian Occupational Therapy Journal, 48,* 66–74.

McEneany, J., McKenna, K. & Summerville, P. (2002). Australian occupational therapists working in adult physical dysfunction settings: What treatment media do they use? *Australian Occupational Therapy Journal, 49,* 115–127.

McKnight, J. (2001). *A procrastinator's guide to simple living.* Carlton: Melbourne University Press.

Melamed, S. & Meir, E. I. (1995). The benefits of personality-leisure congruence: Evidence and implications. *Journal of Leisure Research, 27*(1), 25–40.

Ostrow, R. (2002, February 9–10). Joyous days, childish ways. *The Weekend Australian*, p. R31.

Passmore, A. E. (2001). The relationship between leisure and mental health in adolescents. *Australian Occupational Therapy Journal, 48,* 50.

Primeau, L. A. (2003). Play and Leisure. In E. B. Crepeau, E. S. Cohn, & B. A. B. Schell (Eds), *Willard and Spackman's occupational therapy* (10th ed.), pp 567–570. Philadelphia: Lippincott, Williams & Wilkins.

Roberts, K. (1999). *Leisure in Contemporary Society.* New York: CABI Publishing.

Schor, J. (1999). *The overspent American.* New York: HarperCollins.

Siegenthaler, K. L. (1997). Health benefits of leisure. *Parks and Recreation Journal, 1,* 24–32.

Smith, R. W., Perry, T. L., Neumayer, R. J. Potter, J. S. & Smeal, T. M. (1992). Interprofessional perceptions between therapeutic recreation and occupational therapy practitioners: Barriers to effective interdisciplinary team functioning. *Therapeutic Recreation Journal, xxvi*(4), 31–42.

Specht, J., King, G., Brown, E. & Foris, C. (2002). The importance of leisure in the lives of persons with congenital physical disabilities. *American Journal of Occupational Therapy, 56,* 436–445.

Stebbins, (1996). Casual and serious leisure and post-traditional thought in the information age. *World Leisure and Recreation, 38*(3), 4–11.

Stormann, W. (1989). Work: True leisure's home? *Leisure Studies 8,* 25–33.

Sussenberger, B. (2003). Socioeconomic factors and their influence on occupational performance. In E. B. Crepeau, E. S. Cohn & B.A.B. Schell (Eds), *Willard and Spackman's occupational therapy* (10th ed.), pp 97–109. Philadelphia: Lippincott, Williams & Wilkins.

Townsend, E. & Wilcock A. (2003). Occupational justice. In C. H. Christiansen & E. A. Townsend (Eds), *Introduction to occupation: The art and science of living*, 243–272. New Jersey: Prentice-Hall.

Turner, H., Chapman, S., McSherry, A., Krishnagiri, S. & Watts, J. (2000). Leisure assessment in occupational therapy: An exploratory study. *Occupational Therapy in Health Care, 12*(2/3), 73–85.

Unsworth, C. (1999). Living with epilepsy: Safety during home, leisure and work activities. *Australian Occupational Therapy Journal, 46,* 89–98.

Veal, A. J. & Lynch, R. (2001). *Australian leisure* (2nd ed.). Pearson Education Australia Pty Limited.

Wilding, C.B.H. (2003). *Integrating occupation, spirituality and mental illness: A journey through life of meaningful being and doing.* Unpublished master's thesis, University of South Australia, Adelaide, South Australia, Australia.

CHAPTER TWENTY

The Legislative and Policy Context of Practice

Anita Barbara
Gail Whiteford

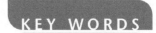

KEY WORDS

Legislation
Policy
Resourcing
Practice opportunities and constraints
Activism

Chapter Profile

This chapter, one of the final in the book, describes how state and federal legislation influence everyday practice decisions and actions. While other chapters in this book have explored the more immediate impacts of contextual influences such as social practices and codes of ethics, the legislative and policy context of practice is less obvious, but highly significant. The impact of governmental platforms and attendant policy development are in fact absolutely relevant to everyday practice and in many respects, may be viewed as a "double-edged sword" for many health professions with respect to mandates and constraints in service provision. For example, many legislative developments in health and human service related areas have provided a mandate for the employment of professionals such as occupational therapists. In practice though, health professionals may actually be seriously constrained in their clinical reasoning and subsequent actions by policy and legislative directives that are more rhetorical than actual because of a lack of concomitant resourcing.

The chapter introduces the theoretical frameworks for understanding the influences of policy and legislation on professional practice. Examples and "case stories" of policy influences on occupational therapists are presented for consideration, highlighting some discrete areas of practice and the tensions between legislation, stated policy and ideal practice. The chapter concludes with reflections on the need for health professionals to increase levels of awareness, responsivity and activity in relation to policy at both an individual and a collective level.

Introduction

The legislative and policy context of practice can appear to have a broad and inaccessible influence on the work of health and human service professionals. In the immediate environment of providing services to clients and consumers, it is a challenge for a busy practitioner to reflect and consider the "who" and "how" of legislation and policy. Indeed, some practitioners may have little awareness of the administrative processes that influence their position and service delivery, while others have an in-depth understanding of the policy context in which they work, yet are frustrated at the constraints that the policies they interact with on a daily basis have on their professional autonomy.

As outlined in Box 20.1, the legislative and policy environment that governs the directions and decisions of a health professional at any given moment is complex. Legislative influences range from the broad legislation that may have created a practitioner's position in the first place through to more directive policy, which guides the specifics of daily practice.

This chapter discusses broad practice implications of working within a legislative and policy context and presents some challenging case examples for reflection. The real context of the state of New South Wales, Australia, is used to highlight the interaction of state and federal legislation and policy. However, much of the legislation and policy discussed is very similar to other states and developed countries. Readers are encouraged to consider the comparative policy and legislation environment of their own specific state, provincial or national context.

Legislation or policy?

It is important to establish some clear definitions of what is meant by legislation and policy. Although the two terms are often used in tandem, there is a significant difference that affects how practitioners experience their influence. Legislation refers to the action of making or giving laws (*The New Shorter Oxford Dictionary*, 1993) within a highly formalised system of parliament. Laws can be made or given at international, national and state levels. Box 20.2 outlines some examples of legislation at all three levels.

Although parliamentary systems vary, in principle, the legislative process involves the making of laws through bill presentation and voting in houses of parliament with final approval being given by the head of government. In Australia and the state of New South Wales, a Westminster style of parliament exists.

CASE STUDY

Box 20.1: The multi-layered nature of the legislative and policy context of practice

In order to understand how complex the legislative and policy environment of practice is, let's consider Terry's position. Terry is an occupational therapist working in a large urban centre in vocational rehabilitation for a government agency. The position involves being a case manager and providing occupational therapy services to people who are returning to work or seeking work who have a disability or have sustained a workplace injury. The job also involves occupational health and safety consultation to organisations. A busy morning in the office involves phoning a client's doctor, reviewing a client's return to work plan, communication with an insurance company and planning for a manual handling training session for a local industry.

Does Terry know of or understand the range of legislation and policy that is influencing his daily practice? The very existence of his job is guided by the Federal *Disability Discrimination Act 1992* and the NSW *Disability Services Act 1993*. The development and review of a client's return to work plan is guided by the NSW WorkCover Rehabilitation Providers Standard and Conditions of Accreditation, while the NSW *Occupational Health and Safety Act 2000* mandates the approach from a local industry to seek manual handling training and the provision of this training. How and why the therapist communicates with other agencies, such as a client's doctor, is guided by the NSW *Privacy and Personal Information Protection Act 1998*.

All of this impacts on Terry's everyday work: the processes he follows; the ways in which he interacts with others; and the form of the outcomes of his intervention. In this context, Terry would not be deemed competent without an in-depth knowledge of all these legislative drivers.

Broadly, a bill is proposed in one house, passes to the second house (which acts as a house of review) and, if agreed upon, passes to the Governor or Governor-General for approval (NSW parliament website, 2002).

The concept of policy, however, is much less defined and clear in definition. A policy is any course of action or principle adopted or proposed by a government, party or individual (*The New Shorter Oxford Dictionary*, 1993). The term can vary greatly, to range from a statement of intent through to a clear set of standing rules for action (Palmer & Short, 2000). Health professionals, therefore, can work within policy established at the highest level of government and organisational structures through to "micro" policy created at the point of service delivery. For example, government policy may mandate the delivery of occupational therapy services to specific groups such as people with disabilities, while policies on exactly

Box 20.2: Levels of Legislation

International Law — The International Bill of Human Rights

> All human beings are born free and equal in dignity and rights. They
> are endowed with reason and conscience and should act towards one
> another in a spirit of brotherhood.
>
> > From the Universal Declaration Of Human Rights (Art 1),
> > adopted by General Assembly Resolution 217 A (III) of
> > 10 December 1948.

The International Bill of Human Rights consists of the Universal Declaration
of Human Rights, the International Covenant on Economic, Social and
Cultural Rights and the International Covenant on Civil and Political Rights
and its two Optional Protocols (Office of the High Commissioner for Human
Rights, 1996). Both International Covenants on Human Rights, by which
states accept a legal as a well as a moral obligation to human rights, have
been ratified by 132 states including Australia, New Zealand, the United
Kingdom and the United States of America (Office of the High Commissioner
for Human Rights, 1996). The Bill of Human Rights remains the fundamental
source for the promotion and protection of human rights and freedom
throughout the world.

Federal Law — The Australian *Disability Discrimination Act 1992*

This Australian Commonwealth Act was passed in 1992 to protect and
promote the rights of people with disabilities in all facets of life. The Act's
objectives are to eliminate discrimination on the grounds of disability in the
areas of work, accommodation, education, access to premises and in the
provision of goods and therapists (*Disability Discrimination Act 1992*). A
therapist working in an education system supporting students with
disabilities, or a therapist providing consultation on public access, would be
working within the guidelines of the *Disability Discrimination Act*.

**State Law — The New South Wales *Privacy and Personal Information
Protection Act 1998***

This Act introduces a set of privacy standards for the NSW public sector that
regulate the way public sector agencies deal with personal information
(Lawlink NSW, 2002). It also provides a mechanism for complaints and
investigations regarding breaches of the Act. The Act provides standards for
the provision of personal information within and between agencies and a
system to ensure permission and approval is provided for the sharing of
personal information. For therapists working in the public sector, the Act
provides standards for discussing a person's details with other service
providers, referring a person to another service provider and in the
distribution of records or reports about a person.

Box 20.3: Translating vision into policy, policy into action

"At the heart of this policy is a commitment to putting children first, and supporting them within their family and community. This means planning supports and resources so that children/young people with a disability are surrounded by responsive support that begins within the family, moves to the extended family (relatives, friends and carers), to professional service providers (doctors, teachers, therapists) and wider community organisation (community transport, voluntary, recreational organisations)."

("Putting Children First" Policy, NSW Department of Ageing, Disability and Home Care, 2002)

---

what these services are, who is given priority and how long services are provided for, may be decided by the occupational therapist delivering the service.

Box 20.3 provides an example of some opening statements of a NSW state policy relating to children with disabilities. Note the emphasis on principles, vision and human rights in these statements. Later in this chapter, we explore the challenges associated with matching stated objectives to everyday actions. Many therapists may relate to the "vision" as expressed in the statement in Box 20.3, but experience real struggles in achieving this vision in actual service delivery.

Do we experience legislative or policy changes differently? The definitions provided suggest that policy can and does change at a faster rate than legislation. Policy changes relate to the priorities or direction of a government and are implemented through programs and strategic documents. With concepts of policy being so broad, the remainder of this chapter will refer predominantly to policy developed at a government or higher organisational level. Of particular interest is how policy, while created at a distance from practitioners, still influences their practice and professional decision-making in real and immediate ways.

Do practitioners understand the policy environment? Occupational therapists examined

Viewing yourself or your profession as a political entity is probably a concept many practitioners are not familiar or comfortable with. The many challenging roles of being a health professional in current health and human settings can feel overloaded already. Many health professionals are juggling roles as a clinician, manager, administrator, supervisor and educator, and the idea of political activism can appear removed from core work and everyday demands.

Ironically though, while practitioners may be reluctant to engage with the political context that influences their practice, they theoretically acknowledge the importance of the broad social, economic and political environment upon the consumers of their services. Occupational therapists for example, are continually engaged in a multi-layered, environmentally-driven view of their clients. Contemporary theoretical models such as the Occupational Performance Model (Australia), the Canadian Model of Occupational Performance and the Model of Human Occupation, all stress the need to view clients with an understanding of the world in which they live (Chapparo & Ranka, 1997; Law, Polatajko, Baptiste & Townsend, 1997; Kielhofner, 2002). Given this theoretical milieu in which the impact of environment and context is centralised with respect to the "other", it is interesting to note a seemingly inconsistent lack of active engagement by occupational therapists with the environments and contexts that drive their practice. In the face of increasing political and legal changes that affect health-care delivery, many occupational therapists apparently maintain an image of themselves as apolitical (Hocking, Nicholson & Horsford, 1997).

As with a number of other health professions, there have been some consistent efforts to make the profession of occupational therapy more aware of legislative and policy contexts. The challenge has been firstly to inform therapists that changes in social policy can have a direct impact on professional practice (Cameron & Masterson, 1998; Hocking, Nicholson & Horsford, 1997; Scott Lee, 1999). The challenge has also been to enthuse and empower therapists to become more involved to policy and legislative feedback. Instead of feeling removed and isolated from policy, involvement in strategic planning can allow the profession to promote its holistic view of health and particularly environmental influences on people's health (Godfrey, 2000). Practising therapists, as well as managers, researchers and educators, need to understand and address the importance of policy and legislation. Occupational therapy, like other allied health professions, is a valuable resource for modern health care, but is not greatly involved in health-care policy and planning. The fact that therapists have often been restricted mainly to implementing the decisions made by others can contribute to feelings of frustration, detachment and powerlessness (Cameron & Masterson). The three stories of occupational therapists that follow in this chapter provide an insight into this experience by contemporary practising therapists.

Examples of occupational therapists influencing policy and legislation are traditionally published in association newsletters, informal journals and conferences. Articles submitted and published in national and international journals are limited, which doesn't allow therapists to appreciate the global importance of being involved in policy review and development. Hocking, Nicholson and Horsford (1997) provide some small but significant examples of occupational therapists involved in political lobbying in New Zealand. Standards developed by the New Zealand Association of Occupational Therapists regarding assessment and treatment of people who have had a cerebrovascular accident were endorsed by the Stroke Foundation of New Zealand. In another example, feedback was provided by therapists about problems in working with school children regarding the delineation of funding between the Ministry of Education and the Regional Health Authorities. These situations may well be consistent with lobbying occurring in similar settings in other countries, however the profession still needs greater promotion of its achievements and influences.

Cameron and Masterson (1998) refer to the "policy gaze" as new outlook or approach for occupational therapists to be more aware of the macro sociopolitical context in which they work. To "gaze" upon something suggests a serious, although often slightly removed, look at something. It may be a useful analogy for therapists' initial interaction with policy and legislation by acknowledging the difficulty many health professionals face in feeling isolated and removed from serious policy development.

Legislation and policy: A double-edged sword

Since policy affects practice in real and significant ways, it is hoped that, in general, legislative and policy developments support quality practice and best outcomes for service recipients. Indeed, our professional expectation is that governmental policy is formulated, implemented and evaluated through a rigorous system aimed at accountability and outcomes on key indicators. But how sure are we that much of the policy and legislation we implement will ensure the best outcome for us and our clients? In practice, the complexity of formulating and analysing policy can mean the distance between policy intent and the actual implementation of policy with our clients, can be vast. The need to include numerous perspectives, including economic, political, sociological and epidemiological, in policy developments makes it a challenging process (Palmer & Short, 2000).

What is proposed is that many policy developments create a double-edged sword for health practitioners. Even though much policy is designed with clear intent that supports consumers, the implementation of policy and especially the constraints of limited funding, can negate or neutralise initial visions and objectives. Box 20.4 provides some examples of overarching objectives of government legislation or policy relevant to the practice of occupational therapy in a variety of fields. On initial reading, these statements appear to support many of the principles of occupational therapy practice, such as inclusiveness and the right to participate. However, a critical orientation is required here in order to interrogate the potential rhetoric embedded in them: exactly how "translatable" are these statements in everyday practice? Is it, in fact, a case of "good intentions overruled" as Townsend (1998) suggests, wherein the gap between intent and delivery becomes untenable in the face of numerous pragmatic constraints?

Outlined below are the stories of three occupational therapists who interact with a range of policies in their work. At least one of them interacts with each of the policies introduced in Box 20.4 as examples of the statements of intent we often see in policy documents and publications. Note the positive and encouraging objectives and aims of these policies in their intent.

Stories from practice

Story 1 — Policy in vocational rehabilitation

The area of employment in vocational, or occupational rehabilitation has been a growth area for occupational therapists and other health professionals over the past

Box 20.4: Acts with good intentions

The NSW PADP Program

The NSW Program of Appliances for Disable People aims to assist eligible residents who have a life-long or long-term disability to live and participate within their community by the provision of appropriate equipment, aids and appliances.

(NSW Health Department, 2000)

The NSW *Mental Health Act 1990*

The objectives of the Department of Health under this Act in relation to mental health services are to establish, develop, promote, assist and encourage mental health services which:

(a) develop, as far as practicable, standards and conditions of care and treatment for persons who are mentally ill or mentally disordered which are in all possible respects at least as beneficial as those provided for persons suffering from other forms of illness, and

(b) take into account the various religious, cultural and language needs of those persons, and

(c) are comprehensive and accessible, and

(d) permit appropriate intervention at an early stage of mental illness, and

(e) support the patient in the community and liaise with other providers of community services.

(NSW Parliamentary Counsel's Office, 2004a)

The NSW *Disability Services Act 1993*

The objects of this Act are:

(a) to ensure the provision of services necessary to enable persons with disabilities to achieve their maximum potential as members of the community, and

(b) to ensure the provision of services that:

(i) further the integration of persons with disabilities in the community and complement services available generally to such persons in the community, and

(ii) enable persons with disabilities to achieve positive outcomes, such as increased independence, employment opportunities and integration in the community, and

(iii) are provided in ways that promote in the community a positive image of persons with disabilities and enhance their self-esteem, and

> **Acts with good intentions** — *continued*
>
> (c) to ensure that the outcomes achieved by persons with disabilities by the provision of services for them are taken into account in the granting of financial assistance for the provision of such services, and
>
> (d) to encourage innovation in the provision of services for persons with disabilities, and
>
> (e) to achieve positive outcomes, such as increased independence, employment opportunities and integration in the community, for persons with disabilities, and
>
> (f) to ensure that services or persons with disabilities are developed and reviewed on a periodic basis through the use of forward plans.
>
> (NSW Parliamentary Counsel's Office, 2004b)

twenty years. Occupational therapists have assumed roles of providing tertiary rehabilitation, case management to people entering or re-entering the workforce as well as occupational health and safety consultation. The premise of vocational rehabilitation is consistent and supported by the core concepts of occupational therapy. Paid work, as a productive occupation, is a means by which people make a social or economic contribution to their community or provide economic sustenance (Law, Polatajko, Baptiste & Townsend, 1997). Like other occupations, paid work is an important source of purpose, meaning and satisfaction in our lives as well as generating income.

Vocational rehabilitation is an area that surrounds therapists with a growing amount of policy and legislation. State and federal legislation provides significant rules and procedures for this area of employment which therapists must understand and work within. In the state of New South Wales, Australia, a range of legislation and policy development greatly influences the daily work of occupational therapists in vocational rehabilitation. The story of Kate in Box 20.5 outlines the positive and negative influences legislation and policy has on her practice in vocational rehabilitation. This area of employment is unique in the roles policy and legislation have had in mandating the employment of therapists, but also in the restrictions they can place on professional decision-making and independence.

Story 2 — Policy in assistive equipment schemes

Prescribing or recommending assistive equipment (or aids) has a long historical association with the occupational therapy profession. A key task of therapeutic practice is using tools or equipment to enhance clients' performance (Hocking & Wilcock, 1997). To prescribe equipment such as wheelchairs, an occupational therapist establishes a clear picture of the client's occupational needs, their abilities and environmental factors. Such an intervention can be seen as quite an intimate

CASE STUDY

Box 20.5: Kate

Kate is an occupational therapist who has worked in vocation rehabilitation in the government and private sector for eight years. Kate describes her daily activities as greatly influenced by a range of federal and state legislation as well as formal documents such as Codes of Practice and Rehabilitation Provider Guidelines.

> Over my eight years in this area, although things such as the basics of OH & S legislation haven't changed greatly, it is the little things that change that get to you. Who you can see and when, how long you can work with a client, you really have to know what the rules are and how this changes what you can do.

Kate is clear about the positive influences policy and legislation have on her work:

> Policy gives you guidelines and creates outcomes and aims for clients. I like this about this area of work. In NSW for example, WorkCover sets very strict policy and procedures about what services will be offered, so you can be very clear with your clients. I also think the basic premise of the *Disability Services Act* and Occupational Health and Safety Legislation is the acknowledgement of the role of work in our community. I think it is great that somewhere "on high" it is known that enabling people to work improves their quality of life and helps them to feel like a worthwhile person.

Kate also outlines what are the negative influences of legislation on her work:

> Some aspects of legislation doesn't allow you to view a person holistically, it addresses work in isolation and doesn't allow you to acknowledge enough the affect an injury has on home life. For example, I was working with a teacher who needed much more support in their home life to help them to return to work, but this intervention couldn't be provided by my service under the Act.

Does Kate feel like she can influence policy and legislative directions in vocational rehabilitation?

> I think some feedback gets passed on to working parties and I know our association has done some lobbying to do with payment issues for occupational therapists? I think somehow we do make an influence, it is just hard to trace how that happens exactly?

Kate — *continued*

Kate's final comments summarise her relationship with the policy and legislative context in which she works:

> Although we need policy, it can be frustrating when it restricts your individual practice as an occupational therapist. Sometimes I can't "be" an occupational therapist and I don't always think that is the best thing for a client.

---

or individual process, wherein the therapist and client work together to make the final decision.

It is the reality of funding that instantly places this common task of occupational therapists into the legislative or policy sphere. Due to the enormous cost of many items, many clients have access to some form of funding scheme, whether government or private in origin. In NSW, the scheme to provide state funds for assistive equipment is the Program of Appliances for Disabled People (PADP). Situated within the Department of Health, this scheme aims to assist people who have a life-long or long-term disability to live and participate within their community by the provision of appropriate equipment (NSW Health Department, 2000). Research suggests that despite these enabling policy directions articulated at a state level, people are being denied timely and appropriate access to funds to meet their equipment needs (Dowling, 2003). Further, the persisting medical interpretation required to define or validate need may restrict the acknowledgment of the social aspects of equipment needs (Dowling). The narrative of Heather (Box 20.6) explores some of these issues.

Story 3 — Policy in mental health

In Australia and many other Western countries, our understandings of mental health and approaches to service delivery have undergone great change during the end of the last century. Movements towards community-based care, consumer empowerment, early intervention and health promotion have provided a rich opportunity for health practitioners to play a significant collaborative role (Lloyd, Kanowske & Maas, 1999). Significant legislation and policy development in mental health in Australia have created a number of key documents that guide mental health service development and provision. The National Mental Health Policy and National Mental Health Plan aim, where possible, to prevent the development of mental health problems, reduce the impact of mental health problems on our community and ensure the rights of people with mental disorders (Lloyd, Kanowske & Maas, 1999). In the state of NSW, the *Mental Health Act* is the significant legislation that mandates and directs service delivery. For practitioners working in mental health services, the influences of policy and legislation are obvious and increasing. The story of Jan (in Box 20.7) is that of an

CASE STUDY

Box 20.6: Heather

Heather is an occupational therapist working in medical rehabilitation in NSW. She described the principle of PADP as "excellent" and the scheme as "brilliant, when it works". But for Heather, her interactions with the scheme are many and varied in regard to meeting the needs of her clients. She talked of "fluking it" in reference to having a client's equipment approved and funded in a timely manner. She also talked of "working the system":

> You have to outline very carefully in your application the level of care the person needs and frame it in a way that makes it sound very serious for the person to have the equipment ... no you don't use terms like quality of life much.

Of greater concern was Heather's discussion of how limited funds in PADP influences her clinical recommendations. Heather outlined:

> ... always having PADP in the back of my mind ... I sometimes think straight away about second hand options, or whatever I know is in the store room, you know sometimes that funding is so tight it is not even worth applying for what you really think is needed.

Realism about funding is a constant factor for therapists such as Heather and can mean not applying for equipment that the therapist's clinical reasoning would suggest is needed. As Heather reflects:

> Not enough money in the scheme is a bigger issue than just for occupational therapy.

occupational therapist who has worked in mental health service delivery for many years and who reflects on the legislative and policy influences on her work during that time.

The policy context for Kate, Heather and Jan

The stories of Kate, Heather and Jan reflect ideas presented in the literature in relation to how practitioners, in this instance occupational therapists, work with policy. Interestingly, all three were very aware of what policy and legislation affects their daily work. Their stories also illustrate the diverse range of work occupational therapists are engaged in, and therefore the broad range of policy and legislation the profession interacts with.

The three practitioners also demonstrated an understanding of how policy and legislation impact on potential outcomes for their clients. Heather's words support

CASE STUDY

Box 20.7: Jan

Jan is an occupational therapist who works in a community-based adult mental health service. She has many years' experience in mental health in Australia, New Zealand and the United Kingdom in both hospital and community-based services. Jan outlines a range of legislation and policy that directs her work as an occupational therapist:

> I can name a range of policy and legislation I am aware of. There is of course the national mental health policy plus in the state of NSW the *Mental Health Act*. But then we also need to be aware of things like privacy legislation, child protection, Workcover, suicide management documents and things like the NSW Families First Policy which is rolling out. Overriding all of that is policy on how we assess, triage and document, we have to make sure we follow the rules there.

How does all this policy influence Jan's practice? She describes it thus:

> In many ways it is business as usual, but you have to be aware of these changes. But look at the size of these documents. Ten years ago you would receive a circular, maybe six or seven pages long, but now you receive these huge booklets and manuals and somehow you have to read and them and know what is going on.

Jan acknowledges the positive influences all the policy development has on her work:

> What it does do for you as a worker, and I think for experienced workers in this age, is keep you moving in the right direction. Policy makes sure you do things as you should, such as highlighting the role of family needs in mental health or guiding your documentation. It also outlines the expectations for the client. We talk about partnerships now and policy has helped create that idea.

On negative aspects of policy and legislation, Jan outlines how mental health policy developments have restricted some aspects of assessment, clinical independence and professional individualism:

> Policy governs you alright, and it takes away, or at least, hinders some of my legitimate tools as an occupational therapist. You have to follow the rules in assessment, even if it interferes with your therapeutic rapport. It also erodes yourself as a professional. In our pool we all have to be a little bit of an occupational therapist and a little bit of a psychologist, even if that is not the best way to work.

Jan — *continued*

Jan is unsure of exactly what impact she has had, or could have, on policy development in her area of work. She states she has never had an official position where she felt she had been involved in "serious" policy development, but has made efforts to feed information and ideas up through the organisation. Jan expresses some concerns about policy development in her organisation:

> It almost seems like we have a group of experts come in and tell us how to do our job and to a certain degree you need objectivity because you don't want to perpetuate bad practice. But at the same time if you want change in the workplace, or change in any place, whether it's community or whatever, you need to involve all the parties and you need to have them feeling that their contribution is being heard.

Jan is aware of her professional association's involvement in policy review and consultation but feels the profession could have even wider consultation with experienced practitioners:

> You need to use your skilled workers and have them feeling that they are senior and that they can contribute through the profession. If we are going to be involved in policy development we need to be knocking on the door, we need to be there as an association. We may be only able to squeak, but you know we can squeak quite loudly.

---

the impact that equipment policy has on the practice of occupational therapy and on the lives of people with disabilities (Dowling, 2003). As discussed previously, the objectives of the PADP scheme, as outlined in Box 20.5, suggest a policy compatible with occupational therapy philosophy. At the operational level of clinical practice however, funding pressures and priority systems can constrain rather than enable occupational therapists' practice. The double-edged sword then, is evident in this scheme, which in principle enables clients to access equipment, but in reality actually impairs or delimits opportunities for occupational engagement due to a paucity of adequate resourcing. The three stories also support another key aspect of practitioners' interaction with policy and legislation: the need for lobbying. Kate, Heather and Jan all understood that their profession or organisation was attempting to influence policy directions. However, none of them had a clear picture of how and why they would be involved, but were hopeful that somehow the message was getting through.

The stories presented above are indicative of some of the realities faced by practitioners as they go about delivering their services in different environments and contexts. The common thread to them is both the opportunities and constraints encountered in attempting to best serve clients while working within the parameters of federal and state legislation and policy. What their stories ultimately suggest however, is the need for health professionals to mobilise at both an individual and collective level to more effectively co-create the policy environment in which operate rather than being passive recipients of "good intentioned", but pragmatically and ethically unsustainable, policy directives.

Future directions

> For health professionals and their patients to shape health care practice, education and research by influencing policy and funding, it will be necessary to change power relations between practitioners and their patients ... and between practitioners/patients and policy/funding decision makers both locally and nationally.
>
> (Titchen & Higgs, 2001, p 223)

Throughout this book, the theme of the practitioner working in different contexts to deliver appropriate and sustainable services to different client populations effectively has been explored from numerous perspectives. In particular, Chapter 5 dealt with some of the challenges presented by hegemonic practice, that is in which dominant ideologies and discourses become tacit to everyday actions and, in this way are reproduced and reinforced despite the fact that they may be at odds with the belief system of the individual professional and his or her profession as a whole. Becoming aware of these often intangible influences, whether they take the form of policy directives or funding decisions, is the first step, but action is requisite to change and transformation. Indeed, enacting agency and the role of activist has been described as a central to what it means to be a professional (Kemmis, 2004; Titchen & Higgs, 2001; Wilcock, 1998).

What forms can activism take to address the legislative and policy context of practice? Individually, the practitioner has a number of means through which to interact with those policies that shape his or her everyday work. At an organisational level, it is possible for an individual to lobby key decision-making bodies that influence client services. Critiquing policy at this level, with an orientation to local context and local needs, for example in a socioeconomically depressed or rural community, can result in significant improvements from the service recipients' perspective. At a professional level, an individual practitioner can become involved in action groups that actively promote a policy framework based on key principles (for occupational therapists, for example, this may include the principle of occupational justice) and which advocates and responds to submissions to policy reviews. Individual practitioners can also express their professional autonomy through self-directed representation to state and federal members of parliament, ombudsmen and regulatory authorities such as health services commissioners in either a proactive or "whistle-blowing" capacity.

While such activity can influence the policy terrain of everyday practice and therefore the lives of people that professionals serve, collective action can be more powerful and rapid in its impacts. To this end, professional bodies, especially the health professions, can mobilise themselves to a far greater extent than historically has been the case. Directly lobbying politicians, political parties and funding agencies is an important activity, however, it needs to result from a well-articulated and prioritised policy agenda, developed through member consultation. If not, the risk is fragmented and potentially inconsistent policy developments. One of the major challenges facing professional bodies in being more proactive in shaping the policy environments in which their members work is a concomitant change to management infrastructures and resourcing. Many professional groups struggle to respond quickly to policy-related opportunities, for example through media releases, due to a lack of adequate staffing or expertise. This will be an area of urgent need if professional groups are to be acknowledged as agents of change and social transformation through both "bottom up" and "top down" processes in the future.

Conclusion

In today's world, health professionals work in complex, multidimensional contexts. One of the often invisible, but highly significant, contextual influences on their practice is that of federal and state legislation and policy. Legislation and policy can be described as a double-edged sword in that, while enabling the existence of a service through an articulated commitment to principles of social justice, it may also serve to severely delimit or constrain practice due to a lack of adequate detail to enable translation to specific environments or due to a lack of adequate resources. In this chapter we have explored and discussed what legislation and policy are, how they are created and what the impacts can be on practitioners. Case examples, drawn from practising occupational therapists in different fields, were presented for consideration and to bring a narrative, experiential dimension to the discussion. Central to the narratives were the common themes of opportunity and constraint, along with a seeming uncertainty as to how to act effectively to stimulate debate, dialogue and potential change to cogent pieces of legislation and policy frameworks. In closing, a reflection on key activities in which individuals and professional bodies can collectively engage have been presented as future imperatives.

Acknowledgments

Thank you to the three occupational therapists (real names not used) who were interviewed for this chapter.

References

Cameron, A. & Masterson, A (1998). The changing policy context of occupational therapy. *British Journal of Occupational Therapy, 61*, 556–560.

Chapparo, C. & Ranka, J. (1997). The Occupational Performance Model (Australia): A description of constructs and structure. In C. Chappara & J. Ranka (Eds), *Occupational Performance Model (Australia): Monograph 1*, pp 1–22. Sydney: Occupational Performance Network.

Dowling, L. (2003, July). *Equipped for life, a very private public issue: Policy and equipment in the lives of children and families.* Paper presented Australian Social Policy Conference, Sydney, Australia.

Godfrey, A. (2000). Policy changes in the National Health Service: Implications and opportunities for occupational therapists. *British Journal of Occupational Therapy, 63*(5), 218–224.

Hocking, C., Nicholson, A. & Horsford, M. (1997). Editorial: To be or not to be political. *New Zealand Journal of Occupational Therapy, 48*(1), 3–4.

Hocking, C. & Wilcock, A. (1997). Occupational therapists as object users: A critique of Australian practice 1954–1995. *Australian Occupational Therapy Journal, 44*(4), 167–176.

Kemmis, S. (2004, March). *Knowing practice: Searching for saliences*. Paper presented at Participant Knowledge and Knowing Practice Conference, Umea, Sweden.

Kielhofner, G. (2002). *A model of human occupation: Theory and application*. (3rd ed.). Baltimore: Lippincott Williams & Wilkins.

Law, M., Polatajko, H., Baptiste, S. & Townsend, E. (1997). Core concepts of Occupational Therapy. In E. Townsend (Ed.), *Enabling Occupation: An occupational therapy perspective*, pp 29–56. Ottawa: CAOT Publications ACE.

Lawlink NSW. (2002). *The Privacy and Personal Information Protection Act 1998*. Retrieved 3 March 2004 from http://www.lawlink.nsw.gov.au/pc.nsf/pages/briefguide

Lloyd C., Kanowske H. & Maas F. (1999). Occupational therapy in mental health: Challenges and opportunities. *Occupational Therapy International, 6*(2), 110–125.

NSW Department of Ageing, Disability and Home Care. (2002). *Putting Children First*. Retrieved 30 October 2003 from http://www.dadhc.nsw.gov.au

NSW Health Department. (2000). *NSW Health Policy on the Program of Appliances for Disabled People (PADP): Circular No 2000/103*. Sydney: NSW Health Department Health Services Policy Branch.

NSW Parliamentary Counsel's Office. (2004a). *Mental Health Act 1990*. Retrieved 3 March 2004 from http://www.austlii.edu.au/au/legis/consol_act/mha1990128/s6.html

NSW Parliamentary Counsel's Office. (2004b). *Disability Services Act 1993*. Retrieved 3 March 2004 from http://www.austlii.edu.au/au/legis/consol_act/dsa1993213/s3.html

New South Wales Parliament Website. (2002). *Stages on Passing a Law in New South Wales*. Retrieved 30 October 2003 from http://www.parliment.nsw.gov.au

Office of the High Commissioner for Human Rights. (1996). *Fact Sheet No. 2 (Rev. 1), The International Bill of Human Rights*. Retrieved 30 October 2003 from http://wwwunhchr.ch/html/menu6/2/fs2.htm

Palmer, G. R. & Short S. D. (2000). *Health care & public policy: An Australian analysis*. Melbourne: Macmillan.

Scott Lee, S. J. (1999). Lobbying for occupational therapy. *OT Practice, 4*(8), 5, 12.

The New Shorter Oxford English Dictionary on Historical Principles. (1993). Oxford: Clarendon Press.

Titchen, A. & Higgs, J. (2001) A dynamic framework for the enhancement of health professional practice in an uncertain world: The practice-knowledge interface. In J. Higgs & A. Titchen (Eds), *Practice knowledge and expertise*. Oxford: Butterworth-Heineman.

Townsend, E. (1998). *Good intentions overruled: A critique of empowerment in the routine organization of mental health services*. Toronto: University of Toronto Press Inc.

Wilcock, A. (1998). *An occupational perspective of health*. New Jersey: Slack.

CHAPTER TWENTY-ONE

Globalisation and the Enabling State

Gail Whiteford

Global context

Cultural impacts

Communications

Political responses

Chapter Profile

As a conclusion to this book, this chapter introduces the concept of globalisation, an inescapable context of contemporary life and professional practice. Key features of globalisation, both positive and negative, that have impacted on individuals in every nation are discussed and impacts on communities and forms of practice are highlighted. Additionally this chapter will consider the emergence of the "Third Way" and the concept of the "Enabling State" as a political response to the challenges of globalisation and critique its stated objectives. The chapter concludes with reflections on how globalisation as a current and future context of practice may impact on the forms of service delivery and community interactions and the potential of the Enabling State as a means through which to address them.

Introduction

That societies globally have undergone radical transformation in the last fifty years is evident. The biggest changes that have impacted on national states and communities have been the rise of individualisation, increasing social fragmentation, loss of faith in government, environmental degradation and globalisation (Jacob, 2002).

Of these changes, globalisation if most often discussed as the basis of numerous social and economic problems, and while there may be some truth to such assertions, in itself, it remains a poorly-understood concept. In order to understand some of the impacts on individuals, communities and professionals, some background discussion chronicling the emergence of globalisation is requisite.

Globalisation: An overview

> One of the striking features of globalisation is just how readily and plentifully all manner of implications seem to flow from it. It is an extraordinarily fecund concept in its ability to generate speculations, hypotheses and powerful social images.
>
> (Tomlinson, 1999, p 2)

Despite commentary from numerous quarters and a range of perspectives, there is little agreement as to what globalisation is. Such a lack of consensus may reflect the fact that globalisation is a term that seems to have variable meanings dependent on the perspective from which it is viewed. Despite differing standpoints, there is some agreement however, that rather than being viewed as an end point, or outcome, globalisation should be regarded as a process (Eslake, 2001; Harris, 2002; Pot, 2000). The focus on process tends to be described either fairly specifically as a trade-related phenomenon or more broadly as a cultural one. Eslake, for example, defines globalisation as "a logical extension of the process through which barriers to the exchange of goods and services are being either dismantled or overcome" (p 61), while Pot describes globalisation as "the social process in which the constraints of geography on social and cultural arrangements recede" (p 47). An additional perspective linked to cultural processes is that of citizenship and the interaction between the individual and society. This is reflected in the definition of globalisation as a "series of processes that help to create a cosmopolitan democracy" by Wiseman (1988, p 117) and in the suggestion that globalisation is an aggregate of all those processes which bring people together in a single world society in which interdependence is a defining feature (Holton, 1997).

Given that globalisation has been defined as those processes which bring the world closer together in a mutually interdependent way and which have economic, cultural and societal impacts, it is no wonder that it is a hotly contested phenomenon with both staunch advocates and strong critics. Critics of globalisation focus on several key issues, namely that globalisation increases inequality, that it is a process resulting in cultural erosion and that it ultimately leads to the decline of the nation state (Holton, 1997; Streeton, 2001). Defenders point out firstly that globalisation is not new; rather it is an extension of international trade practices dating back to the mid 1800's (Harris, 2002; Eslake, 2001). Additionally, they suggest that the inequities so commonly focused on by critics of globalisation have actually been diminished through participation in world trade, with the suggestion by Eslake that globalisation has actually lead to poverty reduction for the majority of the world's poor. As to cultural convergence, the threat of the creation of a bland world monoculture (Whiteford, 1995) is countered by those who argue that while international cultural icons exist, local traditions and practices are actually resilient to change (Holton), and that local responses to the threat of cultural imperialism have been vigorous. As to the erosion of national sovereignty, Held (2001) argues that while globalisation has transformed the nature of the political community and has impacted on the power of the state, "any description of this as a simple loss or diminution of national power distorts what has happened" (p 394). Eslake reinforces this view, adding that governments have not, in real terms, had their powers eroded but are being increasingly forced through global scrutiny to be more accountable for their policy decisions.

Clearly, the arguments for and against globalisation are more complex and wide ranging than what may be reasonably presented within the limitations of this chapter. Perhaps the statement, with respect to globalisation, that "most gain, many lose and probably more lose for other reasons and blame it on globalisation" (Harris, 2002, p 10) approximates the reality of the impacts of globalisation. It is a reality that has also been noted as representing as many possibilities as threats (Latham, 2001), particularly to those everyday social practices that constitute the very fabric of societies and collective identities. The inescapable reality is, ultimately, that globalisation has led to change on an unprecedented scale. In the following sections, this chapter will explore some of the impacts on everyday practices and social interactions.

Globalisation and everyday practices

> What must be remembered is that the imponderable aspects of culture like images of knowledge, attitudes to religion and the modern phenomenon of fundamentalism(s), styles of modernity and political regimes, have also become globalised.
>
> (Elkana, 2000, p 283)

I remember some years ago talking with a colleague who had been working as a volunteer abroad in Kalimantan telling me an interesting story about going to a particularly remote part of Kalimantan, travelling to the depths of the jungle by canoe and entering a tiny hut on the river. In the hut, happily playing on the floor next to his mother was a little boy. When he looked up, she saw that he was wearing a Bart Simpson t-shirt. This, said my colleague, made her feel despondent: there was no escaping "Western" culture, no matter how you travelled.

Cultural practices and images

While such a story points to a perceived erosion of difference between national and cultural boundaries and identities, the cultural impacts of globalisation are in fact, far more complex than a cross fertilisation of genres and images (Capra, 2003). Indeed, the concept of culture itself, which has traditionally been associated with time and place (Tomlinson, 1999), begins to seem more problematic in a context of the borderlessness created by mass media and the adoption of English as the international language of trade (Appiah, 2000). If we return to definitions of culture as being systems of shared meanings (Whiteford, 1998), then the greater the exposure to other languages, images and lifestyles, the more diffuse and potentially conflicting these systems of meaning become.

One of the most cogent descriptions of the negative cultural impacts of globalisation comes from Ife (2002) who suggests that:

> The imposition of a global culture, sometimes referred to as the "McDonaldisation" or the "Disneyfication", has been noted by many commentators and can be seen in everyday life. People in different parts of the world are increasingly wearing similar clothes, eating similar food, watching the same movies, listening to the same music and playing the same games. The imposition of a culture, based on mainstream American consumer culture … has a devastating effect on local communities and cultural diversity. (p 143)

As Ife suggests, the impacts of increased levels of consumption of imported goods on local communities can be negative on numerous fronts (environmentally, culturally, economically) and has been described as a relationship between consumers and multinational corporations that is reminiscent of that between serfs and feudal landlords (Klein, 2001). There are however, differing perspectives on the topic of consumerism and globalisation. Legrain (2003), for example, argues that painting a global picture of passive, mindless consumers is patronising. He argues that, in fact, consumers are aware of the hype that surrounds brand images and are far more conscious of value for money and quality in their purchasing decisions. Alternatively, it has been suggested that we have entered into a global context in which consumption has actually become a dying trend, one in which the orientation will not be to the ownership of objects but to the purchase of experience:

> In the Age of Access one buys access to lived experience itself … experience industries, which include the whole range of cultural activities from travel to entertainment, are coming to dominate the new global economy.
> (Rifkin, 2000, p 145)

Communications practices

This so called "Age of Access", in which people increasingly consume "paid for" chunks of experience, has of course been made possible through the global technological innovations we now come to accept as "givens" in many countries. Indeed, in their assertion that the global economy itself has actually been fuelled by the growth in the telecommunications industry (worth an estimated $1 trillion USD), Rechenbach and Cohen (2002) point to the growth in long distance and wireless services, cable television and internet access as being foundational to the telecommunication boom. The single most important impact of such globalised telecommunication links has been the creation of the "network society", a society in which powerful interests come together, sharing information and power across national borders (Ife, 2002). This network society is one in which "the generation of new knowledge, economic productivity, political and military power and communication through the media are all connected to global networks of information and wealth" (Capra, 2003, p 130).

While such scenarios describe the means of interaction of those in multinational corporations and other globalised operations (including organised crime), how has technology impacted on everyday practices at individual and community level? Certainly there are arguments in favour of the burgeoning cyber-communities that highlight the potential emancipation of groups of citizens otherwise disenfranchised by distance, lack of mobility, disability, socioeconomic status or sexual orientation (Spender, 1995). A more cautionary, and indeed critical, view has been presented by Walmsley (2000) in his work on community place and cyberspace. In his thorough critique of the impacts of cybercommunities on social and professional practices, he identifies 12 reasons why cyber-interactivity may fail to produce social transformation and emancipation. These include the:

- inherent inequity of access to communications and the emergence of electronic "ghettos" (p 10);
- transitory nature of cybercommunities;
- risk of cybercommunities being characterised by superficiality;
- risk of diminishing levels of real human interaction;
- potential invasion of the privacy of the individual as a by-product of electronic surveillance; and, finally
- lack of concomitant organisational change relative to telecommunications advances.

Work and work-related practices

Organisational change, or lack thereof, is also implicated in the impacts of globalisation on work and work-related practices. The preceding two decades have witnessed significant impacts on the way we think about work, interact with work colleagues, access full-time employment or otherwise and interact with employers and/or unions.

Globalisation has meant that companies have increasingly had to compete internationally. Ironically, doing this in turn leads to a more competitive globalised environment (Streeton, 2001). Competing in a more competitive, globalised context has several major consequences. First, companies look to rationalise their production in an attempt to be as "lean" and efficient as possible. Second, because labour force regulations such as occupational health and safety standards, working conditions, employment rules and pay rates are nationally determined, international competitiveness may be seen as negatively influenced by more demanding standards. This, in turn, leads to pressure to downgrade nationally-determined standards, or as Pot (2000) suggests, a process in which governments come under pressure from the corporate sector to regulate the labour market in order to increase international competitiveness.

Such a drive towards international competitiveness has in turn had significant impacts on labour markets internationally. Unemployment has been identified by numerous commentators as one of the most serious and pervasive by-products of globalisation (Capra, 2003; Johnson, 2002; Prigoff, 2000; Stigliz, 2002; Streeton, 2001) with massive social impacts on whole communities and nation states. As Capra points out, the main group at risk are unskilled or semi-skilled workers who, as a labour pool, move in and out of jobs with the risk of being "replaced at any moment either by machines or by generic labour in other parts of the world depending on the fluctuations in the global financial networks" (p 125). Underemployment then, in the form of casualisation, short-term and temporary contract work becomes another serious consequence of globalised work practices, especially when the requirements of contemporary social arrangements such as getting a loan or a mortgage are dependent upon demonstrable full-time employment income. In this respect, like the long-term unemployed, the chronically underemployed become relegated to the hinterland of society and may become increasingly excluded from taken-for-granted social practices such as having a holiday or engaging in other leisure pursuits. Conversely, it has been argued that shifts in global work practices have actually had a net beneficial impact on labour markets, with more people being employed in service industries, as opposed to manufacturing industries, than ever before (Legrain, 2003). However interpreted though, globalisation has led to increased activity in the labour movement and unions internationally, with workers becoming increasingly mobilised with respect to the perceived erosion of minimum rights and conditions in the workplace. Indeed, it seems that "conditions appear right for the re-emergence of labour as a social movement" (Johnson, p 237).

Conditions may appear right for a re-invigorated labour movement that will address workplace practices internationally, but what of the political backdrop to such significant social phenomena? A critical appraisal of the emergence of a new political paradigm that supposedly transcends the traditional divide of Left and Right, the Third Way, follows.

Political responses: Politics' Third Way

The Third Way, its supporters claim, is the only political movement that faces up to the realities of globalisation and social change on a massive scale (Botsman, 2001). Originally a term used by Pope Pius XII who called for a third way between socialism and capitalism at the end of the nineteenth century (Halpern, 1998), the Third Way has been described variously as "an attempt to develop a left of centre political philosophy that responds to the big changes transforming the world" (Giddens, 1999, p 1), a "sharp break in political continuity which may render many political certainties obsolete" (Gamble & Kelly, 1998, p 5) and "the only game in town" (Botsman, p 17). It has been well received by feminists who point to its potential to address past inequities through structural change and the centralising of gender issues as opposed to treating women as another special interest group (Hancock, 2000). There also seems to be some support for the philosophical orientation of the Third Way from indigenous quarters (Pearson, 2001) who embrace its apparent commitment to community capacity building which is primarily concerned with issues of self-determination (Fitzgerald, 2002).

One of the best descriptors, perhaps, comes from Paul Kelly (2000) who posits the suggestion that:

> The Third Way is based upon a recognition that the first way, social solutions based by state intervention won't suffice anymore. It is based upon the recognition that the second way — solutions based upon individual wealth and economic libertarianism — won't suffice anymore. A new synthesis is required (p 1).

If an innovative synthesis in the form of a new political paradigm is indeed required, then it is necessary to evaluate what constitutes its core agenda and the description of how such an agenda is translated into everyday policies and practices. An overview of the core agenda of the Third Way is presented in the next section and is followed by a description of the concept of the Enabling State, the Third Way's blueprint for social change geared to the specific context of globalisation.

Agenda item 1: Education and lifelong learning

An investment in education and a prioritisation of education policy appear to be central to the values underpinning the Third Way. Viewing education as a vehicle to the creation of stronger societies with greater resilience to change, the focus is on "mobilising learning resources to all parts of society" through reinvigorating adult education, creating new community schools, developing re-skilling programs and introducing new funding systems such as "lifelong learning accounts" (Botsman, 2001, p 20). The clear aim is to keep the workforce educated, skilled and responsive to labour market changes in order to enhance employability.

Agenda item 2: Social partnerships

Key themes in this area of concern are cross-sectorial collaboration, the creation of partnerships between community and business sectors and multidisciplinarity. As Botsman (2001) suggests, the questions that policy-makers should ask are:

> ... in tackling social problems, how many alliances and partners can we draw into the work of government ... the public sector needs to discover the skills of networking and collaboration. (p 21)

The key idea here is that the business sector engage with communities beyond models of passive consumerism into more active patterns of occupational engagement at the most local level.

Agenda item 3: Service devolution

In this, one of the more challenging agenda items of the Third Way, nothing short of a minor revolution is being suggested with respect to governance. As is evident in many countries globally, national governments spend vast amounts of money to deliver services to groups of people yet ultimately fail to "get it right" from the perspective of service recipients. In this new model of governance, the power of bureaucratic structures is minimised with greater control over service delivery and co-ordination occurring at a community level. Botsman (2001) stresses that in this model, where the government becomes a clearing-house for service delivery, it does not abrogate its responsibility both to fund and monitor public services including health, housing, welfare and education. Ultimately, it seems this model represents a movement towards greater levels of self-determination in communities and an ability to respond to specific social issues within specific, regional contexts.

Agenda Item 4: Fostering social entrepreneurship

Social entrepreneurship is constructed within the value system of Third Way politics as the appropriate response to welfare systems that have, ultimately, disempowered people and contributed to social isolation. Social entrepreneurs are concerned with developing occupational potential in people and communities, not in the creation of bureaucratic structures. Botsman (2001) summarises the orientation as one in which "communities tend to grow inside-out ... generating social capital and normalising poor neighbourhoods. With this social platform in place, employment and training programs of governments are likely to achieve their best results" (p 24).

Agenda item 5: Communitarian politics and the reinvention of democracy

The Third Way seeks to re-engage disenchanted populations of people in active dialogue with government about important moral and ethical issues in an attempt to construct social policy collaboratively. What has been dubbed "internet democracy" is wholeheartedly embraced by Third Way supporters who see electronic communications as a means of direct input into decision-making processes. Internet democracy is the means by which people can "re-engage in the political process by giving them more information and more democratic power". (Botsman, 2001, p 26)

Agenda Item 6: Encouraging increased levels of corporate responsibility

Third Way visionaries predict that the future environment for commerce will be one in which corporations will be rewarded for ethical behaviour in the marketplace by consumers and governments alike. Policy initiatives that would provide the vehicle for this scenario include tax incentives for corporate philanthropy, mandatory corporate reporting on social and environmental responsibilities and the "badging" of good and bad corporate citizens. The "openness" of the e-environment and the relative ease with which consumers can assess information regarding corporate activities is seen as one of the major factors that will expedite such increased corporate responsibility and social responsiveness.

Agenda item 7: Addressing economic governance and spatial economics

Globalisation is the key to understanding the economic agenda of the Third Way. In particular, the European Union is representative of Third Way economic values, standing for cross-national regulation of trade and investment. However, unlike the traditional polarised positions of Left and Right with respect to labour and trade regulations, the Third Way is supposedly about enabling free trade while maintaining social standards; in other words, maintaining an orientation to the "social investment state" (Giddens, 1998, p 99). On the geographic/spatial front, globalisation can impact negatively at local levels "ghettoising" at risk communities and increasing levels of unemployment and underemployment. Third Way politics seeks to redress this through the diversion of private sector investment into such areas.

Given that the areas identified above describe the core agenda of the Third Way, it is important to consider what this agenda means within the concept of the "Enabling State", a descriptive term used by Third Way strategists. More importantly, what the Enabling State represents in real terms — that is, to real people engaging in everyday activities and social practices in real communities — requires some discussion.

Translating the Agenda of the Third Way: The Enabling State

> The linking of the global and the local is ... a major challenge to community development. In order to see how this may be achieved, it is useful to examine the idea of globalisation from below.
>
> (Ife, 2002, p 146)

The concept of the Enabling State is founded in the values of the Third Way and may be seen as the translation of those values into a model of governance. As described by Latham (2001), the Enabling State model is the only appropriate model in the context of postmodern society as it transcends the rigid policies and practices of traditional Right and Left politics. Most importantly, it purportedly represents a new way of understanding the relationship between government, business and community as well as an opportunity not to have to choose "between the Old Left and the New Right" (Tanner, 1999, p 15). Originally, these ideas were what Giddens (1998) labelled the "Social Investment State". This has more recently been renamed the "Enabling State" (Botsman & Latham, 2001).

While many would support the view that innovative responses to global and community challenges are indeed necessary, is there adequate substance to the Enabling State as a model of governance? More importantly, does it represent a model through which new occupational opportunities can be created in communities in a "bottom up" manner to enhance levels of community participation? This particularly needs to be examined when, in its own assertion, the Enabling State seeks to be a "facilitator of community projects and social outcomes ... it seeks to foster the mutual interests and creative talents of people rather than bureaucratic rules and structures" (Latham, 2001a, p 249) .

The basis for focusing on community-led solutions to the pressing problems of unemployment, underemployment and welfare dependence is based on a view that traditional leftist politics was too state oriented and that traditional right wing parties were too market oriented and that, ultimately, communities were the losers (Hancock, 2000). If, as the Enabling State promises, resources are mobilised at a government level but responsibility for utilising them to address social and occupational issues rest at a community level, there are several advantages. First, community-led solutions, such as job clubs, green exchanges and so on, that are supported by state and federal funding are, from an occupational perspective, far superior to those devised by bureaucrats. This is because they address the context in which specific occupational issues arise.

Devolution of decision-making to the level of communities which respect to the creation of employment and training initiatives, in the presence of a clear line of accountability, is occupationally sound and reflects the principles of "bottom up development" so crucial to sustainable community development (Ife, 2002 p 148). Scanlon (2001) however, offers a more critical perspective suggesting that, while the commitment of the Third Way to community development and community capacity building is noteworthy, it will ultimately prove too difficult to reconcile with the model's free market orientation.

An area in which community *in*capacity is seemingly reinforced is through the delivery of traditional welfare systems into indigenous communities (Pearson, 2001). The Enabling State emphasises a specific need to re-think indigenous community structures, focusing primarily on the development of social capital. Emphasising self-help, reciprocity and innovation, programs are conceptualised and developed within the socioeconomically depressed communities in which they occur and are then supported/subsidised by government funds. A crucial belief here is that the process of disestablishing traditional welfare systems requires a transformative approach towards welfare-dependent communities. This means understanding the importance of access to education and training opportunities to enhance the range of choices available to redress the negative consequences of the poverty trap (Mawson, 2001).

If we consider the impacts of such an approach to levels of occupational participation, the principles are sound. Latham (2001b) points to numerous examples in Australia and the UK: community gardens in housing estates; churches transformed into community-owned and operated health clinics; and car parks and cafes created and run by unemployed youth. On the issue of reciprocity, we need to be more critically cautious of concepts such as "mutual obligation" currently enshrined in legislation in Australia. Mutual obligation systems require recipients of government benefits such as the unemployment benefit or supporting parent benefit to engage in community work schemes. While this may, at one level, seem reasonable, issues of autonomy, choice and power are omnipresent and must be addressed to prevent the exploitation of what could prove to be a cheap pool of labour. To prevent this, in-depth consultative processes with community members are requisite. This means focusing on developing understandings of what the aspirations of individuals and communities are, and how they can be realised contextually.

The Enabling State is one in which attention is apparently directed at "place", an arena often traditionally overlooked in politics. Third Way theorists, as previously noted, seek to address the problems of geography; of dehumanised urban environments and ghettoised housing estates which delimit opportunities for occupational and social interaction. The Enabling State seeks to focus on location and tackle the fact that "disadvantaged places" are the problem, not characteristics of the people who reside within them (Hunter, 1995).

All social activities are situated in place, time, society, culture and history. This notion is supported by Walmsley (2000) who also reminds us that the concept of community is as much to do with the interactions between people and with institutions as it is with actual locations. This fact notwithstanding, the homes, parks, businesses, cafes, schools, institutions as spaces in which people engage in everyday activities and occupations, are of primary importance. Focusing government attention and resources to address space and place to enhance opportunities for active engagement through community-funded initiatives can, therefore, only been seen as a positive response to a real and significant problem. Fitzgerald (2002) cites an example of such attention to space and place and capacity building in his description of the "Schools as Communities" program in Australia. This program has apparently brought together young people, families and a range of community members in an attempt to strengthen the local community through engaging in mutually-valued occupations together.

In order to achieve such successes, the vehicle required in the Enabling State is enhanced intersectoral collaboration. In this model, education and health providers, housing services, businesses and community groups would need to be able to move more freely, enhance their "portability" (Giddens, 1998) and work in multidisciplinary, skill-mixed ways. Clearly, this constitutes a challenge to current constructions of professional knowledge boundaries and established modes of practice and would require a real and concerted effort to break down bureaucratic structures that currently preclude such interaction. Whether or not this is achievable is not only dependent on structural forces, but the collective will of professionals to negotiate the power relationships that would ultimately be impacted upon by such moves. An orientation to the end user of professional services, the client or consumer, may be seen as the most essential perspective to inform such developments into the future.

Conclusion

Globalisation is a phenomenon that has, arguably, impacted structurally on every nation state around the world and has stimulated a range of responses both critical and supportive. It has impacted on social and cultural practices, communication practices and work and workplace practices in every country of the world. It has led to change on such a massive and unprecedented scale that governments and multinational corporations alike have sought new paradigms to inform and guide policy and practice. In this context, new political models seeking to transcend traditional polemic and entrenched modes of governance have emerged.

The Third Way is such a new model and is a self-described response to the limitations of traditional Left and Right wing political systems that fail to acknowledge either the realities of global change in the information area, or the desperate requirement for investment in the social capital of communities in order to save them. The Enabling State is a model of governance which has developed from the principles which underpin the Third Way:

- the de-bureaucraticisation of government;
- the combining of a free market approach and globalisation with a requirement for responsible and ethical corporate practice; and
- the creation of social partnerships to address community problems.

Accordingly, the litmus test of Third Way politics and the Enabling State as an entity will be their ability to:

- address past inequities with respect to levels of participation of minority groups;
- build the capacity of local communities in response to some of the threats of globalisation such as underemployment and unemployment;
- facilitate greater accountability of the business sector and its contribution to the "triple bottom line" (that is, financial, social and environmental); and, finally, as its name suggests,
- enable people to engage in a truly participatory democracy.

Whether this is the paradigm most appropriate to address the significant challenges that globalisation presents us will need to be judged in the international arena in the years ahead.

References

Appiah, K. (2000). Enlightenment and cultural dialogue: Lessons. In W. Krull (Ed.), *Debates on issues of our common future*, pp 263–282. Germany: Velbruck Wissenschaft.

Botsman, P. (2001). Master to servant state. In P. Botsman & M. Latham (Eds), *The enabling state: People before bureaucracy*, pp 3–13. Sydney: Pluto Press.

Botsman, P. & Latham, M. (2001). *The enabling state: People before bureaucracy.* Sydney: Pluto Press.

Capra, F. (2003). *The hidden connections.* London: Flamingo.

Elkana, Y. (2000). Rethinking — not unthinking — the Enlightenment. In W. Krull (Ed.), *Debates on issues of our common future*, pp 283–313. Germany: Velbruck Wissenschaft.

Eslake, S. (2001). What is globalisation? Fact vs fiction. *Policy,* Summer 61–64.

Fitzgerald, R. (2002). *Capacity building: The agenda for community services.* Sydney: Community Services Commission.

Gamble, A. & Kelly, G. (1998). *The third way debate: Summary of the NEXUS on-line discussion.* From http://www.netnexus.org/library/papers/3way.html.

Giddens, A. (2002). *Interview with Guy Lodge.* From http://www.geocities.com/Athens/bridge/8651/Giddens.htm.

Giddens, A. (2000). The Third Way and its critics. Cambridge: Polity Press.

Giddens, A. (1999). *The Goodman lecture*. From http://cafonline.org/goodman/go_speech99.cfm.

Giddens, A. (1998). The third way: The renewal of social democracy. Cambridge: Polity Press.

Halpern, D. (1998). *The third way debate: Summary of the NEXUS on-line discussion*. From http://www.netnexus.org/library/papers/3way.html.

Hancock, L. (2000). Women's policy interests and the Third Way. *Southern Review, 33*(2), 196–211.

Harris, S. (2002). Globalisation in the Asia Pacific context. *Research Paper 7, 2001–2002*. Canberra: Parliament of Australia.

Held, D. Regulating globalisation? The reinvention of politics. In A. Giddens (Ed.), *The global Third Way debate*. Cambridge: Polity.

Holton, R. (1997). Four myths about globalisation. *The Flinders Journal of History and Politics, 19*, 141–156.

Hunter, B. (1995). Is there an Australian underclass? *Urban Futures* 18–20.

Ife, J. (2002). *Community development*. Sydney: Longman.

Jacobs, M. (1998). *The third way debate: Summary of the NEXUS on-line discussion*. From http://www.netnexus.org/library/papers/3way.html.

Johnson, P. (2002). Citizenship movement unionism: For the defence of local communities in the global age. In B. Nissen (Ed.), *Unions in a globalized environment*, pp 236–260. Armonk: Sharpe.

Kelly, P. (2000). National disgrace. *The Australian*, 19 February 21–23.

Klein, N. (2001). No logo. London: Flamingo.

Latham, M. (2000). Mutualism: A Third Way for Australia. *Quadrant, March* 9–14.

Latham, M. (2001a). The enabling state: From governments to governance. In P. Botsman & M. Latham (Eds), *The enabling state*, pp 245–262. Sydney: Pluto Press.

Latham, M. (2001b). The new economy and the new politics. In P. Botsman & M. Latham (Eds), *The enabling state*, pp 13–35. Sydney: Pluto Press.

Legrain, P. (2003). *Open world: The truth about globalizsation*. London: Abacus.

Marquand, D. (1998). *The third way debate: Summary of the NEXUS on-line discussion*. From http://www.netnexus.org/library/papers/3way.html.

Mawson, A. (2001). Making dinosaurs dance. In P. Botsman & M. Latham (Eds), *The enabling state*, pp 148–172. Sydney: Pluto Press.

Pearson, N. Rebuilding indigenous communities. In P. Botsman & M. Latham (Eds), *The enabling state*, pp 132–147. Sydney: Pluto Press.

Pot, F. (2000). *Employment relations and national culture*. Cheltenham: Edward Elgar.

Prigoff, A. (2000). *Economics for social workers*. Belmont: Brookes Cole.

Rechenbach, J. & Cohen, L. (2002). Union global alliances at multinational corporations: A case study of the Ameritech alliance. In B. Nissen (Ed.), *Unions in a globalized environment*, pp 76–102. Armonk: Sharpe.

Rifkin, J. (2000). *The age of access*. New York: Putnam.

Scanlon, C. (2001). A step to the left? Or just a jump to the right? Making sense of the Third Way on government and governance. *Australian Journal of Political Science, 36*(3), 481–498.

Spender, D. (1995). *Nattering on the net*. Melbourne: Spinifex Press.

Streeton, P. (2001). *Globalisation: Threat or opportunity?* Copenhagen: Copenhagen Business School Press.

Stiglitz, J. (2002). *Globalization and its discontents:* London: Penguin.

Suter, K. (2000). *In defence of globalisation*. Sydney: University of New South Wales Press.

Tanner, L. (1999). *Open Australia*. Sydney: Pluto Press.

Tomlinson, J. (1999). *Globalization and culture*. Cambridge: Polity.

Walmsley, D.J. (2000). Community, place and cyberspace. *Australian Geographer, 31*(1), 5–19.

Whiteford, G. (1995). Thinking globally, acting locally. *New Zealand Journal of Occupational Therapy, 4*(2), 2–3.

Whiteford, G. (1998). Intercultural occupational therapy: Learning, reflection and transformation. *British Journal of Therapy and Rehabilitation, 5*(6), 299–305.

Whiteford, G. (2001). The Occupational Agenda of the Future. *Journal of Occupational Science, 8*(1), 13–16.

Wiseman, J. (1998). *Global nation?* Cambridge: Cambridge University Press.

Index